The Sick Newborn Baby

In memory of our fathers

——SECOND EDITION——————————————

The Sick Newborn Baby

Christopher J. H. Kelnar

MD, FRCP, DCH
Consultant Paediatrician
The Royal Hospital for Sick Children
and the Simpson Memorial Maternity Pavilion, Edinburgh
Senior Lecturer, Department of Child Life and Health
University of Edinburgh

David Harvey

MB, FRCP, DCH, DObstRCOG
Consultant Paediatrician
Queen Charlotte's Maternity Hospital, London
Senior Lecturer in Paediatrics
Institute of Obstetrics and Gynaecology
University of London

With the assistance of
Karissa Man-Ying Jowaheer

SRN, SCM, FETC
Clinical Teacher
Queen Charlotte's Maternity Hospital, London

Anna Preston-Jones

SRN, SCM
Sister, Special Care Baby Unit
St Thomas' Hospital, London

and a Foreword by
Margaret E. Adams

SRN, SCM, MTD, DN(London)
Senior Midwifery Tutor
Queen Charlotte's Maternity Hospital, London

Baillière Tindall   London Philadelphia Toronto
Mexico City Sydney Tokyo Hong Kong

Baillière Tindall   33 The Avenue
W. B. Saunders   Eastbourne, East Sussex BN21 3UN, England

West Washington Square
Philadelphia, PA 19105, USA

1 Goldthorne Avenue
Toronto, Ontario M8Z 5T9, Canada

Apartado 26370—Cedro 512
Mexico 4, DF Mexico

ABP Australia Ltd, 44–50 Waterloo Road
North Ryde, NSW 2113, Australia

Ichibancho Central Building, 22–1 Ichibancho
Chiyoda-ku, Tokyo 102, Japan

10/fl, Inter-Continental Plaza, 94 Granville Road
Tsim Sha Tsui East, Kowloon, Hong Kong

First published 1981
Second Edition 1987

Typeset by Inforum Ltd, Portsmouth
Printed and Bound in Great Britain by
Biddles Ltd, of Guildford and King's Lynn

British Library Cataloguing in Publication Data

Kelnar, J.H.
  The sick newborn baby. — [2nd ed.]
  1. Infants (Newborn) — Diseases
  I. Title   II. Harvey, David, *1936–*
  618.92′01   RJ254

  ISBN 0-7020-1185-1

Contents

Foreword

The need for a comprehensive textbook of neonatal care has long been a concern of mine. Dr David Harvey is a popular and committed teacher of both junior medical staff and nursing students undertaking the Neonatal Intensive Care Courses. Dr Kelnar was formerly a junior colleague of Dr Harvey at Queen Charlotte's. Both authors are thus well suited to fulfil this need and show their awareness of educational requirements as well as the needs of parents and their babies.

This book puts neonatal care into historical perspective. It encourages a critical approach to modern technology and treatment. In the past these have sometimes created problems as serious as those they have sought to prevent. Tiny, low birth weight babies, on the borders of viability, are entirely dependent on their caretakers for their life support. The knowledge and attitudes imparted by this book will be of vital importance in the diminution of morbidity.

Because of their clarity and depth, the chapters on resuscitation, respiratory problems, jaundice and infection will benefit all those involved in caring for newborn babies. It is good that both the feelings of parents and ethical problems are considered as this counterbalances the extended knowledge in this second edition.

This book should prove even more useful to the specialist neonatal nurse, midwife and junior medical staff now that it has been extensively updated.

August 1986   *Margaret E. Adams*

Preface to First Edition

Infant mortality has improved greatly over the last eighty years, so that deaths in the neonatal period now form a larger proportion of the total. It is therefore not surprising that the last ten to twenty years have seen an explosion of interest in the newborn baby, particularly the ones who are born early and liable to die from respiratory disorders. The perinatal mortality in the United Kingdom is now dropping faster than at any time since it was first recorded; however, the rate could be much lower—fewer babies die in many European countries than in the UK.

The House of Commons Select Committee on Social Services recently issued a report on perinatal mortality. They estimate that the deaths of about 5000 newborn babies could be avoided every year, if existing knowledge about illness in the newborn was applied in practice. The enormous discrepancy between centres with intensive care units for the newborn and other hospitals, without modern facilities, shows that many lives could be saved.

We have all been concerned about the long-term outlook for babies who survive today but would have died in the past. Recent follow-up studies suggest that babies weighing over 1000 g have an extremely good outlook if death from respiratory distress or intraventricular haemorrhage can be prevented. This is probably true also for babies under 1000 g although there is still a question mark over those as small as 600 g. The first day of life is the most dangerous and good care at birth and subsequently can prevent many deaths.

There are a number of books on the very simple care of newborn babies and also on highly intensive care. This book aims to be between those two extremes and to provide a guide to the care of both normal babies and those requiring special care. Some aspects of more intensive care (for example mechanical ventilation) have also been included where this has seemed appropriate. We have tried to be as practical as possible but it is not always sufficient to know how to do something unless you also know why it is being done. We have been very lucky in Britain in having the advice of physiologists, who have shown us the basic principles of care from careful physiological research on newborn babies. It would be a shame not to have included some of this information as a guide to our work.

Modern care of the newborn depends on building up a multidisciplinary team of doctors, nurses, social workers and laboratory staff to provide expert technical care for the many physical disorders of newborn babies, as well as to give them and their families as much loving care as possible, and we have tried to emphasize this team approach to the care of the newborn.

We hope therefore that the book will interest many different members of this team. It is very important that special and intensive care units and postnatal wards throughout the country should be staffed by those with experience and understanding of newborn babies and their problems. The Joint Board of Clinical Nursing Studies has drawn up syllabuses for nurses training in special and intensive care of the newborn. Course 402 is for those planning to work in special or intensive care; Course 400 is for those who expect to take charge of such units. We hope that this book will be of particular use to nurses on these courses.

We constantly recognize the difficulties of a new houseman or nurse faced with the intensive care of the newborn. It is a very frightening experience, because the babies seem so fragile and precious. They are not able to explain what symptoms they have and the principles of their care can often mystify. Many young doctors have told us how traumatic it is to work for the first few weeks in a neonatal special or intensive care unit. Our aim in this book is to give a basis for such doctors by including information on important techniques that are now used, perhaps for only short periods, in district general hospitals. For instance, it is now common for a baby to need mechanical ventilation for several hours before a team can come from the regional intensive care unit to collect the baby for more prolonged care. Every young paediatrician must know the basic principles of neonatal care, both for normal babies and for those who are ill, and we hope that this book provides both a practical and readable guide.

Laboratory technicians and social workers do not always have the background medical knowledge to disentangle the complicated jargon that many doctors use. It is our hope that this book will also help them to understand what is being said on the ward rounds so that they can ask questions more frequently without feeling embarrassed. It is only by a constant stream of discussion that our care of the newborn will improve.

We do not think that undergraduates need spend very much time in a neonatal intensive care unit but should spend more time on the ordinary postnatal wards understanding problems such as jaundice or the establishment of breast feeding. Our aim has been to make this section of the book sufficiently straightforward to interest them.

Most of the people reading this book will plan to work in an industrial society. However, most babies are born in rural societies or in the sprawling cities of the third world, and tetanus is probably more important as a cause of neonatal death worldwide than all the conditions we see in our unit. We believe that the principles of neonatal care can be adapted to any society or situation if the right priorities are recognized; we have included one chapter on care in the developing world where it is

x   Preface to First Edition

vital not to become too dependent on modern technology but to do the most possible with few resources.

We are grateful to Miss M. Adams for writing the foreword and to her and her staff for their constructive criticisms, and to Dr Eric Hurden for his survey of the literature on drugs in breast milk. We thank all those who have provided illustrations (acknowledged in the text), Miss Barbara Hulme for typing the manuscript; and the staff of Baillière Tindall for their encouragement.

C. J. H. Kelnar
David Harvey

Preface to Second Edition

Since the first edition of this book there has been further progress in the care of sick newborn babies. The perinatal mortality rate is even lower than five years ago and it is now not unusual to see the survival of a baby weighing less than 700 g at birth. The management of sick newborn babies continues to increase in complexity. We must always look critically at the possible effects of new treatments and strive to support parents during this very stressful period.

This book was intended to be an introduction for nurses and house officers to the care of newborn babies and we have been very pleased that many have found it useful. We hope that the changes we have made reflect the trends of the last few years and will allow it to be used for the English National Board Course 405 which has replaced the two previous neonatal nursing courses.

We are grateful to Karissa Jowaheer and Anna Preston-Jones for their help with this edition and to our colleagues in Edinburgh and in London for their suggestions and corrections.

August 1986   *Christopher Kelnar*
David Harvey

—1————————

The Challenge for Perinatal Care

Causes of Death

The end of pregnancy and the first few days of independent life are a dangerous time for a baby. Many deaths occur then and an illness can easily lead to serious consequences, such as brain damage, which may affect the whole of the baby's life. Many couples now expect to have only two children and it is important for them and their families that the children should be born alive and should be left without disability; this is the reason for the great concentration of medical and nursing care in the perinatal period. It is essential that any newborn baby should have a careful examination shortly after birth and should receive good basic care during the first few days. A baby who is ill, or is born very early, will need special or even intensive care. We find it useful to review the newborn baby's needs and problems with a problem list (Table 1.1).

There have been major changes recently both in the numbers of children born in Great Britain and other developed countries and in the frequency of their deaths. The number of deaths is measured as the perinatal mortality rate (PMR), which includes all stillbirths and live-born babies dying within the first seven days (the definitions of mortality rates are given at the end of this chapter). This rate has dropped remarkably since it was first recorded in the 1920s; in fact, it has fallen by a third since the first edition of this book. Even so, of all the deaths of those under 15 years in the United Kingdom, about one in five still occurs within the first 24 hours after birth. The present perinatal mortality is about 7500 deaths each year. Not all the survivors are normal: any disability, whether physical, intellectual or emotional, may cause significant handicap in adult life.

In Britain there has been a trend to smaller families, although the reduction in birth rate has not been as great as in some European countries. Fig. 1.1 shows the birth rate in selected years from 1961 to 1984. We are very nearly at the point where births only just replace deaths and there may be a decline in population by the end of the century. However, there was an increase in the birth rate in the 1970s.

Fig. 1.2 shows the PMR in Great Britain over the last 50 years. The scale is logarithmic, and therefore shows the increasing rate of fall of perinatal mortality in the last few years. The PMR in England and Wales in 1984 was 10.1. One can be very proud of figures such as these, but there has been concern that mortality figures are not as low as those in

Table 1.1 Problem list for reviewing the needs of a newborn baby.

General	Special
1 Food	1 Respiratory
2 Warmth	2 Cardiovascular
3 Comfort	3 Fluid balance and renal function (urea, electrolytes,
4 Love	input/ output)
	4 Weight, nutrition and intestinal function
	5 Haematology
	6 Infection
	7 Bilirubin
	8 Glucose
	9 Calcium
	10 Neurology
	11 Parents
	12 Drugs
	13 Other

some other countries. PMR has dropped as fast, or even faster, than in most developed countries; it is infant mortality, particularly the deaths after the neonatal period, that shows a lagging Britain. Fig. 1.3 shows how infant mortality (deaths of live-born children within the first year of life) has fallen more slowly than in other countries. However, there is still room for improvement in perinatal care.

The consultative document of priorities for Health and Personal Social Services in England, published by the Department of Health and Social Security in 1976, suggested that 'the first priority should be the improvement, in places where facilities are currently inadequate, of special care for newborn babies, where there is a potential both to save lives and to improve greatly the quality of life by preventing life-long handicap at relatively small cost'. The aim of this book is to help in the reduction of such deaths and handicap.

The British Perinatal Mortality Surveys of 1958 and 1970 helped considerably in the identification of causes of perinatal mortality and the effect of social conditions and other factors. Table 1.2 sets out the major

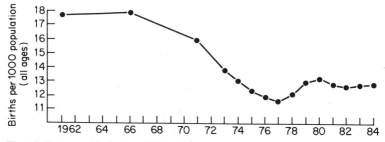

Fig. 1.1 Birth rate (England and Wales) for selected years since 1961. (OPCS)

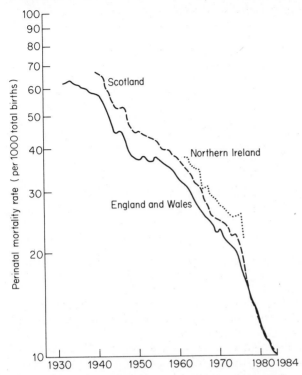

Fig. 1.2 Perinatal mortality in Great Britain 1931–1984. (OPCS)

findings in perinatal deaths in the two surveys. There were remarkable changes in the 12 years between the two surveys; deaths caused by birth trauma dropped by 87% and this was probably due to better obstetrics: difficult forceps deliveries are now extremely rare and have been replaced by caesarean sections. Pneumonia also became less common; it is difficult to be certain of the reason for this, but the use of antibiotics probably played a part. There are some causes of death which did not change at all. It is not surprising that congenital malformations produced the same number of deaths in 1970. In the UK, neural tube defects were the commonest fatal congenital malformations. They now account for a smaller proportion of perinatal mortality, partly because more terminations of pregnancies are performed as a result of detection of these abnormalities by screening tests in mid-pregnancy (Fig. 1.4).

It is, however, worrying that there was no reduction in the number of deaths from respiratory distress syndrome (RDS). Babies should die only rarely from RDS provided it is managed properly. Recent advances in the care of premature labour and the use of betamethasone and

Table 1.2 Major findings about perinatal deaths (British Births Survey 1970; Perinatal Mortality Survey 1958)

Major findings	Singletons and twins 1970			Singletons and twins 1958		
	% All deaths	Incidence per 1000 deliveries	Order	% All deaths	Incidence per 1000 deliveries	Order
Stillbirths with intrauterine asphyxia	26.3	6.1	1	29.9	10.0	1
Congenital malformation	21.5	5.0	2	15.1	5.0	3
Stillbirths without anatomical lesions	14.9	3.4	3	15.4	5.1	2
Respiratory distress syndrome	13.7	3.1	4	9.1	3.1	4
First-week deaths with intrauterine asphyxia	7.6	1.7	5	4.3	1.4	6
Immaturity	6.8	1.6	6	–	–	–
Blood group incompatibility	2.8	0.6	7	4.0	1.3	7
Intracraneal birth trauma	1.8	0.4	8	8.9	3.0	5
Intraventricular haemorrhage	1.8	0.4	9	2.4	0.7	11
Massive pulmonary haemorrhage	0.8	0.2	10	2.7	0.9	10
Pneumonia	0.5	0.1	11	4.0	1.3	8
Extrapulmonary haemorrhage (first-week deaths)	0.5	0.1	12	0.3	0.1	12
No anatomical lesions	–	–	–	2.7	0.9	9
Miscellaneous	1.0	0.2	13	1.2	0.3	13
Total	100.0	23.0		100.0	33.1	

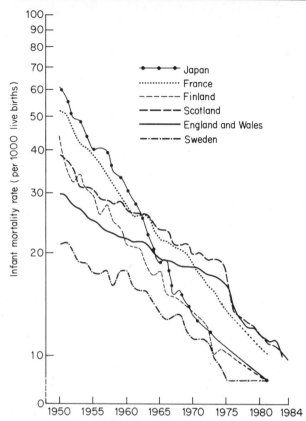

Fig. 1.3 Infant mortality in various countries 1950–1984

salbutamol, together with ventilation after birth (see Chapter 6), have reduced the death rate from RDS since 1970. The causes of perinatal death
in developing countries are often very different from those seen in Europe
and North America. The PMR is much higher and is dominated by death
from trauma and infection; respiratory distress syndrome appears to be
less common. Neonatal tetanus, which is hardly ever seen now in Britain,
is the major cause of perinatal mortality in some parts of the world. The
use of tetanus toxoid, and the instruction of village midwives in the use of
clean instruments to cut the cord and the avoidance of dirty dressings on
the umbilicus would save more babies than most of the sophisticated
techniques mentioned in this book.

Small babies are more likely to die than normal sized babies. The 1970
survey showed that 68% of first-week deaths occurred in babies weighing
2500 g or less. In addition, immaturity, which was used as a term to
describe infants of 1000 g or less at birth but in whom no abnormality
could be demonstrated at post-mortem, was responsible for 15% of

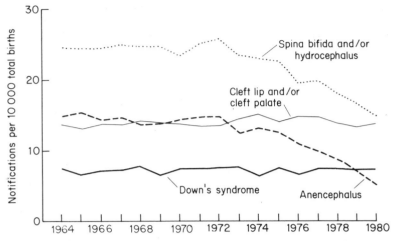

Fig. 1.4 Notifications of congenital malformations, England and Wales, 1964–80

first-week deaths. These infants were regarded as 'near abortions' and many lived only a very short time after birth. There is evidence that in some areas the number of registered live births under 1000 g has increased recently, probably because babies of 24 weeks or more are now seen as having a chance of life. Intensive care may actually increase the PMR if small babies are kept alive for a short while and then die. A baby born dead before 28 weeks gestation is at present counted as an abortion and does not enter mortality figures, but if the baby is born alive, and then dies, it does. It is clear that short gestation and low birth weight are major factors in death during the first week. These will be discussed further in Chapter 2.

PMR varies not only from one country to another, but also within the United Kingdom. This is shown by an analysis of the figures for perinatal mortality from the different Regional Health Authorities (RHA). In 1980, Northern Ireland had a PMR of 15.6 per 1000 compared with only 13.4 per 1000 in England. There were wide variations between the different regions in England, from as high as 15.3 in the North Western RHA to as low as 10.8 in South West Thames. Some of the differences might result from differing standards of medical care, but it is more likely that they arise from social differences; it is well recognized that PMR is higher in lower socio-economic groups. The social class classification based on the occupation of the chief wage earner of the family is shown in Table 1.3. The extent of the drop in birth rate varies in different parts of our community. Fig. 1.5 shows the changes in birth rates in different social classes. In 1975, the number of births in social classes I and II was 96% of the number in 1970; in contrast, there was a

Table 1.3 Classification of social classes (Registrar General).

Class	Definition
Non-manual	
Class I	Professional occupations (e.g. lawyers and doctors) (5.5%)
Class II	Managerial and lower professional occupations (e.g. sales managers, teachers and nurses) (18.5%)
Class IIIN	Non-manual skilled occupations (e.g. clerks and shop assistants)
Manual	
Class IIIM	Skilled manual occupations (e.g. bricklayers and underground coal miners) (37.5%)
Class IV	Partly skilled occupations (e.g. bus conductors and postmen) (18%)
Class V	Unskilled occupations (e.g. porters, ticket collectors and general labourers) (8.5%)

NB The percentages in each social class in the 1971 census are shown in parentheses.

major drop in births in social classes IV and V as they were only 67% in 1975 of the number in 1970, and the rise since then has widened the gap. Social changes such as these underlie the recent improvement in PMR since the babies who might have been born in social classes IV and V would have been at greater risk than those in social classes I and II (Fig. 1.6). Many other factors may affect perinatal mortality (see Chapter 2).

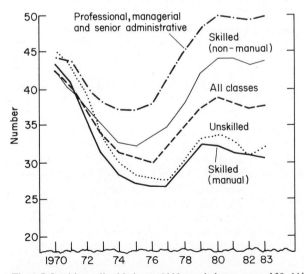

Fig. 1.5 Legitimate live births per 1000 married women aged 30–44 by social class of husband (England and Wales). (OPCS)

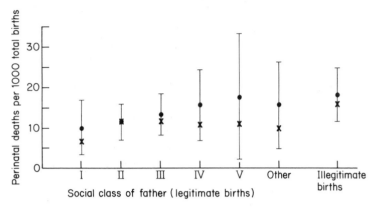

Fig. 1.6 Comparison of perinatal mortality rates by social class (Kensington, Chelsea and Westminster Area Health Authority 1979–80). (Key: X, Mortality rate for Kensington and Chelsea AHA; ☀, Mortality rates for England and Wales with 95% confidence limits based on numbers of total births in Kensington and Chelsea and Westminster AHA)

The persistent high levels of unemployment might be expected to increase the gap between the deprived and wealthier sections of the community (Cole et al., 1983). Seventy per cent of perinatal mortality and morbidity is associated with the 7% of infants who are of low birth weight.

Organization of Perinatal Care

The last 15 years have shown a continuation of the major trend away from home births; 99% of babies are now born in hospital (see Table 1.4). It is difficult to produce figures which show convincingly that hospital births are safer than births at home. The Netherlands have one of the lowest PMRs in the world despite a high proportion of home deliveries, but even in that country there has been a trend towards hospital delivery.

Analysis of perinatal mortality of different parts of Great Britain according to the proportion of deliveries which occurred at home suggested that the mortality of small babies was heavily influenced by their place of birth and there should be no excuse for knowingly delivering a preterm baby at home. The best place for the birth of a preterm baby is in a hospital with a fully equipped intensive care unit. There is, perhaps, an argument in favour of the home delivery of full-term babies since they are at very low risk. It seems reasonable that women should be delivered at home if that is their wish and provided they know that there is a slightly higher risk for their own lives and for their babies' lives. There are clearly some emergencies such as a prolapsed cord in the first stage of labour which could not be successfully managed at home since it would be impossible to do a caesarean section there. A reasonable compromise is delivery in hospital and discharge home after only a few hours. Hospitals should be as comfortable and as homely as possible.

A major obstacle to the improvement of perinatal care is the shortage of skilled paediatric nursing and medical staff and of training posts for them to gain experience in the care of tiny and ill newborn babies. This is particularly important because of the difficulty in recognizing the significance of early signs of illness in newborn babies and the rapidity with which they can become ill and die without treatment.

The lessons for perinatal care have not always been well learned in the past. In the 1950s many harmful treatments were used for newborn babies. An editorial in the *Lancet* in 1974 said 'this period must surely be regarded as the one in which modern neonatal iatrogenesis reached a peak'. For example, the widespread use of intravenous nikethamide during resuscitation was not only useless but harmful; the common use of intragastric oxygen was useless; hypoglycaemic convulsions and brain damage were common because small babies were not fed for up to five days, in order to reduce the risks of aspiration; babies were not kept warm enough; some developed kernicterus following high doses of synthetic water-soluble analogues of vitamin K and the indiscriminate use of sulphonamides in the newborn period; and unnecessarily high and frequent doses of chloramphenicol caused death due to circulatory collapse from the 'grey baby' syndrome.

The greatest harm to babies was caused by the swings in fashion in the use of oxygen therapy. Liberal amounts of oxygen in the 1940s led to many blind children with retrolental fibroplasia and, following this, the refusal to allow babies to have anything more than 40% oxygen in the

Table 1.4 Place of confinement: 1964, 1974 and 1984 (OPCS).

Year	Maternities (thousands)	Percentage distribution of maternities by place of confinement		
		NHS hospitals	Home	Other
1964	890.5	67.1	28.4	4.5
1974	640.8	94.0	4.1	1.9
1984	634.0	97.8	1.0	1.2

1950s led to many unnecessary deaths and much handicap from hypoxia in hyaline membrane disease.

The handicaps seen in the survivors of neonatal care in 1950s led many people to feel that the intensive or special care of newborn babies would only increase the number of handicapped survivors. There is now reasonable evidence that many of the disabilities resulted from medical and nursing methods then in vogue. Improvement in our knowledge of the physiology of the newborn baby has increased the number of survivors; follow-up studies suggest that the prevalence of major handicaps is quite low. More than nine out of ten babies surviving with a birth weight of 1500 g or less are likely to be normal; this is three times more than 30 years ago. The baby who weighs less than 1000 g at birth now has more than a 50% chance of survival, as high as that for babies weighing between 1000 and 1500 g 20 years ago (Stewart et al., 1981). In attempting to improve survival rates we must be careful not to introduce techniques which could damage the baby's brain or other organs. This means that in every centre which has an intensive care unit careful follow-up studies must be done to ensure that harm is not being caused. There is some evidence that the number of children with cerebral palsy and chronic lung disease has increased recently as the techniques of intensive care are applied to smaller and smaller babies.

A major priority in a developed country must be to ensure a good standard of medical care throughout the whole country. This should be done carefully so that the consumer's wishes are followed. For instance, it may be necessary to arrange a regional centre for the care of women of very high risk, but this may result in long journeys during the antenatal period. Because some women need to travel to special centres, it does not follow that every woman needs such care. Attention should be paid to the convenience of individual women and their families and financial help should be given where there is need.

Adequate arrangements must be available in every country for home and hospital delivery of normal pregnant women. An obstetric and paediatric flying squad should be available where a sudden emergency occurs, so that specialist medical help is immediately available. In 1984 a document on categories of neonatal care produced by the British Paediatric Association and the British Association for Perinatal Paediatrics (see Appendix) included a summary of the resources required for neonatal care.

The following seem sensible recommendations for improving our perinatal mortality rate and the quality of surviving babies:

1 Special care nurseries should be available in all obstetric units. It is usually suggested that the unit should have six cots per 1000 deliveries per year. This may be a high estimate as less than 10% of all newborn babies should need admission to the special care unit (see Chapter 4). A

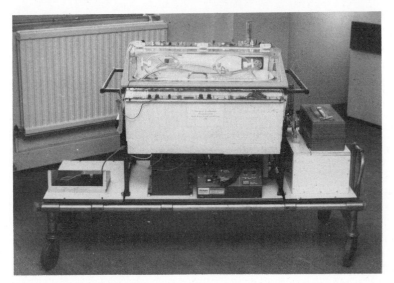

Fig. 1.7 A portable incubator

unit of 20 cots is an efficient size; this implies that obstetric units should
be of a reasonable size (about 2000–3000 deliveries a year) in order to
have a special care baby unit and sufficient staff. The unit should be
within the maternity unit and, if possible, attached to a children's
hospital or a general hospital with a paediatric unit. There should be an
efficient system to allow mildly ill babies or small babies to be transported
from general practitioner units or from home if they need special care and
for their mothers to be transferred with them whenever possible.

2 There should be sufficient, adequately trained, experienced resident
paediatric staff and nurses constantly available. They must be trained in
special care of the newborn.

3 There should always be adequate equipment; there must be piped
oxygen, air and suction and a laboratory with microtechniques to assay
chemicals in blood and urine. There should be apparatus in the special
care baby unit, or very near it, for measuring blood gases. Monitoring
equipment is essential and every hospital should have a technician to
keep it in working order.

Every region should have at least one intensive care unit to serve a total
population of about three million people. This should certainly be in a
maternity hospital; one or two intensive care cots per thousand deliveries
are needed. Ill babies can be transported to the unit in a portable
incubator by a paediatric team of doctors and nurses who can collect a
baby by ambulance or helicopter (Fig. 1.7). All women in premature

labour (at a gestation less than about 33 weeks) or who are likely to have a very ill baby should be advised by their doctors to be transferred for delivery to a hospital with an intensive care unit. This may mean that a woman is very far from her home and family. It is important that, in the future, money and transport should be provided so that members of the family, friends and, most important, the woman's other children can be with her and the ill newborn baby.

Every country should organize its neonatal services so that ill babies can receive skilled care. Clearly, this must be done within the resources available, which means that countries without much money and with very high mortality rates may need to pay attention to basic neonatal care before moving on to a more sophisticated system. Neonatal special and intensive care is expensive. It is particularly expensive to train skilled personnel, both paediatricians and nurses, and also to buy, run and service elaborate equipment. But this cost is insignificant in comparison with the cost of not providing adequate perinatal care. The total expense of caring for one severely handicapped individual in Great Britain through a lifetime of 50 years is at present in the order of £½ million. This takes no account of the stress and suffering of the individual family concerned. It may be that neonatal intensive care is not as expensive as once believed, since babies need less space and less laundry than other patients in hospital. The cost of one intensive care cot is equivalent to an ordinary bed in a general hospital in the United Kingdom, not to the cost of a bed in an adult intensive care unit.

It is vital that every maternity hospital should develop a team for perinatal care. There is a lot to be gained from close liaison between the obstetricians and paediatricians. Regular perinatal mortality conferences allow mistakes to be identified and corrected. We hope that local confidential enquiries into perinatal mortality will allow maternity and neonatal services to be better planned in future.

Definitions

Many terms which need defining will be used throughout this book. For convenience, these definitions are given here. They conform to the *WHO International Classification of Disease (1977)*.

Live birth   the complete expulsion or extraction from its mother of a product of conception, irrespective of the duration of the pregnancy, which, after such separation, breathes or shows any other evidence of life, such as beating of the heart, pulsation of the umbilical cord, or definite movement of voluntary muscles, whether or not the umbilical cord has been cut or the placenta is attached; each product of such a birth is considered live-born.

Fetal death   the death prior to the complete expulsion or extraction from its

Table 1.5 Definitions of stillbirth and infant mortality rates.

$$\text{Stillbirth rate} = \frac{\text{Stillbirths} \times 1000}{\text{Live births} + \text{stillbirths}}$$

$$\text{Perinatal mortality rate} = \frac{(\text{Stillbirths} + \text{deaths at 0--6 days after live birth}) \times 1000}{\text{Live births} + \text{stillbirths}}$$

$$\text{Early neonatal mortality rate} = \frac{\text{Deaths at 0--6 days after live birth} \times 1000}{\text{Live births}}$$

$$\text{Late neonatal mortality rate} = \frac{\text{Deaths at 7--27 days after live birth} \times 1000}{\text{Live births}}$$

$$\text{Neonatal mortality rate} = \frac{\text{Deaths at 0--27 days after live birth} \times 1000}{\text{Live births}}$$

$$\text{Postneonatal mortality rate} = \frac{\text{Deaths at 1--11 months after live birth} \times 1000}{\text{Live births}}$$

$$\text{Infant mortality rate} = \frac{\text{Deaths under the age of 1 year after live birth} \times 1000}{\text{Live births}}$$

mother of a product of conception, irrespective of the duration of pregnancy; death is indicated by the fact that after such separation the fetus does not breathe or show any other evidence of life, such as beating of the heart, pulsation of the umbilical cord, or definite movement of voluntary muscles.

Birth weight   the first weight of the fetus or newborn obtained after birth. This weight should be measured preferably within the first hour of life before significant postnatal weight loss has occurred.

Low birth weight   less than 2500 g (up to and including 2499 g). (NB This is not yet the formal definition in the UK as, at present, the definition includes babies weighing exactly 2500 g.)

Gestational age   the duration of gestation is measured from the first day of the last normal menstrual period. Gestational age is expressed in completed days or in completed weeks (for example, events occurring 280–286 days after the onset of the last normal menstrual period are considered to have occurred at 40 weeks gestation). Measurements of fetal growth, as they represent continuous variables, are expressed in relation to a specific week of gestational age (for example, the mean birth weight for 40 weeks is that obtained at 280–286 days of gestation on a weight for gestational age curve).

Preterm   less than 37 completed weeks (less than 259 days).

Term   from 37 to less than 42 completed weeks (259–293 days).

Post-term   42 completed weeks or more (294 days or more).

The definitions of mortality rates are shown in Table 1.5 and Fig. 1.8.
   Terms or concepts not included here are defined when they are first mentioned in the text.

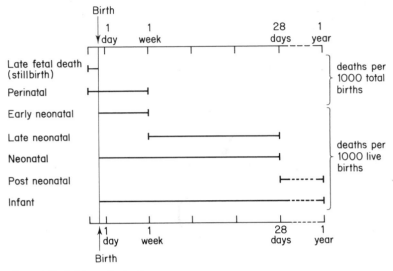

Fig. 1.8 Definitions of mortality rates

The World Health Organization (WHO) made some recommenda-tions about perinatal mortality rate. The problem is that a baby born at less than 28 weeks gestation is at present included in perinatal mortality figures if he is born alive but later dies, but is not included if he is born dead. Practice varies from country to country and some of the differences in PMR from one developed country to another may be the result of a local rule to exclude some babies from statistics. The WHO now recommends that two different sets of statistics should be kept. One set of national figures would include all babies weighing at least 500 g (or at least 22 weeks gestation or 25 cm crown–heel length when a weight is not available), whether the baby was alive or dead at birth. The second set of statistics would be produced for international comparison, these would include only those babies weighing 1000 g at birth (with a gestational age of 28 weeks or 35 cm crown–heel length when weight had not been recorded. (If one subtracted babies weighing under 1000 g from British perinatal mortality figures in 1970, it would have reduced the PMR from 23.7 per 1000 to around 20 per 1000.) The deaths of babies under 1000 g become proportionately even more important with a lower perinatal mortality; the British PMR is now around 10 per 1000; it is possible that it could be as low as 7.5, if one excluded the tiny babies.

Further Reading (including general texts)

Avery, G.B. (1981) *Neonatology*, 2nd ed. Philadelphia: Lippincott.

BPA/RGOG Liaison Committee (1978) *Recommendations for the Improvement of Infant Care During the Perinatal Period in the United Kingdom*. London.

Ciba Foundation (1978) *Major Mental Handicap: Methods and Costs of Prevention*, Symposium 59 (new series). Amsterdam: Elsevier.

Davis, J.A. & Dobbing, J. (1981) *Scientific Foundations of Paediatrics*. 2nd ed. London: Heinemann Medical.

Fletcher, M.A., MacDonald, M.G. & Avery, G.B. (1983) *Atlas of Procedures in Neonatology*, Philadelphia: Lippincott.

Grant, J.P. (1984) *The State of the World's Children*. Geneva: UNICEF.

Hurt, H. (ed) (1984) Continuing Care of the High Risk Infant. In *Clinics in Perinatology*, *11*, 1–247. Philadelphia: W.B. Saunders.

Kitzinger, S. & Davis, J.A. (1978) *The Place of Birth*. Oxford: Oxford University Press.

Klaus, M. & Fanaroff, A.A. (1979) *The Care of the High Risk Neonate*, 2nd ed. Philadelphia: W.B. Saunders.

Korones, S.B. (1981) *High Risk Newborn Infants: The Basis for Intensive Nursing Care*, 3rd ed. St Louis: C.V. Mosby.

MacFarlane, A. & Mugford, M. (1984) *Birth Counts (statistics of pregnancy and childbirth)*. London: HMSO.

Philip, A.G.S. (1980) *Neonatology: A Practical Guide*, 2nd ed. London: Henry Kimpton.

Philip, A.G.S. (ed) (1985) Non-invasive neonatal diagnosis. In *Clinics in Perinatology*, *12*, 1–304. Philadelphia: W.B. Saunders.

Potter, E.L. & Craig, J.M. (1976) *Pathology of the Fetus and Infant*, 3rd ed. Chicago: Year Book Medical Publications.

Roberton N.C.R. (ed) (1986) *Textbook of Neonatology*. Edinburgh: Churchill Livingstone.

Sheldon, R.E. & Dominiaki, P.S. (1980) *The Expanding Role of the Nurse in Neonatal Intensive Care*. New York: Grune & Stratton.

Thomas, R. & Harvey, D. (1985) *Neonatology* (Colour Aids Series). Edinburgh: Churchill Livingstone.

Trade Union Congress (1981). *The Unequal Health of the Nation*. Summary of the *Black Report*.

World Health Organization (1977) *Manual of International Statistical Classification of Diseases, Injuries and Causes of Death*, vol. 1. Geneva.

— 2 —

Prenatal Influences on the Baby

Causes of Prematurity

Seventy per cent of perinatal mortality occurs in the 7% of infants of low birth weight. Those countries with more small babies have a higher infant mortality (Fig. 2.1). Clearly, if we are to improve survival and quality of life, we must reduce the number of babies who are born early. We are still far from understanding the causes of prematurity in most cases. Nevertheless, if all the knowledge now available were put into practice, significant benefits would follow. Some factors we can do something about; there are many that for political, social, emotional, or financial reasons are difficult to change.

In an individual pregnancy, there is sometimes an obvious cause when the baby is born too small or too early. For example, the mother may have pre-eclampsia or an antepartum haemorrhage; she may have twins; the fetus may be abnormal. In most cases there is no simple explanation;

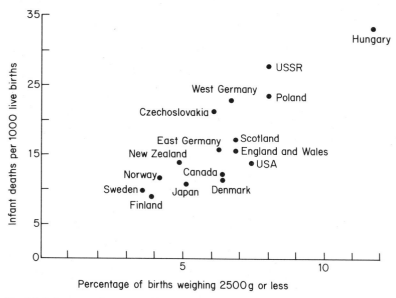

Fig. 2.1 Infant mortality rates and incidence of low birth weight for selected countries (1972–77). From MacFarlane & Mugford (1984)

16

Table 2.1 Factors influencing the length of gestation or fetal growth.

Gestation	Fetal growth
Shortened	*Reduced*
1 Previous obstetric history	1 Maternal illness during pregnancy
2 Maternal illness during pregnancy	2 Chronic maternal disease
3 Chronic maternal disease	3 Maternal age
4 Maternal age	4 Parity
5 Fetal disease	5 Maternal height
6 Social class	6 Ethnic group
7 Multiple pregnancy	7 Genetic factors
8 Major life events	8 Birth weight of other family members
	9 Social class
Lengthened	10 Smoking
1 Drugs	11 Poor nutrition
2 Anencephaly	12 Alcohol
	13 Weight gain in pregnancy
	14 Multiple pregnancy
	15 Altitude
	16 Fetal disease
	17 Fetal abnormalities
	Increased
	1 The baby of the diabetic mother
	2 Beckwith's syndrome
	3 Transposition of the great arteries

it is likely that the result was the end-product of many genetic and environmental factors.

Very often, a baby is born early and is also found to be smaller than expected for the gestation because he has grown too slowly in utero. Many of the factors which are associated with pre-term delivery are also associated with slow growth, so that there is a lot of overlap between the two. It is very important that gestation should be measured as accurately as possible. Women should keep an accurate record of their menstrual history and attend an antenatal clinic early in pregnancy so that a clinical and ultrasound assessment of gestation can be made. When the baby is born he should be weighed and measured accurately and his weight plotted on a birth/weight gestational age chart to show whether he is small-for-dates (see Chapter 5). Table 2.1 summarizes the factors known to influence the length of gestation or fetal growth which are discussed in more detail below. It is often very difficult to be certain whether a factor is associated with short gestation or produces slow fetal growth; in many cases the factors are intermingled. More detailed information on many of them can be obtained from Chamberlain et al. (1975). A baby may be born small because of short gestation, because he has been growing slowly in utero or for both reasons. The care of small·babies is discussed in Chapter 5.

Factors which alter the length of gestation

Short gestation

Previous obstetric history. It is common experience that women who have had mid-trimester miscarriages tend in a subsequent pregnancy to have a preterm delivery or another mid-trimester miscarriage. In many of these cases there is cervical incompetence which is often treated by cervical suture.

There has been considerable controversy about the effect of therapeutic abortion on subsequent pregnancies. Some workers have suggested that it is more likely to lead to mid-trimester miscarriage and preterm births, whereas a large study in the Far East suggested that it has no effect. It seems likely that the chance of a subsequent preterm birth depends on the type of operation used for therapeutic abortion. If the cervix has been greatly dilated during the operation then it is more likely to be incompetent in a later pregnancy.

Intrauterine infection. There have been reports that bacterial infections of the amniotic cavity can lead to premature rupture of the membranes and preterm delivery. In developing countries, zinc deficiency may lead to amniotic infection by reducing the antibacterial defences of the fluid.

Maternal illness during pregnancy. A pregnancy may have to be terminated because of serious illness in the mother: the commonest indications are the hypertensive disorders and antepartum haemorrhage from either placenta praevia or accidental haemorrhage (placental abruption). Very often labour is induced at term, or just before, because of only mild illness in the mother; to allow the pregnancy to continue longer might increase the risk to both mother and fetus. It is therefore common to see labour induced at term for mild hypertensive disorders associated with other high-risk factors such as the mother's age or previous obstetric history.

Chronic diseases in the mother. Some disorders such as chronic renal disease or essential hypertension are often complicated by pre-eclampsia during pregnancy; they lead to therapeutic interruption of the pregnancy and, therefore, a shorter gestation. It is thought that other disorders such as tuberculosis and urinary tract infection are more likely to lead to spontaneous premature labour.

Maternal age. This appears to have very little effect on the length of gestation; the longest pregnancies occur in women during their 20s and gestation is shorter in those women over 35 or under 20 years.

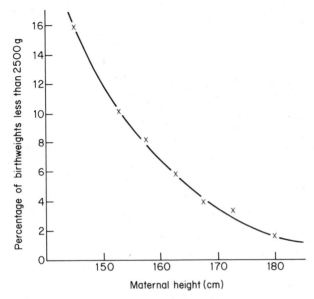

Fig. 2.2 Percentage of low-birth-weight babies in relation to the mother's height. From MacFarlane & Mugford (1984)

Fetal diseases. Labour is often induced when it would be dangerous to leave the fetus in utero, for example induction of labour for rhesus disease.

Congenital abnormalities are sometimes associated with short gestation, as well as with failure to grow normally in utero. We know that many fetuses with chromosomal abnormalities are rejected by the mother in early pregnancy; this is also common when an abnormality is complicated by hydramnios.

Major life events. Recent evidence supports the view that a sudden emotional upset can precipitate preterm labour. Major life events, such as bereavement, are more common in the recent past of women in preterm labour than those at term. Certainly, our grandmothers would have believed in it.

Social class. It is common experience that the families of babies in special care baby units have more social problems than do those of normally sized babies.

There is a suggestion from the British Births Survey that babies born into social classes IV and V have a shorter gestation than those in the middle class. The difference appears to be greater for unsupported mothers.

Multiple pregnancy. This frequently leads to premature labour. It is common to see twins in a special care baby unit. In many cases the labour occurs spontaneously and in some countries much attention has been paid to these pregnancies by using beta-mimetic drugs to prevent premature labour. Pre-eclampsia and other disorders of pregnancy are commoner in multiple pregnancies and labour may need to be induced.

Long gestation

Drugs. It is thought that certain drugs may prolong pregnancy. There is some evidence that women who take aspirin freely during pregnancy are more likely to go into spontaneous labour after term because of the drug's antiprostaglandin effect.

Congenital abnormalities. Some women bearing abnormal fetuses, for example anencephalics without pituitary glands, often fail to go into labour spontaneously at the appropriate time. This may be the result of poor fetal adrenal function.

Factors affecting fetal growth

Some of these factors appear to affect growth throughout pregnancy but most of them only have an effect towards term.

Reduced growth

Maternal illness in pregnancy. In many of the common disorders of pregnancy, such as pre-eclampsia or antepartum haemorrhage, the baby is smaller than one might expect. It is thought that maternal blood supply to the placenta is decreased in many of these disorders.

Chronic disease in the mother. Chronic hypertension and renal disease are notorious for producing very small-for-dates babies. Cyanotic congenital heart disease is another cause.

Maternal age. The heaviest babies are born to women in their late twenties and early thirties. There is a lower mean birth weight in babies whose mothers are under 20 or over 35. This effect is more obvious at term.

Parity. First-born babies are generally lighter than those born subsequently. Again, this effect is more obvious as term approaches.

Maternal height. Short women have smaller babies than tall women (Fig. 2.2). The mean birth weight in the British Births Survey was 3.16 kg for women under 157 cm (62 in) and 3.41 kg in those 165 cm (65 in) or more.

Ethnic group. This is one of the most important factors influencing the incidence of low birth weight. Studies from the USA have shown that nearly one in eight babies born to black mothers weighs 2500 g or less; this is about twice as many as those born to white mothers, even allowing for the positive correlation with low maternal income and poor education. Paradoxically, before 35 weeks gestation, black fetuses are heavier than white and black children are taller than their white peers at the age of two years. There are many studies of birth weight around the world and, in general, babies born in developing countries are lighter. This is particularly marked in babies from the Indian subcontinent; the birth weight of babies there is lower than European babies at term, but there is very little difference between the two groups before 32 weeks. It seems that the babies are small-for-dates because of some factor constraining growth towards the end of the pregnancy. A study in a London borough showed that Indian babies were, on average, 250 g lighter than white babies and West Indian babies were intermediate. It is difficult to be certain what factor is being exerted through the mother's race. It might be a genetic factor; on the other hand it might be a reflection of poor nutrition or short stature; it is probably a result of both.

Genetic factors. Work before the Second World War on the size of foals at birth showed that genetic factors have an important influence on the size of the newborn animal. A pure-bred foal from a large variety is larger than the pure-bred foal from a small variety of horse. A cross breed between a large and a small horse is intermediate in size, but the size depends on whether the mare is from the large or small variety: in the horse, it is the *mother's* size that largely determines the rate of intrauterine growth in a cross between two extremes of adult size.

Birth weight of other members of the family. The birth weight of a baby is significantly related to the birth weight of the last child born to the same mother. Some women have several children who are small at term; there is a significant correlation between the mother's own birth weight and those of her children, which is much stronger than that between the baby's and the father's birth weights. This may be because a woman who is small at birth tends to be a small adult and therefore has a smaller uterus and placental site.

Social class. The mean length of gestation is hardly different in the different social classes, but the mean birth weight is significantly lower in social classes IV and V when compared with social classes I and II. This indicates that there are more small-for-dates babies in the lower social

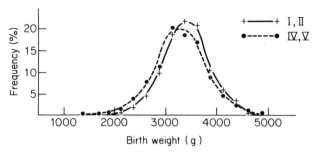

Fig. 2.3 Distribution of birth weight for social classes I, II, IV and V (singletons, LNMP certain). From Chamberlain et al. (1975), by permission of the authors and the National Birthday Trust Fund

classes. It is probable that a multitude of factors, including ethnic group, nutrition, maternal height and smoking, play an important part in influencing this. Fig. 2.3 shows the distribution of birth weight in social classes I and II, compared with social classes IV and V.

Cigarette smoking. This has been shown to be a major influence of fetal

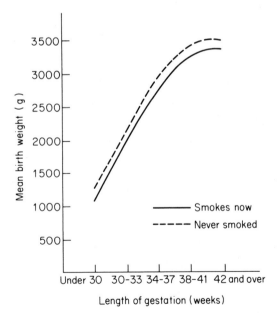

Fig. 2.4 Mean birth weight for length of gestation according to maternal smoking habits (singletons, LNMP certain). From Chamberlain et al. (1975), by permission of the authors and the National Birthday Trust Fund

size. Fig. 2.4 shows the mean birth weight for length of gestation in women who smoked in pregnancy and those who had never smoked. Babies are about 200 g lighter in women who smoke. There is also a lower reading age in later childhood in those children whose mothers smoked during pregnancy.

Smoking seems to have a direct effect on the fetus and the reduced fetal growth is not due to smoking mothers eating less well. Women who smoke inhale nicotine and also have higher carbon monoxide levels in their blood. As a result, the fetus obtains less oxygen and grows less well. For this reason the effect on birth weight is more or less uniform at all stages of gestation (see Fig. 2.4).

Nutrition during pregnancy. It was shown in the 1939–45 war that a period of starvation during pregnancy reduced the size of the baby at birth. This was shown in Leningrad and also during a period of starvation in Holland during the winter of 1944–5 when perinatal mortality and the incidence of low birth weight increased in women starved during the third trimester of pregnancy. Studies from Guatemala suggest that energy (calorie) supplements given to pregnant women who had chronic under-nutrition in pregnancy increased the birth weight of their babies. This is very important for developing countries, as a simple energy supplement during pregnancy may improve the size of the fetus. This may cause problems at delivery because a small woman, when she moves to an area with better nutrition, may have a larger fetus and will therefore develop cephalopelvic disproportion.

Alcohol. The fetal alcohol syndrome has been described in babies born to chronic alcoholic women. The features of the syndrome include low birth weight and short length, microcephaly, irritability in infancy, a low IQ in later childhood and a number of minor dysmorphic features. This syndrome has been increasingly recognized but it is not yet clear whether small quantities of alcohol taken regularly during pregnancy might reduce the size of the fetus. It seems that a consumption of more than 60 ml of absolute alcohol a day could damage a fetus; perhaps six spirit drinks a day could cause fetal abnormality while birth weight might be reduced by only half that amount of alcohol (see Chapter 5).

Weight gain during pregnancy. This is an important clinical sign, since women who gain very little weight in pregnancy have smaller infants. Of course, one may sometimes be led astray by an abnormally large weight gain which is a reflection of oedema from pre-eclampsia or hydramnios when the baby is abnormal and therefore small.

Multiple pregnancy. It has long been known that this leads to small-for-dates babies. In general, the more babies in one pregnancy the lighter

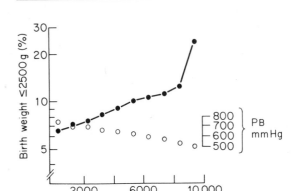

Fig. 2.5 Frequency of low birth weight related to altitude in the USA mountain states, 1952–57. Adapted from Grahn & Kratchman, 1963

they are. The mean birth weight of twins tends to deviate from the mean for singletons at about 32 weeks and that of triplets deviates at about 28 weeks.

Altitude. This has a major effect on the growth of the fetus in utero. Those women who spend their pregnancies at a higher altitude have smaller babies (Fig. 2.5). Presumably this reflects the amount of oxygen which reaches the fetus, since the oxygen tension in the atmosphere is lower at high altitudes.

Fetal disease. Congenital infection, particularly rubella, leads to slow intrauterine growth. There are usually other signs that suggest the diagnosis, such as purpura and hepatosplenomegaly.

Fetal abnormalities. Many of these are associated with low birth weight. This is particularly striking in chromosomal abnormalities such as the autosomal trisomies. However, many babies with other congenital abnormalities tend to be small-for-dates; one of the major exceptions is transposition of the great arteries where the babies are larger than expected. It is striking that babies who are small-for-dates and have congenital abnormalities are symmetrically small; this means that their head circumference is in keeping with low birth weight. Babies who are small-for-dates because of other causes of slow growth in utero, however, often have a relatively large head in comparison to the rest of the body (see Chapter 5).

Any of these factors may come together to influence the size of the baby. The incidence of low birth weight is a major factor in the perinatal mortality rate. Many countries with low PMRs, such as the Scandinavian

Table 2.2 Aspects of the antenatal history to be noted.

1 Maternal age
2 Occupations of mother and father
3 Marital status
4 Mother's medical history
5 Ethnic group
6 Family history
7 History of previous pregnancies
8 Record of antenatal care
9 Mother's menstrual history
10 Estimate of gestation
11 Blood group and serology of mother

nations, have a lower incidence of low birth weight babies than the United Kingdom. The reasons for this are not clear, but it does seem that better social conditions and taller mothers lead to larger babies who are healthier at birth and less likely to die. Information from China is interesting because a Chinese woman there seems to be at only low risk of having a small or preterm baby. This may account for the surprisingly low PMR in China, which is a developing country.

We are still almost entirely ignorant of the factors in individual women that lead to repeated low birth weight. Clearly, we still have a long way to go before our knowledge of the various factors affecting the length of pregnancy and growth of the fetus can be used in the large-scale prevention of the birth of small babies and thus in a major improvement in perinatal mortality.

Increased growth

Factors associated with increased growth in utero are discussed in Chapter 15.

Antenatal Care

There are many aspects of antenatal care which are of importance to paediatricians. Whenever he assesses a baby, the paediatrician should read the antenatal notes carefully. Note the following (summarized in Table 2.2) and enter them in the baby's notes when relevant.

1 *Maternal age.*
2 *Occupations of mother and father.* These will help in assessing the social class of the family and will prevent the nurse or doctor from falling into the trap of talking at too sophisticated a level for the parents, or

conversely, talking down to a mother, such as a nurse, who is already well informed about medical matters. It is best to encourage questions to ensure that the parents have grasped the information given.

3 *Marital status.* An unsupported mother is much more likely to have difficulties in looking after her child and special help may have to be organized.

4 *Mother's medical history.* In particular, note any history of tuberculosis which would mean that the baby should have BCG in the neonatal period.

5 *Ethnic group.* Certain illnesses are commoner in some groups than others. For instance, cystic fibrosis is common among the English but is rare in black people. Ashkenazy Jews have a much higher incidence of some inborn errors of metabolism, e.g. Tay–Sachs disease.

Parents who were born outside Europe and North America have a higher incidence of tuberculosis. There may therefore be a good reason for giving BCG to their babies in the neonatal period.

6 *Family history.* Note any diseases which could be inherited and any record of consanguinity, for instance cousin marriages.

7 *History of previous pregnancies.* This should be studied in great detail since there may be a recurring history of abnormalities such as preterm births or of an important inherited condition for which a special examination must be made. Any previous perinatal deaths are bound to cause anxiety at subsequent deliveries.

8 *Record of antenatal care.* Read the notes about the number of visits during pregnancy. Women should attend the antenatal clinic early in pregnancy but it is common for them to book late; this complicates the assessment of the gestation and may mean that a number of vital tests are done late or not at all (such as serological tests for syphilis). Poor attenders at the clinic do seem to have a greater risk of perinatal death. A history of irregular attendance in the antenatal period may give you a warning that there will be difficulties with the child's care. A glance through the antenatal record makes certain that no abnormalities have been noted during the antenatal period.

9 *Mother's menstrual history.* The date of the last menstrual period is very important, but a proper assessment of gestation can be made from the date only if the mother has regular periods, with a standard cycle. It is wise to recalculate the expected date of delivery to be certain that it is accurate. It is very common to find that the period of gestation on the notes has been rounded up. You may well find that a baby who is only 36 weeks gestation and five or six days has been been called 37 weeks. There is an appreciable difference in mortality rate between one week of gestation and the next; weeks of gestation refer to *completed* weeks.

10 *Estimate of the length of pregnancy.* Record the estimate of the length of gestation and any special observations made during pregnancy. The initial basis for determining the baby's maturity is the mother's men-

strual history. Look at the history of the cycle and the last menstrual period; recalculate the estimated date of delivery. Did the obstetrician's assessment at the first visit correspond with the dates? Is there any record that the mother felt movement at the expected time (18–20 weeks for the first baby or 16–18 weeks in subsequent pregnancies)?

The dates that are obtained from the menstrual history and from clinical examination are wrong in up to 25% of cases. Many women have only a shaky memory of the date of the last menstrual period and some will be embarrassed to mention this; they may say a date is certain when it is not. The use of the contraceptive pill has led to further confusion about dates as periods may be quite irregular after stopping the pill.

For all these reasons, careful assessment of gestation is needed during a pregnancy and ultrasound has made this much easier. An ultrasound reading of the biparietal head diameter between 10 and 20 weeks of a pregnancy, or of the crown–rump length before 10 weeks of pregnancy, gives an estimate of the expected date of delivery that is even better than the date obtained from menstrual dates. The estimate is accurate within a week either way. It seems that ultrasound is a safe method of examining the fetus and no complications have been reported so far. For gestational assessment in the newborn, see p. 348.

11 *Mother's blood group and serology.* Note the blood group of the mother, and in particular, the rhesus group. Note the results of the serological tests for syphilis: congenital syphilis should be totally prevented by careful serological testing in pregnancy. The test for rubella is especially important in assessing a small-for-dates infant. The blood should be screened for Australia antigen as carrier mothers could infect their infants at delivery, or the fetus transplacentally, with subsequent development of hepatitis.

Assessment of Fetal Growth and Well-being

Growth

Ultrasound is again very useful in assessment of growth so long as the gestation has been dated accurately by an early ultrasound reading. Serial measurements of the fetal biparietal diameter will show whether the baby is growing properly or whether head growth has slowed (Fig. 2.6). Most small-for-date babies have a relatively large head compared to the rest of the body, so slowing of the growth of the fetal skull indicates severe growth failure. Recent techniques of ultrasonic examination give even more accurate information about fetal growth; for instance, it is possible to compare the head circumference with the thoracic circumference. An increase in the head/upper abdominal circumference ratio indicates slowing of growth and the technique is able to predict birth weight very accurately, to within 200 g.

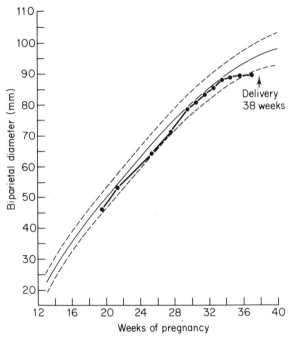

Fig. 2.6 A case of intrauterine growth retardation with cessation of growth of the head late in pregnancy

Antenatal cardiotocography

In a baby who is at high risk, for instance a small-for-dates fetus or the fetus of a mother with a medical disorder such as diabetes, there may be a risk of stillbirth. It is possible to measure the fetal heart rate externally and to look at the changes in heart rate during the painless Braxton–Hicks contractions of the uterus. Slowing of the fetal heart rate during a Braxton–Hicks contraction may indicate hypoxia and a possible risk of death. Many obstetricians use this as a routine method of assessment and deliver the baby when there is any evidence of intrauterine hypoxia. Fetal cardiotocography (FCTG) is further discussed under Care of Labour (see p. 36).

Fetal movements

After 18–20 weeks of pregnancy most women can feel the movements of the baby. There appears to be a relationship between a reduction in the number of movements and hypoxia. There are various methods of assessing this. The simplest is to allow the mother to count up to ten movements after waking and to note the time when the tenth occurs. If there are less than ten movements throughout a day they can be recorded separately. Charts have been prepared in Cardiff to allow the mother to make this assessment herself and to tell the doctor when there are only a few fetal movements. A more objective method of measuring fetal movements is to use the real-time ultrasound scanner which provides a moving picture of the baby. Ultrasonic scanners are now easily portable and much cheaper and so they are becoming a standard method of assessing the health of the fetus.

Urinary oestrogen estimations

A low excretion of oestrogens suggests poor production in the fetus. This investigation is not as popular as it was because of the difficulties of 24-hour urine collections and the wide variability of normal values. Some laboratories now measure plasma oestrogens.

Human placental lactogen

The plasma concentration of human placental lactogen is low in babies of high risk.

Detection of Abnormalities

Many parents who have a family history of congenital abnormalities or who have already suffered the tragedy of an abnormal baby do not want to have another child with such a problem. There are now a number of techniques for detecting abnormalities early enough in pregnancy for a therapeutic abortion to be performed. Unfortunately, most of the techniques can be used in only a small proportion of pregnancies and are unlikely to alter appreciably the number of congenital abnormalities in our community, with the probable exception of spina bifida. The techniques that can be used to detect abnormalities include the following.

Chromosomal analysis

This is usually done at present by culturing amniotic fluid cells and is used for the detection of Down's syndrome (mongolism, trisomy 21), which now accounts for a third of all the severely mentally handicapped persons in the United Kingdom (see also Chapter 8). There is an increased risk of Down's syndrome in the babies of older women: it is about 1 in 1600 when the mother is 22 years old but 1 in 100 if she is 40

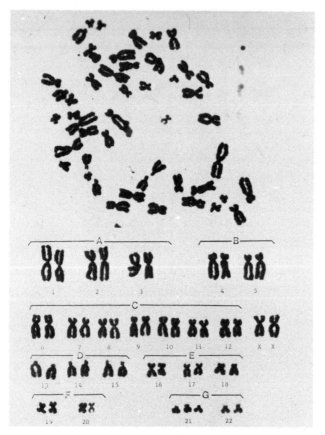

Fig. 2.7 A karyotype of Down's syndrome (trisomy 21)

years. The abnormality is an extra chromosome 21, so the baby has 47 chromosomes instead of the usual 46 (Fig. 2.7). This extra small chromosome usually comes from the mother, but in a third of the cases it comes from the father and there also appears to be an increased risk of the disorder when the father is old. There are other rarer types of Down's syndrome where the extra chromosome 21 is attached to another chromosome (translocation) so that the baby has only 46 chromosomes but has the amount of genetic material equivalent to 47 chromosomes. This can be inherited from either the mother or the father, who can be easily identified because he or she has only 45 chromosomes but is apparently normal. Whenever a baby with Down's syndrome is born the blood should be examined for chromosomes so that these rarer types can be identified and the parents warned of the increased risk of having another child with Down's syndrome. The risk in these translocations is 1 in 5 when the mother is the carrier and 1 in 20 when it is the father.

The usual practice in the United Kingdom is to offer amniocentesis to all women over the age of about 38 years and to those where there is a family history of Down's syndrome. Some centres offer it to women over the age of 35 years. About 50% of Down's syndrome babies are born to women under the age of 30 years, so the number of cases in our community will not be greatly reduced by this policy of amniocentesis, but a number of tragedies in older women will be prevented.

It is unlikely that amniocentesis could ever be offered to all pregnant women, which would be a way of avoiding this condition altogether, because there is an increased risk of miscarriage when an amniocentesis is performed. The increased risk is the order of 1% and there is also an increase in the number of congenital abnormalities in babies born after amniocentesis, mainly talipes equinovarus and congenital dislocation of the hip, and of respiratory distress syndrome.

However, individual women will have their own views about whether they want amniocentesis and some will undoubtedly be prepared to take the extra risk of miscarriage in order to avoid having a child with Down's syndrome. On the other hand, many people have an objection to abortion, which is the only way of avoiding the birth of a Down's baby when it has been discovered in utero. The new technique of chorionic villus biopsy may offer a way out of some of these difficulties. During the first trimester, a small sample of placental tissue is obtained through the cervix. If a serious chromosomal abnormality is discovered from the culture of the material, it is then early enough in pregnancy to do a simple abortion. Unfortunately, the procedure may have a risk of miscarriage as high as 10%, although it has been lower in very recent series.

Amniocentesis is done at about 16 weeks of pregnancy and this means that a late abortion has to be performed, usually using prostaglandins; this can be a traumatic experience for the mother. At amniocentesis, a sample of amniotic fluid is taken, the cells are grown in the laboratory and chromosome analysis is made two to three weeks later. It is possible to identify other chromosome disorders including the rarer trisomies and the disorders of the sex chromosomes. There are some conditions, such as haemophilia, which are inherited in sex-linked recessive fashion and therefore only boys are affected. In these conditions chromosomal analysis can be done on the amniotic fluid cells to detect whether the fetus is a boy or a girl. A boy could then be aborted, but since only one in two is affected it means aborting as many normal fetuses as abnormal ones. Many people find this objectionable although it must be remembered that in the United Kingdom many abortions are done for rubella in pregnancy when we know that many of the children will not have been damaged by the virus. Haemophilia can now be diagnosed in utero in some very special centres.

Biochemical investigations on amniotic fluid or cells

Inborn metabolic errors

There are many, very rare, inborn errors of metabolism which can be diagnosed in utero. They are usually inherited in an autosomal recessive fashion and cause a wide variety of disorders, very often with mental handicap. Since most of them are disorders of metabolism, it is possible to detect the abnormality in the fetal cells grown from amniotic fluid. The absence of an enzyme can be discovered or an accumulation of metabolites shown in the cell. Since these disorders are very rare, the test is performed only when there is a family history of the specific disorder and general screening is not possible. Those which can be diagnosed in utero now number about 60 and are listed in Table 2.3. Occasionally it may be possible to identify parents who could pass on the disease and are therefore heterozygous for the gene. An example is Tay–Sachs disease which is very common in Ashkenazy Jews; there have been screening programmes among Jewish people in the United Kingdom and North America to identify those who might be carrying the condition and to warn them before they have children. The original promise of prenatal diagnosis for Duchenne muscular dystrophy has not been fulfilled,

Table 2.3 Inherited metabolic diseases diagnosable prenatally.

Acatalasaemia
Acid phosphatase deficiency
Adenine phosphoribosyl transferase deficiency
Adenosine deaminase deficiency
Adrenogenital syndrome (21-hydroxylase deficiency)
α_1-Antitrypsin deficiency
Arginosuccinic aciduria
Aspartyl glucosaminuria
Bloom's syndrome
Cerebro-hepato-renal syndrome (Zellweger's disease)
Chédiak–Higachì syndrome
Citrullinaemia
Cockayne's syndrome
Congenital erythropoietic porphyria
Congenital hyperammonaemia Type II
Cystathioninuria
Cystic fibrosis
Cystinosis
Cystinuria
Dihydropteridine reductase deficiency
Fabry's disease
Fanconi's anaemia
Farber's disease
Fucosidosis
Galactosaemia
Galactokinase deficiency

Table 2.3 Inherited metabolic diseases diagnosable prenatally (contd).

Galactose-4-phosphate epimerase deficiency
Gaucher's disease
Glucose-6-phosphate dehydrogenase deficiency
Non-ketotic hyperglycinaemia
Glycogenoses (glycogen storage diseases) Type I–IV
Glutaric acidurias Types I and II
GM_1 gangliosidoses Types I and II
GM_2 gangliosidoses Type I (Tay-Sachs) Type II and III
Haemoglobinopathies
Haemophilia (A and B)
Hartnup disease
Histidinaemia
Homocystinuria
3-hydroxy-3-methylglutaric aciduria
Hypercholesterolaemia
Hyperlysinaemia
Hypervalinaemia
Hypophosphatasia
I-cell disease
Isovaleric acidaemia
Propionic acidaemia (ketotic hyperglycinaemia)
Krabbe's leucodystrophy
Lactosyl ceramidosis
Lesch-Nyhan syndrome (hyperuricaemia)
Lysyl protocollagen hydroxylase deficiency
Mannosidosis
Maple syrup urine disease (branched chain ketoaciduria)
Menke's kinky hair disease
Metachromatic leucodystrophy
beta-Methylchrotonylglycinuria
Methylmalonic acidaemia
Methyltetrahydrofolate methyl transferase deficiency
Methyltetrahydrofolate reductase deficiency
Mucolipidoses Types I–III (includes I-cell disease)
Mucopolysaccharidoses Types I–VII
Multiple sulphate deficiency (mucosulfatidosis)
Niemann-Pick disease
Ornithine-transcarbomylase deficiency
Orotic aciduria
Phosphohexose isomerase deficiency
Pyruvate decarboxylase deficiency
Pyruvate dehydrogenase deficiency
Refsum's (phytanic acid storage) disease
Saccharopinuria
Severe combined immunodeficiency
Sickle cell disease
T-cell immunodeficiency
Thalassaemia (alpha and beta)
Tyrosinaemia Type I
Wolman's disease
Xeroderma pigmentosum
X-linked ichthyosis (steroid sulphatase deficiency)

because the measurement of fetal creatine kinase has proved unreliable. The new, and rapidly developing, techniques of gene mapping may produce a reliable prenatal diagnosis for this condition, and for others like cystic fibrosis, very soon.

Autosomal recessive disorders are commoner in couples who are near relatives because they are more likely to share many genes, including a rare harmful one.

The list of disorders which can be diagnosed is growing every day and Table 2.3 should be checked against the most up-to-date list. The rapid advances in research lead us to hope that the commonest autosomal recessive condition in Great Britain—cystic fibrosis—will soon be diagnosed in utero either by enzyme analysis or the use of a genetic probe.

Other inherited metabolic diseases are being investigated with a view to antenatal diagnosis. In any case of a pregnancy at risk for one of the diseases not listed, provided that the diagnosis of the previous affected child is secure, the Prenatal Diagnosis Group should be consulted for the most up-to-date information, either via the local cyto- or biochemical genetics departments (or see p. 347).

Neural tube defects

Neural tube defects are common congenital abnormalities in the British Isles. About half are fetuses with anencephaly where the brain is exposed and the baby dies; the other half are different types of spina bifida where there is an opening over the spinal cord. The neonatal diagnosis is discussed in Chapter 9. Since severe degrees of spina bifida cause serious mental and physical handicap in later life, there has been a move to make a diagnosis early in pregnancy so that the abnormal fetus can be aborted.

When parents have had a child with anencephaly or spina bifida they have a 1 in 25 chance of having another child with a neural tube defect, although the risk is higher in Wales and Ireland and lower where spina bifida is rare. In anencephaly and the 90% of spina-bifida cases where the neural tube is exposed to amniotic fluid, body fluid from the fetus can escape into the amniotic fluid. The normal fetus produces a protein, known as alpha-fetoprotein, which is present only in fetal life and in one or two rare conditions during later life. It is present in the mother's blood in only a low concentration, but appears to peak during mid-pregnancy. If there is a possibility of a leak of body fluids from the fetus into his surroundings, the concentration of alpha-fetoprotein in amniotic fluid will be much higher than in a normal pregnancy; there will also be a greater concentration in the mother's blood. Since spina bifida produces a leak from the fetus into amniotic fluid, the discovery of this protein has permitted the early diagnosis of neural tube defects during pregnancy. A similar leak is also found in babies with conditions such as exomphalos or congenital nephrotic syndrome, but these are much rarer.

Where there is a previous history of neural tube defect in the family, for instance where one parent has had spina bifida or where the parents have had a previous child with the condition, it is important to manage the pregnancy carefully. An ultrasound examination should be done at about 16 weeks gestation, since this is the best method of diagnosing anencephaly and of confirming the gestational age. At about 16–18 weeks a sample of amniotic fluid can be taken for alpha-fetoprotein analysis. The back can also be scanned by ultrasound to detect a defect in the neural arches which would indicate spina bifida. Unfortunately, a lesion very low in the spine is difficult to diagnose by ultrasound.

The measurement of alpha-fetoprotein in the mother's plasma can be used to screen women who have no history of a baby with neural tube defect. It is best to take the sample between 16 and 18 weeks of pregnancy. At the same time it is wise to do an ultrasound examination to make certain that the gestation is correct, since the commonest cause of an apparently high plasma alpha-fetoprotein is an incorrect estimate of gestational age. At the same time the uterus can be examined by ultrasound for twins or missed abortion since these are other reasons for a high maternal plasma alpha-fetoprotein. If the high alpha-fetoprotein (usually over the 97th centile) is found on two occasions, amniocentesis can be offered.

The first sample of blood should be taken only from women who understand the reason for sampling and wish to be screened. Amniocentesis is done under ultrasound control and the head and back are scanned at the same time. The expertise needed for scanning the back is much greater than when untrasound is used for the measurement of gestation and it seems that this investigation will have to be done only in specialist centres. Undoubtedly, some cases of neural tube defect can be diagnosed early in pregnancy and this method will be used more and more in the future. However, it is possible to miss some cases and this could cause great distress if a woman has been told that her baby will not have spina bifida. The sampling of blood and the examination of the fetus including amniocentesis could also cause considerable anxiety to some pregnant women. This is a reason for making certain that they wish to enter the scheme when the first blood sample is taken.

Fetoscopy

Fetoscopy involves examining the baby through a tiny fibreoptic telescope which is passed into the uterus through the abdominal and uterine walls. The first fetoscopes were fairly large and fetoscopy was often followed by miscarriage. The most recent instruments are much finer and have been used with greater success. The most obvious use of fetoscopy is to look for an external abnormality of the fetus such as a cleft lip or spina bifida. It may be very difficult to use the instrument since

Table 2.4 Indications for fetal blood sampling.

1 Bleeding disorders

2 Haemoglobinopathies

3 Karyotyping

4 Immunodeficiencies

5 Viral infections

6 Metabolic disorders

7 Non-rhesus hydrops

only a small portion of the fetus can be seen at one time, and the procedure should be done in specialized centres under careful ultrasound control.

An even more exciting use of the fetoscope is to take samples from the fetus; it is now possible to take a blood sample from the placental vein and to get a specimen of fetal blood. The blood is examined in a counter to measure red cell size and to confirm that the sample is fetal and not maternal blood. This technique can be used for the diagnosis of a growing list of conditions (Table 2.4) such as thalassaemia and sickle cell disease, or other blood disorders such as haemophilia.

Care of Labour

Good care by an experienced obstetrician is essential if a woman is to be delivered safely of a healthy normal baby. Obstetricians are properly proud that trauma is now a very rare cause of fetal death or morbidity. The death rate from trauma in the 1970 perinatal survey was one-seventh that in the 1958 survey. This reflects the increased readiness of obstetricians to use caesarean section as the method of delivery when damage to the baby otherwise seems likely. A number of recent techniques have been added to the traditional method of assessing the baby's health during labour. It seems that fresh stillbirth from anoxia during labour should now be considered a preventable condition.

Diagnosis of fetal asphyxia during labour

The classic signs of intrauterine asphyxia are meconium staining of the liquor and fetal tachycardia (>180 beats/min) or bradycardia (<100 beats/min). However, clinical assessment is only crude and has therefore

been refined by fetal cardiotocography (FCTG). The principle is continuous recording of the fetal heart rate and the intrauterine pressure
changes, both of which are printed by the machine. There are several
warning signs of asphyxia which are shown by such a record:

1 *Tachycardia.* There is a normal acceleration of heart rate during
contractions and fetal movements. However, a rate continually above
180 beats/minute is sinister.

2 *Loss of base-line variability.* The visual record normally shows an
irregular line and loss of this variation occurs early in asphyxia.

3 *Bradycardia.* Continuous bradycardia is very worrying, although it is
occasionally the result of complete fetal heart block.

The FCTG is mainly used to show any intermittent dips in heart rate.
The dips are often divided into type I and type II (Fig. 2.8). The first
occur during a contraction while the second, which are thought to
indicate asphyxia, occur at the end or after a contraction. Quite often
variable dips are seen. Although type I dips are usually benign, any

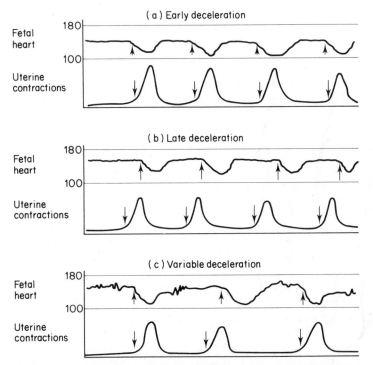

Fig. 2.8 Fetal cardiotocographic tracing. (a) Type 1 or early deceleration, suggestive of
head compression, (b) Type 2 or late deceleration, suggestive of uteroplacental
insufficiency, (c) variable deceleration, suggestive of cord compression. From Forfar &
Arneil (eds), with permission from the editors and Churchill Livingstone

prolonged or deep slowing of the heart may be a danger sign. Some obstetricians measure the area of the dip and use this as a measure of fetal distress. Since dips are common, the fetus should be investigated further by sampling of scalp blood for pH. Asphyxia produces a marked acid-aemia; a pH below 7.25 is usually considered to be sign of hypoxia. The use of the cardiotocograph has now been extended to monitor a high-risk fetus before labour. Regular recordings of fetal heart rate and Braxton–Hicks contractions can be done using external monitors to detect slowing of the fetal heart rate. Any suggestion of hypoxia would probably be an indication for delivery.

Premature labour

A baby who is born early has a much greater chance of dying than one born at term. If one could prevent premature delivery one could greatly reduce perinatal mortality. The methods of stopping premature labour are still not very successful. Where there is clear cervical incompetence, probably from a previous termination of pregnancy, cervical suturing may prevent premature dilatation of the cervix and therefore premature delivery. Some success has been claimed with the use of betasympathomimetic drugs, such as ritodrine. Some studies in central Europe suggest that, when used in multiple pregnancy (a common cause of premature deliveries leading to high perinatal mortality) ritodrine has reduced the likelihood of the babies being born early. The drug is used in premature labour to stop the labour by reducing uterine contractions.

Even when labour cannot be postponed until term, it may be useful to put off premature labour for several days in order to allow steroids such as betamethasone to have an effect on lung surfactant production (see Chapter 6). Controlled trials suggest that where betamethasone has been given to the mother more than 24 hours before delivery, the incidence of hyaline membrane disease in the baby is less.

A not uncommon cause of premature delivery is mistaken dates and induction of labour. It is very important that a careful menstrual history should be taken and that modern methods of assessing the length of gestation, such as ultrasound, should be used.

Drugs in Pregnancy

A number of different drugs and classes of drugs have been shown to be associated with an increased risk of fetal abnormalities when taken by the pregnant mother. The best known example is, of course, thalidomide (Fig. 2.9); but the striking and severe abnormalities produced by the

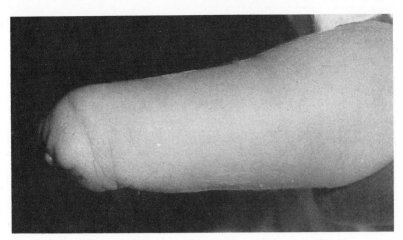

Fig. 2.9 The results of thalidomide: there is no hand on this arm

drug led to its early incrimination and withdrawal. Most drugs have much subtler adverse effects and it is important during pregnancy to avoid using newer drugs whose safety is not well tried and tested, except in exceptional circumstances.

In all cases the value of a drug to the mother must be weighed against possible risks to the fetus. Thus it is reasonable to use high-dose quinine to treat chloroquine-resistant malaria, but not for malaria prophylaxis as it increases the risk of abortion. Similarly one may use frusemide to treat heart disease in pregnancy, but not for physiological ankle oedema when there is a risk of reducing maternal intravascular volume and placental perfusion. As a general rule, all drugs should be avoided during pregnancy unless they are essential. It is convenient to divide pregnancy into two periods: the first trimester and the second and third trimesters.

The first trimester

If dangerous and possibly teratogenic drugs are to be avoided in early pregnancy, it is important for the doctor to assume, when prescribing, that any woman of child-bearing age is pregnant unless she can give specific assurances that she is not. If this rule is not followed, teratogenic drugs may be given inadvertently before either the family doctor or the woman herself knows that she is pregnant.

Small doses of X-rays to the pregnant woman (e.g. for a chest radiograph) are probably not harmful, but larger doses may cause fetal death or abnormalities such as microcephaly or, possibly, childhood leukaemia. There does not seem to be any evidence that clinical ultrasound is harmful to the fetus.

Table 2.5 Drugs which may affect the fetus if given during the first trimester of pregnancy.

Drugs	Use	Proved or suspected abnormalities
19-nor-progestagens (such as norethisterone and norethynodrel)	For treatment of recurrent abortion	Masculinization of female fetus
Isoretinoin (and related drugs)	Acne	Abortion and central nervous system defects
Lithium	Mania	Cardiovascular malformations
Phenytoin	Anticonvulsant	Folic acid antagonist producing cleft lip, finger and toe abnormalities, diaphragmatic hernia. There is increased risk if toxic levels are present and blood levels should be monitored throughout pregnancy
Salicylates (including aspirin)		A possible risk of premature closure of the ductus arteriosus, pulmonary hypertension, and periventrical haemorrhage
Trimethoprim (in co-trimoxazole)	Urinary tract infection	Folic acid antagonist producing congenital malformations; probably a theoretical risk, but folic acid supplements should be given
Warfarin	Anticoagulant	Nasal bone hypoplasia, bony defects in limbs, and punctate epiphyses

Some drugs which may affect the fetus if given during the first trimester of pregnancy are listed in Table 2.5. It must be emphasized that with all these drugs there is only a small increase in risk of the specific abnormalities mentioned when compared with the general population.

Second and third trimesters

Substances with molecular weights of less than about 600 cross the

Table 2.6 Drugs which may affect the fetus if given during the second and third trimester of pregnancy.

Drugs	Effects on fetus or newborn
Antibiotics and related agents	
Tetracyclines	Chelate with calcium and therefore are deposited in tissues undergoing mineralization. Produce yellow teeth and reduce bone growth

Drugs	Effects on fetus or newborn
Antibiotics and related agents	
Sulphonamides and co-trimoxazole	If given shortly before delivery they might possibly displace bilirubin from protein binding sites, leading to neonatal kernicterus
Streptomycin	Poorly excreted by the newborn kidney and toxic to the eighth cranial nerve
Drugs acting on the central nervous system	
Narcotics	Respiratory depression, poor feeding, withdrawal fits (see Chapter 14)
Barbiturates	Produce deficiency of vitamin-K-dependent liver clotting factors leading to haemorrhagic disease. In anticonvulsant doses they may also produce withdrawal fits or apnoeic attacks
Diazepam	Hypothermia, hypotonia, poor sucking, jaundice, withdrawal fits and apnoeic attacks
Salicylates	Low levels of factor XII, platelet abnormalities and prolonged prothrombin time leading to neonatal haemorrhage
Antihypertensives	
Reserpine	Bradycardia, poor temperature control, nasal obstruction, lethargy and respiratory depression
Ganglion blockers	Hypotension and paralytic ileus
Thiazide diuretics	A very small risk of thrombocytopenic purpura
Propranolol	Bradycardia, congestive cardiac failure
Thyroid drugs	
Iodides (e.g. in cough mixtures or contrast media used in radiography)	Goitre, hypothyroidism
Carbimazole or thiouracil	Goitre, hypothyroidism
Anticoagulants	
Coumarins (e.g. warfarin or phenindione)	Fetal or neonatal haemorrhage due to prolonged prothrombin time. Heparin which does not cross the placenta should be substituted for these oral drugs about one month before the expected date of delivery
Steroids	Possible increased risk of intrauterine growth retardation and long-term effect on subsequent growth
Antidiabetic drugs	
Chlorpropamide	Possibility of neonatal hypoglycaemia

placenta easily. Most drugs come into this category, and they are often more toxic to the fetus than to the mother (Table 2.6). This may be because drugs such as barbiturates can enter the brain more easily, or because drugs are less well excreted by the fetal kidneys or liver, for example chloramphenicol, sulphonamides and phenytoin. The persistence of maternally derived drugs in the newborn baby must be considered when prescribing safely in late pregnancy or during labour. In addition many drugs are excreted in breast milk (see Chapter 7).

Further Reading

Action on Smoking and Health (1980) Mothers who smoke and their children, *Practitioner*, *224*, 735.

Anthony, A.N. (1947) Children born during the siege of Leningrad in 1942. *Journal of Pediatrics*, *30*, 250.

Babson, S.G. & Benson, R.C. (1980) *Management of the High Risk Pregnancy and Intensive Care of the Neonate*, 4th ed. St Louis: C.V. Mosby.

Beard, R.W. & Sharp, F. (eds) (1985) Preterm Labour and its Consequences. *Proceedings of the thirteenth study group of the Royal College of Obstetricians and Gynaecologists*, London.

Berry, P.J. (1986) The pathology of the embryo and fetus, *Hospital Update*, *12*, 121.

Brock, D.J.H. (1982) *Early Diagnosis of Fetal Defects*. Edinburgh: Churchill Livingstone.

Butler, N.R. & Alberman, E.D. (1969) *Perinatal Problems*. Edinburgh: Livingstone.

Butler, N.R. & Bonham, D.G. (1963) *Perinatal Mortality*. Edinburgh: Livingstone.

Chamberlain, R., Chamberlain, G., Hewlett, B. & Claireaux, A. (1975) *British Births 1970*. London: Heinemann Medical.

Clarene, S.K. & Smith, D.W. (1978) The fetal alcohol syndrome. *New England Journal of Medicine 298*, 1063–7.

Durward, L. (ed) (1985) *Born Unequal—Perspectives on Pregnancy and Childrearing in Unemployed Families*. London: Maternity Alliance.

Forfar, J.O. & Arneil, G.C. (eds) (1984) *Textbook of Paediatrics*, 3rd ed. Edinburgh: Churchill Livingstone.

Grahn, D. & Kratchman, J. (1963) Variations in neonatal death rate and birth rate in the US and possible relations to environmental radiation, geology and altitude. *American Journal of Human Genetics*, *15*, 329.

Loeffler, R.E. (1984) Chorionic villus biopsy. *British Journal of Hospital Medicine*, *31*, 418–420.

Nicolaides, K.H. & Rodeck, C.H. (1985) Role of fetoscopy in perinatal medicine. In *Recent Advances in Perinatal Medicine 2*, ed. M.L. Chiswick. Edinburgh: Churchill Livingstone.

Reed, D.M. & Stanley, F.J. (1976) *The Epidemiology of Prematurity*. New York: Urban and Schwartzenburg.

Smith, P.A., Chudleigh, P. & Campbell, S. (1984) Ultrasound. *British Journal of Hospital Medicine*, *31*, 421–426.

Wald, N.J. (ed) (1984) *Antenatal and Neonatal Screening*. Oxford: Oxford University Press.

Whitfield, C.R. & McNay, M.B. (1984) Amniocentesis. *British Journal of Hospital Medicine*, *31*, 406–416.

Wigglesworth, J.S. (1984) *Perinatal Pathology*. Philadelphia: W.B. Saunders.

3

Resuscitation and Care of the Baby at Delivery

The use of mouth-to-mouth resuscitation dates from antiquity. Benjamin Pugh in 1754 said: 'If the child does not breathe immediately upon delivery . . . wipe its mouth and press your mouth to the child's, at the same time pinching the nose with your thumb and finger to prevent air escaping; inflate the lungs'. Intubation and ventilation using oxygen was described in 1780 by Chaussier in Dijon; it is very surprising that so many useless methods of treating asphyxia have been used since.

The newborn baby is better able to survive a period of asphyxia than an adult. There are several reasons for this: they include the relatively immature brain with its reduced metabolic requirements; the ability to utilize substrates other than glucose for metabolism, for example glycerol, free fatty acids and ketone bodies; and the ability to metabolize glucose anaerobically.

Nonetheless, a baby who is apnoeic with a slow or falling heart rate represents an extreme emergency. In such a situation, treatment, if it is to be effective, must be applied rationally. Many techniques have been developed over the last century which are irrational. These included intragastric oxygen, analeptic drugs, hyperbaric oxygen or electrical stimulation of the phrenic nerve.

The physiological changes underlying the initiation of respiration are described below. Once they are understood the reasons for active resuscitation can be easily appreciated. There are a number of situations in which problems may be predicted before birth so that a paediatrician may be called in good time to attend the delivery and before an emergency arises. These include:

1 premature onset of labour (35 weeks or less of gestation)
2 abnormalities found at rupture of membranes, e.g. polyhydramnios, oligohydramnios or meconium-stained liquor
3 breech presentation or other malpresentation
4 caesarean section
5 evidence of intrapartum asphyxia shown by type II dips on the cardiotocograph, a large dip area, irregular fetal heart rate, fetal tachycardia, or low fetal blood pH on scalp sampling
6 antepartum haemorrhage
7 prolapsed cord
8 severe pre-eclampsia or chronic hypertension
9 maternal diabetes

10 rhesus isoimmunization

11 heavy maternal sedation

12 history of previous neonatal death or of major congenital abnormalities.

The British Birth Survey showed how common apnoea is after abnormal delivery. Of the 16 000 babies in the survey 4.7% had not breathed by three minutes, but nearly a quarter of babies born by the breech or caesarean section had not breathed by that time. The recent changes in maternal anaesthesia have altered the incidence of apnoea. Thus, it is now uncommon to see apnoea in a baby whose mother has an elective caesarean section at term after an uncomplicated pregnancy. It is not necessary to send a paediatrician to such a delivery; the doctors may be better employed in the neonatal intensive care unit.

In an emergency, the resuscitator must be able to rely on his equipment. Therefore before *every* delivery:

1 Check the resuscitation table and its equipment:

(a) laryngoscope of the appropriate size with bright light, spare batteries and bulb (we find the small curved Penlon 'O' and straight Penlon 'WIS' 'O' most useful)

(b) range of endotracheal tubes and standard connectors (2.5 mm for small babies, 3 mm for most babies; 3.5 mm tubes are particularly useful for large mature babies who have aspirated meconium). Some doctors and nurses like to have an endotracheal tube introducer available

(c) manometer at 30 cm of water, or some other method of limiting the pressure used such as an inflating bag. It is common to use an Ambu, Laerdal or Penlon bag. Masks for inflation without an endotracheal tube are necessary

(d) source of suction which is working and has no loose connections

(e) range of suction catheters (5,6 and 8 FG)

(f) oxygen [check the cylinder (and that a cylinder spanner is available) if piped oxygen is not available]

(g) mucus extractors

(h) clock

(i) umbilical venous catheters (8 and 5 FG)

(j) stethoscope

(k) scissors

(l) equipment for securing an endotracheal tube, so that a preterm baby can be transferred to the neonatal unit on mechanical ventilation

(m) airway.

2 Check drugs:

(a) dextrose 5% and 10%

(b) sodium bicarbonate 4.2%

(c) naloxone

(d) normal saline

(e) adrenalin 1:10 000

(f) syringes and needles in a range of sizes.

3 Check that the labour ward temperature is adequate (close the windows!) and turn on the overhead heater. We suggest a labour ward temperature of about 26°C, but at least 20°C. A fan heater could be used to boost the temperature of the room at the time of delivery.

4 Check that the portable incubator is warm.

5 Check the obstetric notes for problems that may be expected.

6 Check that someone has clean hands and a sterile towel to receive the baby from the midwife or obstetrician. Warm towels must be available.

At birth

1 Turn on the clock.

2 Place the baby on the already warm resuscitation table. Have his head towards you. (Many doctors believe that it is harmful to have the head lower than the feet because pressure on the diaphragm from the liver and other organs could hinder breathing.) Gently apply suction to oropharynx and nostrils.

3 Quickly dry the baby by wiping off vernix and amniotic fluid so as to reduce heat loss by evaporation.

By one minute after birth, an assessment of the baby's condition must be made. Subsequent management will vary according to whether asphyxia is present and, if so, whether it is primary or terminal.

Asphyxia

When a baby has too little oxygen in his blood (hypoxaemia) and has become too acid because of accumulated carbon dioxide and lactic acid (acidaemia) he is described as asphyxiated. Failure to breathe is a consequence of asphyxia and of course it will itself lead to asphyxia.

A baby may be born in either primary or terminal apnoea (Fig. 3.1). This terminology has come from experimental asphyxia in animals. There are four characteristic phases of respiration when any newborn mammal is made anoxic: a period of hyperventilation; a period of apnoea usually called primary or preterminal apnoea; gasping; and finally terminal or secondary apnoea. In the period of primary apnoea the animal will survive if it has air to breathe. In terminal apnoea, it dies unless the lungs are ventilated, with cardiac massage and the reversal of acidaemia with alkalis if necessary. Narcotic drugs such as pethidine will greatly prolong the period of primary apnoea, but this can be reversed by naloxone. Brain damage occurs only during terminal asphyxia as a result of prolonged cardiac arrest.

If a baby is in terminal apnoea he will have passed through the stage of

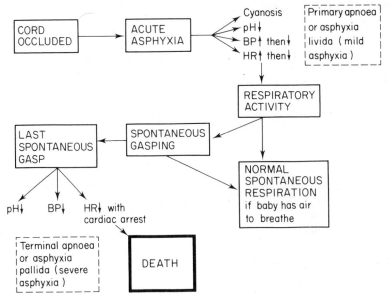

Fig. 3.1 The sequence of events following umbilical cord occlusion

Table 3.1 Differential diagnosis of asphyxia livida and asphyxia pallida.

Primary apnoea (asphyxia livida)	Terminal apnoea (asphyxia pallida)
Apnoea or gasping	No respiratory effect
Cyanosed	Pale and grey
Muscle tone normal or increased	Reduced muscle tone
Heart rate greater than 100/min or less than 100 but rising	Heart rate less than 100/min
Reflex grimacing on stimulation	No response to stimulation
The stage of primary apnoea lasts longer if the mother is given narcotic or anaesthetic drugs. It is shorter if gentle peripheral stimulation or pharyngeal suction is given. This stage is followed by either (*a*) onset of regular respiration or (*b*) more severe asphyxia (terminal apnoea)	If unduly prolonged, may produce brain damage followed *inevitably* by *death* unless: *intervention* by endotracheal (ET) intubation and intermittent positive pressure ventilation (IPPV)

Table 3.2 Causes of neonatal asphyxia.

Immaturity

Respiratory
Obstruction, such as mucus or choanal atresia
Aspiration of blood or meconium
Pneumothorax, usually produced by overenthusiastic resuscitation
Congenital pneumonia
Hypoplastic lungs, as in renal agenesis
Surfactant deficiency, which will later lead to hyaline membrane disease
Diaphragmatic hernia

Metabolic
Acidaemia from antenatal hypoxia
Hypoglycaemia

Cerebral
Congenital cerebral abnormalities
Drugs, such as those given to the mother for sedation
Reflex apnoea, often caused by deep suction of the pharynx
Shock caused by serious blood loss
Severe infection such as Group B streptococcal septicaemia
Traumatic birth

primary apnoea and the last spontaneous gasp by the time of birth. As the management of these two types of asphyxia is quite different, it is important to be able to recognize them clinically. The terms of asphyxia livida (blue) and asphyxia pallida (white) have been out of fashion for some time but are useful when a shocked baby needs active resuscitation. In general, asphyxia pallida is the same as terminal apnoea when the heart rate is very slow and the baby is shocked. The differentiation of these conditions is summarized in Table 3.1, and the causes of neonatal asphyxia are shown in Table 3.2.

The assessment of the baby's condition was formalized by Dr Virginia Apgar by assigning a score of 0 to 2 for each of five facets of the baby's state (Table 3.3). The assessment at one minute is important for the further management of resuscitation. However, it has been shown that an assessment at five minutes is more reliable as a predictor of the risk of death during the first 28 days of life and of the child's neurological state and risk of major handicap at the age of one year. It is therefore customary to do both one-minute and five-minute Apgar scores. The five signs are not equally important—heart rate and respiratory effort are crucial—but each factor is relevant in the differentiation of mild from severe asphyxia. The score identifies high-risk infants in both the short and the long term. The higher the score the better; if the five-minute score is 7 or less it should be repeated at 10 minutes (Table 3.3).

Table 3.3 Apgar scoring.

	Score		
	0	1	2
Heart rate	absent	less than 100/min	more than 100/min
Respiratory effort	absent	gasping or irregular	crying or rhythmic breathing
Muscle tone	flaccid	some flexor tone	good with movement
Response to stimulation	none	poor (with a facial grimace)	good (with a cry)
Colour of tongue or abdominal skin	pallor	cyanosis	pink

The one-minute check

Normal baby: spontaneous respiration established

1 Dry the baby and keep him warm.
2 Check for obvious abnormalities such as spina bifida or imperforate anus; abrasions, fractures, or haemorrhage due to trauma; listen to the heart and lungs; palpate the abdomen for masses or enlarged viscera; examine the genitalia.
3 Put on an umbilical cord clamp about 3 cm from the umbilicus and cut off the rest of the cord. Check for the presence of two arteries (small, thick-walled) and one vein (large, thin-walled).
4 Give the baby to the mother. It is nice for him to be in skin-to-skin contact with her (Fig. 3.2) with a blanket to cover both of them. The baby can then take his first feed.
5 Transfer mother and baby together to the postnatal ward.

The infant with primary apnoea

Action can be taken in the following order:
1 Gentle pharyngeal suction. This provides reflex stimulation of the posterior pharyngeal wall and produces a powerful stimulus for respiration.
2 Blow oxygen over the face (too fast a jet merely cools the baby).
3 Flick the feet—lightly!
4 IPPV by bag and mask if the baby has not breathed by about two minutes.

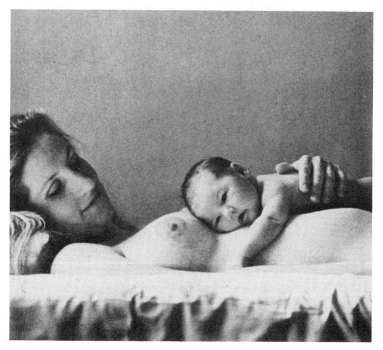

Fig. 3.2 Skin-to-skin contact in a warm labour ward. By courtesy of Professor J. Hedgecoe

If the heart rate falls or the baby remains unresponsive, proceed with the schedule for terminal apnoea.

The infant with terminal apnoea

1 Inspect the vocal cords with a laryngoscope; aspirate liquid under direct vision.

2 Intubate with the largest possible endotracheal tube (ET) (3 mm diameter for the average baby); do not advance more than 1–1.5 cm beyond the glottis (for technique see below).

3 The endotracheal tube should already have a connector attached to it; this can then be fitted on to an inflating bag. The alternative technique is to attach the side limb of a Y connector down which oxygen can flow at approximately 2 l/min.

4 Do not allow the pressure to exceed 30–35 cm of water (a pressure valve may need setting manually or a water manometer may provide automatic blow-off). When a bag is used it is safe to use higher pressures since the volume is controlled.

5 Occlude the open end of Y connector with your thumb and release rhythmically at about 30 times per minute or inflate with the bag; ensure that all connections are tight.

6 Check that both sides of the chest move and there are breath sounds on both sides; the heart rate should gradually increase to normal, and the baby should become pink.

7 Maintain artificial respiration until the baby has started breathing spontaneously and this has become well established (for several minutes).

8 Extubate the baby.

9 Give the baby to mother.

10 Do *not* transfer to the special care baby unit unless there are other indications (see Chapter 4).

NB If the baby is obviously in terminal apnoea, do not wait for one minute before starting resuscitation. A preterm baby should be intubated if he is in any respiratory difficulty, and it is common to use routine intubation for babies under 30 weeks gestation.

If in doubt as to whether apnoea is primary or terminal, proceed as for terminal apnoea—intubate.

Management of cardiac arrest

Press the upper sternum sharply but gently downwards with two fingers once per second (preferably get an assistant to do this); intubate and ventilate as above; if single-handed give ten beats of external cardiac massage before intubating; check efficacy of massage by feeling femoral pulses; discontinue massage when the heartbeat is established; too heavy a pressure or pressure too low down on the sternum may rupture the liver with possible fatal haemorrhage.

Use of drugs in apnoea

Use of drugs, even when indicated, should never delay intubation and artificial ventilation if this is necessary.

1 *Alkali.* A baby who has been apnoeic for some time develops metabolic acidaemia. The best way to correct this is to treat the hypoxia which causes it—by intubation and ventilation with added oxygen. In the most severely affected babies alkali may be given. It must be given *slowly* and *sparingly* as 8.4% sodium bicarbonate (which contains 1 mmol in 1 ml) diluted in an equal volume of 10% dextrose or as 4.2% $NaHCO_3$, which is probably better stocked, instead. Not more than 3 mmol/kg body weight should be given at a rate of not more than 1 mmol/min. A useful rule is to give sodium bicarbonate if the baby has not breathed spontaneously by five minutes. It can be given through a needle into the umbilical vein at the base of the cord, but some paediatricians feel happier to give it

through an umbilical venous catheter. If possible it is valuable to isolate a
section of umbilical cord between two clamps so that a blood gas analysis
can be done to estimate the severity of acidosis before alkali is given.

2 *Naloxone.* If the mother has been given pethidine or morphine within a
few hours of delivery *and* the baby is slow to breathe adequately after
resuscitation, naloxone may be given intravenously, 0.01 mg/kg once
only to counteract the respiratory depression that they cause. Naloxone
has the advantage over previously used narcotic antagonists that it has no
respiratory depressant action of its own. It may be useful to give an
additional 0.01 mg/kg intramuscularly because it will have a longer-
lasting effect.

3 *Analeptics* (e.g. nikethamide). These drugs should *not* be used: they
are unnecessary in primary apnoea and dangerous in terminal apnoea as
they will not effect respiration and may cause fits and hypotension.

Some techniques used in resuscitation

Laryngoscopy and endotracheal intubation (Fig. 3.3)

1 Lay the baby on his back.
2 Hold head with right hand so as to keep the neck slightly flexed and
the head extended on the neck.
3 Hold a laryngoscope in the left hand and pass the blade along the
right side of the mouth, displacing the tongue to the left.
4 Advance blade until it rests in the vallecula between the epiglottis and
base of tongue.
5 Tilt tip of blade slightly upwards so as to bring the glottis (top of
trachea) into view.
6 If necessary, pressure on the cricoid cartilage in the throat with
another finger of the left hand will produce a better view.
7 The glottis may be obscured by fluid. If so, a fine suction catheter is
used to reveal it as a black slit with the vocal cords on each side.
8 An appropriate size of endotracheal tube is taken in the right hand
and passed through the glottis under direct vision.
9 It should not go further than 1–1.5 cm beyond the glottis otherwise
one main bronchus will be entered, so occluding the other and causing
collapse of that lung.
10 Check the position by auscultation over both lungs and the stomach.
11 Air entry should be equal on both sides of the chest.

Mask and bag ventilation (Fig. 3.4)

For new medical staff or nurses and midwives who are inexperienced in

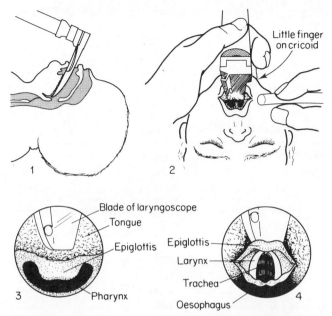

Fig. 3.3 How to intubate. 1, Lie the baby on his back if possible, with the head tilted slightly downwards. Extend the neck so that the chin points upwards. 2, Take an infant laryngoscope with a straight blade and insert the blade into the infant's mouth, gently lifting the tongue. 3, The epiglottis can be seen at the base of the tongue; it hangs down obscuring the entrance to the larynx. 4, Slide the laryngoscope to the base of the epiglottis and tilt the tip of the blade upward. At the same time press gently on the cricoid cartilage with the little finger. The entrance to the larynx will then come into view. An endotracheal tube can then be guided carefully into the trachea. From S. Wallis & D. Harvey (1979) *Nursing Times*, by permission of the authors and editors

resuscitation and when no immediate skilled help is available, this is probably a safer method of resuscitating an asphyxiated baby than unskilled endotracheal intubation.

Great care must be taken not to squeeze the bag too hard otherwise large volumes of oxygen or air may rupture the baby's lungs. A given volume pumped into unexpanded lungs inevitably results in a higher pressure than if pumped into the same lungs when fully expanded. The inclusion of a hole in the inflating valve of such equipment as the Cardiff Infant Inflating Bag (Penlon) allows air to escape to the atmosphere, making it impossible to maintain inappropriately high pressure for more than a fraction of a second.

Chest movement should be the method of judging the efficacy of resuscitation. Make sure that the baby is on his back with his neck slightly flexed and the head extended on the neck. The neonatal face-mask should be positioned so as to produce a good seal over the mouth and nose.

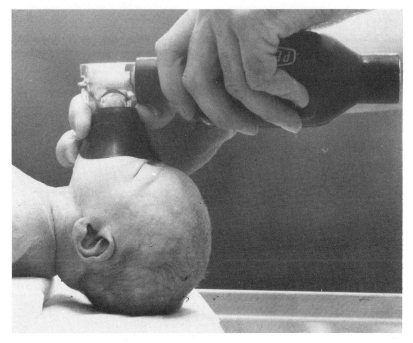

Fig. 3.4 The Cardiff infant inflating bag and mask. (By courtesy of Penlon Ltd)

Insertion of umbilical venous catheter

This is the most reliable way of administering drugs.
1 Fill a 8 or 5 French gauge polyvinyl catheter with normal saline via a three-way tap.
2 Close the tap so that no air may get to the baby on insertion.
3 Cut cord with sterile scissors or scalpel blade to about 2 cm from umbilicus.
4 Grip cut end with Spencer Wells forceps and insert catheter under sterile conditions 5–10 cm into umbilical vein (the large, single, thin-walled vessel).
5 Drugs may be given through the side limb of the three-way tap.
6 *Never* open the umbilical venous catheter to air.

Obtaining cord blood

It has been common to allow blood to drip from the placental end of the cord, but the blood is easily contaminated with Wharton's jelly and it is better to collect the blood with a needle and syringe. It can be taken from a vein on the cord itself or on the fetal surface of the placenta.

It has now been shown that arterial pH at birth is a better measure of asphyxia than the Apgar score. In any birth where this is necessary, such as intrapartum hypoxia or preterm delivery, two clamps can be put on the cord. A sample of arterial blood for gas analysis can be obtained with a needle and syringe.

Complications of endotracheal intubation

Unskilled resuscitation may be dangerous. Errors usually stem from lack of experience and lack of understanding of the physiological mechanisms underlying the onset of respiration. Examples include:

1 Advancing the laryngoscope blade too far, obscuring the glottis and revealing the oesophagus which may be intubated in error. Withdraw the blade slowly and point the tip slightly upwards. The glottis will then come into view.

2 Overextension of the baby's head: this precludes a good view. The neck should be slightly flexed and the head extended on the neck.

3 Insertion of the endotracheal tube too far beyond the glottis (see above).

4 Overenthusiastic use of drugs: the establishment of respiration by artificial ventilation must precede the use of alkali or naloxone. In addition, alkali should not be given unless there is adequate circulation as it will remain in the liver and not progress further.

The techniques of resuscitation cannot be learnt from a book. It is useful to practise on models or stillborn babies, but there is no substitute for constant practice in the company of someone experienced in these techniques. The most important rule is that you must see the larynx before you intubate. It is easy to become agitated and to push the tube in blindly. When this happens it is possible to lose the tube down the oesophagus.

Examination of the Placenta

The placenta should be examined after every delivery because of its relevance to fetal growth. Conditions in which this is particularly useful include ascertaining the zygosity of twins, fetal haemorrhage, intrauterine infection with chorioamnionitis, birth asphyxia with retroplacental clots and placental infarcts, and intrauterine growth retardation (associated with a small placenta). Any abnormal placenta, including those from multiple pregnancies, should be sent to the pathologist for an opinion.

Indications for Transfer to
Special or Intermediate Care Baby Unit

These indications are listed fully in Chapter 4. In summary, babies who have been born by caesarean section or forceps delivery or those who have minor abnormalities should *not* routinely be transferred to the special baby care unit. It is much more difficult for a mother to form an attachment to her baby on a special care baby unit and also more difficult for her to establish breast feeding.

Other Emergencies

There are a number of conditions which require urgent treatment in the labour ward.

Meconium aspiration

This condition is commonly seen in term babies, particularly those who are small for dates or who have had acute intrapartum asphyxia. It is rare in the preterm. It is also discussed in Chapters 5 and 6. If meconium is inhaled into the fine bronchial during delivery a chemical pneumonitis ensues. This may often be complicated by secondary bacterial pneumonia or pneumothorax.

The most important prophylactic procedure is to aspirate the mouth and pharynx throughly as soon as the head is born. Although it is no longer considered good practice to aspirate the pharynx deeply in a normal delivery, it is essential when there is thick meconium in the liquor amnii. It is useful to prevent respiration while this is being done. Some units have a policy of holding the chest firmly to stop the first breath but this is very difficult to do. It seems more practical to do the aspiration while the body is still inside the birth canal.

If thick meconium is aspirated from the mouth, it is then essential to inspect the larynx with a laryngoscope. If meconium is seen on the larynx itself, an attempt should be made to aspirate the trachea. This can be done either by passing a suction catheter through the glottis, or by passing a large endotracheal tube and passing the catheter through that, or by applying it directly. Of course, it is necessary to start ventilation when the suction has been performed. It is not helpful to perform bronchial lavage.

If meconium is aspirated into the lungs, the baby develops respiratory distress because of pneumonitis and plugging of bronchioles with skin debris, mucus and meconium. Affected babies show signs of respiratory distress with tachypnoea, indrawing and sometimes cyanosis. A chest radiograph (Fig. 5.9) at this time is characteristic, showing irregular areas of subsegmental atelectasis with associated hyperaeration. Such babies may need increased inspired oxygen concentrations to maintain normal arterial oxygen tensions. Arterial oxygen levels should be monitored and inspired oxygen concentrations adjusted appropriately. Such babies should also be screened for infection and started on antibiotics because of the high incidence of secondary bacterial pneumonias.

Diaphragmatic hernia

Embryologically, the diaphragm develops from several tissues. Sometimes there are defects where these tissues have not properly fused. Most commonly there is persistence of the left pleuroperitoneal canal through which bowel herniates. This produces an acute emergency as the lung is unable to expand. Air entering the bowel following delivery causes increasing dyspnoea and cyanosis and displacement of the heart to the right. Other signs include bowel sounds audible in the chest and a scaphoid abdomen due to absence of bowel. Treatment is by endotracheal intubation and IPPV until surgery can be arranged to replace the bowel in the abdomen and repair the diaphragmatic defect. It is useful to sedate the baby heavily with an opiate to suppress respiration and thus allow adequate mechanical ventilation. Many surgeons now feel it is better to delay operation for a day or two. Oxygen should never be given by face-mask as air will be swallowed and the bowel will distend and increase the dyspnoea. For this reason, it is useful to pass a gastric tube and empty the stomach of air with a syringe. Associated abnormalities are common, and the prognosis is poor because there is usually pulmonary hypoplasia. This is another reason why it is difficult to expand the lungs (Fig. 3.5).

Pneumothorax

Pneumothorax (see also Chapter 6) is a common complication in the newborn, particularly following meconium aspiration, ventilator therapy, or staphylococcal pneumonia. It may complicate overenthusiastic resuscitation in the labour ward. If a tension pneumothorax develops, the situation may be extremely dangerous. The diagnosis should be considered in any baby who suddenly deteriorates or in whom resuscitation proves particularly difficult. In this situation, there is usually no time for radiographic confirmation (Fig. 3.6). Action should be taken on the basis of clinical signs, but these may be very difficult to detect and so transillumination has proved very valuable. It is necessary to use a very strong fibreoptic source of light. The chest glows brilliantly when a pneumothorax is present, but the investigation is not so useful for babies over 34 weeks gestation as the chest wall is thicker.

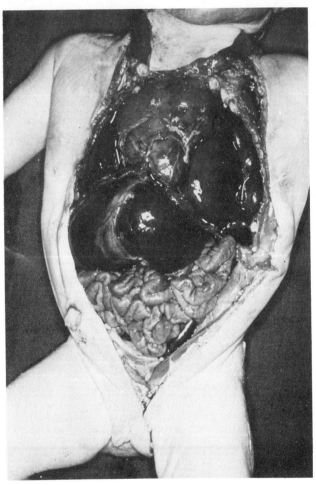

Fig. 3.5 Diaphragmatic hernia. Appearance at autopsy showing gut and liver in the left chest

Emergency treatment is by aspiration of the pleural air. This is conveniently done by using a 21 gauge butterfly needle filled with sterile water. The free end of the tubing is then placed a few centimetres under the surface of sterile water in a sterile container. The needle is then inserted at the fourth intercostal space in the anterior axillary line. If there is a pneumothorax on that side, air will be seen to bubble out from the tubing under the surface of the water on inspiration. This emergency treatment is usually adequate in the early stages. Care must be taken not to insert the metal needle too far so that the underlying lung is not

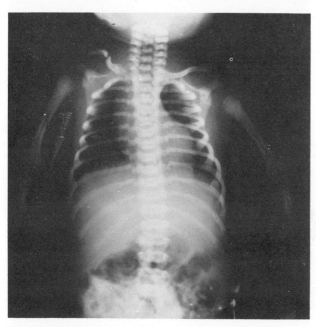

Fig. 3.6 Right-sided pneumothorax

damaged as it re-expands. If there is a large amount of air present, or if the tubing becomes blocked with blood, a more definitive procedure must be carried out inserting a larger polyvinyl tube with a trochar and cannula and attaching it to an intercostal drainage bottle or a valve.

Hydrops fetalis

The signs of hydrops include severe anaemia with a greyish pallor or cyanosis, ascites and generalized oedema and hepatosplenomegaly. The commonest cause of hydrops fetalis in the UK is still severe haemolytic disease of the newborn associated with rhesus isoimmunization although it is much less common than it was. The birth of so severely affected an infant should normally be anticipated before delivery. Treatment is urgent. Clamp the cord immediately: adequate respiration must first be established; laryngeal oedema may be very severe, so do not take the endotracheal tube out too early. Paracentesis to reduce respiratory embarrassment should be performed through the left iliac fossa to avoid an enlarged liver; it is probably easiest to use a polyvinyl intravenous cannula with a central needle. Heart failure should be treated by giving intravenous frusemide 2 mg/kg, and if necessary by venesection (10–20 ml of blood removed from the umbilical vein) and digitalization (see

p. 228). Ventilation is very useful in treating pulmonary oedema. A partial exchange transfusion is then carried out using Group O rhesus-negative packed cells up to a total of 100 ml. Sometimes peritoneal dialysis is required.

Fetal haemorrhage

Fetal haemorrhage may complicate twin delivery (bleeding into the other twin), antepartum haemorrhage, or accidental incision of the placenta by the obstetrician at caesarean section. The baby looks very pale and has tachypnoea and tachycardia. The cord should be tied late and as much blood as possible transferred to the baby before this is done. A transfusion of 20 ml/kg should be given as an emergency. This may be given as Group O rhesus-negative blood; a bottle of blood of this group should always be available in the labour ward for this purpose.

Choanal atresia

The newborn baby is able to breathe mainly through his nose. Any nasal obstruction therefore causes extreme respiratory embarrassment. In choanal atresia, the nasal airway is blocked by a bony or membranous septum across the posterior nasopharynx. The diagnosis should be suspected if there is persistent respiratory difficulty or cyanosis from birth. It is relieved by crying, as it is only in this situation that the baby can get air in through the mouth. The diagnosis is made by inability to pass a feeding catheter down each nostril. Immediate treatment is by inserting an infant oral airway. Elective surgery may then be carried out at a later date.

Exomphalos and gastroschisis

Exomphalos (see also Chapter 8) occurs in about 1 in 10 000 births. The abdominal contents have herniated through the umbilicus into a sac made up of peritoneum and amnion. There are commonly associated abnormalities of the heart, intestines or genitourinary system. Sometimes the sac has perforated before birth.

In gastroschisis there is a defect in the whole thickness of the anterior abdominal wall, usually just to the right of the umbilicus. A large proportion of the gastrointestinal tract including stomach may prolapse through this defect and there is no covering sac. Both conservative and surgical treatment have been advocated; in each the immediate management in the labour ward is identical:

1 Cover the sac or bowel with saline-soaked gauze or silastic sheeting in the form of a bag.

2 Pass a nasogastric tube and suck out stomach contents at frequent intervals to prevent intestinal distension.

3 Consult a surgeon. (Details about the preparation of babies for transfer to a regional neonatal surgical unit, and for surgery are given in Chapter 8.)

Babies who need Transfer to a Regional Centre for Intensive Neonatal Care

Ideally, if problems can be anticipated, a baby should be transferred in utero. This is not always possible—serious unpredicted problems can arise after delivery which necessitate transfer to a regional centre for intensive neonatal care for specialist management. It is important for the referring hospital staff to maintain the baby in as stable and satisfactory a condition as possible until the transfer. It is better to arrange with the obstetric staff for the mother to go with the baby if at all possible. The referring hospital should have the following specimens ready to accompany the baby: (a) maternal high vaginal swab and clotted blood sample, (b) placenta (in sealed bag), (c) cord blood (if possible), and (d) (from the baby) surface swabs (ear, nose, throat, umbilical, rectal), blood cultures and gastric aspirate—all should be taken before antibiotic treatment is started. (Apart from the ear swab and blood culture, the other cultures are not necessary, but some regional centres require them.)

The team who collect the baby must check that they have all the appropriate equipment. This would include:

1 portable heated incubator with working ventilator and circuit

2 full oxygen and air cylinders and spare full cylinders with spanners

3 portable heart-rate monitor, and transcutaneous Po_2 monitor and syringe pump

4 gamgee, blankets and silver swaddler

5 other equipment including mucus extractors, ambu bag, torch, suction catheters, intubating equipment with assorted endotracheal tubes and connectors, electrodes and cream, artery forceps, oxygen tubing and instant camera and flash

6 drugs.

A check list must be kept with the squad call incubator and equipment used must be replaced immediately on return. All the equipment must be checked daily and kept in optimum working order ready for a flying squad call at any time.

The flying squad team, on arrival at the referring hospital, should be prepared to spend time getting the baby into optimal condition for the journey. For example, the baby may require warming if cold, blood gases should be checked as acidosis or hypoxaemia may need correction and intubation and mechanical ventilation may be needed if he is showing respiratory distress. An umbilical catheter may be valuable.

When the baby is warm and stable, prepare for the journey:

1 Make sure the incubator and wrappings are warmed.

2 Check the oxygen and ventilation settings

3 Place the cardiac electrodes and $P_{tc}Po_2$ monitor probe onto the baby.

4 Place the baby in the incubator and wrap him up with the prewarmed gamgee and insulating bubble sheet.

5 Connect the baby to the ventilator; check the ventilator settings, oxygen concentration and air entry.

6 Connect baby to the appropriate monitors.

7 Make sure baby is comfortable and well padded for journey—in case of emergency stops.

8 Check records and equipment with attached list—make sure the specimens are obtained and consent form is completed.

Before departure make sure that the mother has seen the baby. If she cannot go with him take a photograph (preferably before he is connected up to too many tubes) and leave it for her. Remember to keep her and the referring doctors fully informed of how her baby is progressing.

Further Reading

Abramson, H. (1973) *Resuscitation of the Newborn*, 3rd ed. St Louis: C.V. Mosby.

James, L.S. (1977) Emergencies in the delivery room. In *Neonatal–Perinatal Medicine*, ed. R.E. Behrman, St Louis: C.V. Mosby

—4————————————————————

Care of Normal Newborn Babies

The First Routine Examination

It is usually possible to carry out a quick examination of the baby while still in the labour ward. This may be done by the midwife or doctor and is mainly concerned with the detection of serious abnormalities, for example cleft lip and palate or spina bifida. It is a mistake to attempt a full examination of the infant at that time, as the baby may become very cold.

Within the first 24 hours a full examination must be carried out by the doctor. This is best done by the mother's bedside so that she can watch: in this way she is able to ask questions as the examination proceeds and the doctor is able to provide specific reassurances for any worries that she may have. It is an advantage for the examining doctor to be already aware of any unusual circumstances in the family, social, obstetric or paediatric history. Mothers may be very anxious about what, to the doctor, seems to be a trivial blemish on the baby, e.g. stork bite marks, crumpled ears or milia. The mother's anxieties must always be taken seriously and full explanation given. An over-glib response will only increase the parents' anxiety. Always ask about family illnesses, any abnormalities of pregnancy, the gestation and any family history of tuberculosis.

1 Take a good history. Before a routine examination is done the mother's notes must be read carefully for important clues (see Chapter 2).
2 Emergency conditions should have been excluded by the quick examination at birth, but it is surprising how many conditions can be missed at the first examination and for this reason a routine examination should be very thorough. For example, a cleft palate is easily overlooked.
3 Develop a routine method of examining the baby. There are several schemes for this, but it is probably easiest to examine the baby methodically from fontanelle to toe so that no important points are missed. It may be useful to have a printed examination chart to be filled in for every baby.

Head and skull

The baby may have a large or small skull circumference, or it may be within the normal range but out of proportion to the rest of the body. The occipitofrontal circumference at birth may be misleading because the head can change shape quite markedly within the first three days. A

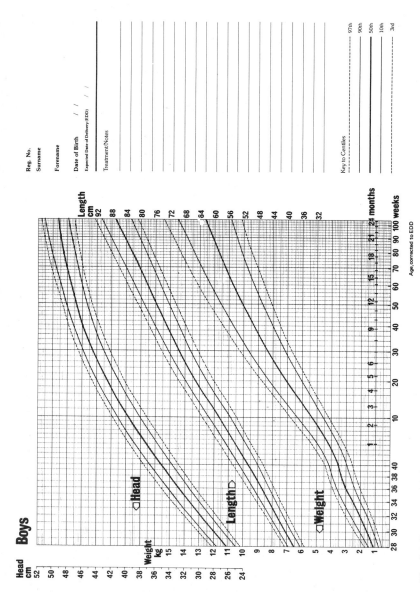

Fig. 4.1 Pearson and Gairdner chart

vertex delivery usually has an elongated head from moulding and this turns to a round shape within a day or so. The doctor should, therefore, always measure the head himself. It is useful to plot the result on a Pearson and Gairdner chart (Fig. 4.1). The baby's head size can be compared with his weight and length. Length is impossible to measure accurately in the newborn period unless it is done with a proper anthropometric instrument such as the neonatometer (Fig. 4.2). It is quite useless to measure the baby with a tape measure. Centile charts for non-caucasian babies are becoming available and will be particularly useful to units serving populations with a high proportion of immigrants.

The fontanelle and sutures should be examined carefully. A small-for-dates baby has a larger anterior fontanelle than a normal baby. If there is any suggestion that the fontanelle is very large or that the sutures are markedly separated, serial measurements of the occipitofrontal circumference should be made, in case the baby is developing hydrocephalus. A third fontanelle between the anterior and posterior fontanelles is one of the supporting signs of Down's syndrome, but it is very inconstant and should not be relied on.

The scalp should be examined carefully because a heart monitoring clip may have been overlooked and be embedded in the scalp amongst the mop of hair. Some babies have marked oedema over the presenting area or bruising where a ventouse cup was applied. A cephalhaematoma is very common (Fig. 4.3) and is a collection of blood between the periosteum of one of the skull bones and the bone itself. It may not be

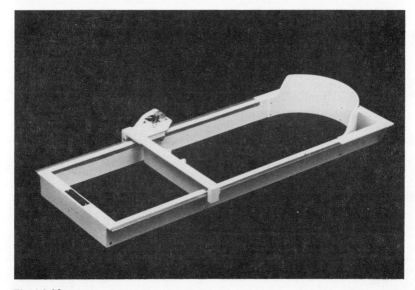

Fig. 4.2 Neonatomer

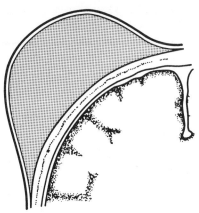

Fig. 4.3 Cephalhaematoma

obvious for a day or two. The fact that the blood is underneath the periosteum means that the swelling is confined to the bone and, therefore, never crosses the midline and thus can be differentiated from oedema or haemorrhage in the scalp itself. The commonest bone to be involved is the parietal bone, but it is also often seen over the occipital bone. The cephalhaematoma is commonly complicated by neonatal jaundice as the blood is absorbed. A cephalhaematoma is often bilateral and one may even see as many as three on one baby if both parietal bones and the occipital bone are involved.

A dangerous haemorrhage is sometimes found under the scalp of black babies (see Chapter 11). The head circumference rapidly enlarges and there is a boggy feel to the whole of the scalp. A baby with this condition needs urgent transfusion if he is not to die from exsanguination.

Microcephaly is shown by a very small head circumference. One should take care before informing the parents about any abnormality of the head circumference because the *rate* of growth of the head is more important that a single circumference reading.

Eyes

Both eyes should be carefully examined. Any discharge or inflammation in the first 24 hours should be investigated urgently as it may indicate gonococcal infection. The baby's eyes are usually open for the first few hours after birth and he seems very alert, but it is common for the lids to become very swollen during the next two days and it may be difficult to see the eye itself. The swelling is probably more common after a difficult delivery. The lids should be carefully separated to reveal the eyeball to make certain that it is present. If the eye itself can be seen the cornea should be observed for size and clarity. A congenital glaucoma causes a cornea which is more than 11 mm in diameter and is cloudy.

There is often a subconjunctival haemorrhage. This disappears within 10 days and is of no significance except that it is upsetting to the parents. It usually appears as a tiny bright red crescent-shaped mark in the white of the eye.

If it is easy to inspect the eye itself it is useful to shine a light or an ophthalmoscope through the pupil. On looking through an ophthalmoscope, the retina appears red and this is called the red reflex. In this way a cataract may be found. The commonest abnormalities of the retina are haemorrhages which again disappear without causing any problem.

Babies often seem to have difficulty in coordinating their eyes during the early weeks of life. They may therefore appear to squint and their gaze sometimes wanders. It should be explained to parents that the baby may have this appearance at this age, but the eyes will become perfectly normal later on. Babies can see very well at birth, and are thought to see things clearly in focus about 25 cm (10 in) away. It is important to remember this when examining the baby as he will enjoy looking at a face; you should be certain that you are the right distance from him and are clearly visible. The parents should be shown how to hold the baby to attract his attention and to get him to look at them, because this is enjoyable for both parents and baby. We are constantly amazed that many parents think a baby is blind at birth and it is useful to tell the parents that the baby can see very clearly.

Ears

The ears should be inspected to ensure that they are not very low set on the head or sticking out abnormally and, most importantly, that there is an auditory meatus. Ears should be considered low set when the helix meets the cranium at a level below that of a horizontal plane with the corner of the orbit. Small lumps of cartilage, usually called accessory auricles, are often found just in front of the ear and may need to be removed if they are very obvious. Some tiny skin tags can be tied off, but larger blemishes should be referred to a plastic surgeon to ensure that all the cartilage is removed.

Marks on the face

A birthmark on the face is usually very obvious, but some of them are entirely benign. The commonest is the simple naevus or 'stork bite mark'. This is usually present as a V-shape mark on the forehead or eyelids (hence the name stork bite since this is supposed to represent the mark of the stork's beak when he carried the baby).

Nose

A baby's nose often appears squashed if there was oligohydramnios. This usually corrects itself within a few days. If the baby has any respiratory difficulty it may be necessary to pass a catheter down each nostril to make certain that there is no choanal artesia (see Chapter 3).

Mouth

A cleft lip is obvious but a cleft palate is not. To be certain that a cleft palate has been excluded, it is necessary both to look at the palate and to feel it. The tongue can be depressed with a wooden spatula to reveal the whole length of the palate; it is possible to have a cleft of the soft palate which cannot be seen without depressing the tongue. A submucosal cleft of the hard palate can be missed by inspection alone. It will become obvious when felt. Other abnormalities in the mouth are usually obvious, such as incisor teeth present at birth, a very enlarged tongue or cysts of the gum.

Some minor abnormalities of the mouth may cause concern to the parents. It is common to see tiny white cysts along the midline of the palate or in the gums. These are often called pearls and disappear without any problem.

Skin of the face

There are a number of common minor abnormalities of the skin. A baby may have tiny blister-like lesions over the face at birth. These are called miliaria crystallina; they burst and disappear spontaneously although it is usually wise to take a swab to ensure that there is no infection.

Tiny white spots on the nose are known as milia (milk spots) and are due to sebaceous gland enlargement. Tiny white cysts are often seen on the face. They are often given long names which are not of great importance.

Neck

It is usually obvious if the neck is abnormally short, but the neck must be palpated to ensure that there are no cysts, webbing or an enlarged thyroid. Occasionally sinuses discharging from the neck can be seen.

Arms

Look at the arms carefully to see if they are the same length. It may be obvious that the baby is moving only one arm, in which case the commonest reasons are brachial plexus palsy (Erb's palsy) (see Chapter

11) or a fractured clavicle or humerus (see Chapter 11). It is embarrassing to miss such common abnormalities as syndactyly or an absent or extra finger; count the fingers on each hand and examine the hand carefully. A single palmar crease is a common physical sign of Down's syndrome. Do not make this diagnosis on the basis of a single palmar crease alone as it occurs in 1% of the normal population.

Heart

Some doctors start the examination with the heart because it is easier to listen to it before the baby starts to cry. Look for cyanosis by inspecting the tongue and look for any breathlessness. Many newborn babies have various soft systolic murmurs but a loud systolic murmur or any diastolic murmur is a reason for immediate cardiac investigation. The femoral pulses should be palpated, but this is usually done later in the examination.

Chest

Look for tachypnoea or retraction of the intercostal spaces or of the ribs or subcostal area. Auscultation of the chest is not very useful but is traditional. It is also useful for junior doctors and midwives to be familiar with normal breath sounds in the newborn so that an emergency (for example an endotracheal tube slipping into the right main bronchus) can be recognized.

Breasts

Assessment of breast size is important as part of the gestational assessment of the baby (see below). Breast engorgement is not usually obvious at the first examination (see below).

Abdomen

Look for marked distension; this may indicate ascites which often occurs in a baby with hydrops. The liver, spleen and kidneys should be felt for. The spleen may normally be palpable just below the costal margin, but it is greatly enlarged in rhesus disease. The liver is most easily felt in the epigastrium; it is usually about half way between the umbilicus and the xiphisternum. A liver edge at or below the umbilicus is abnormal. The kidneys can be palpated by bimanual examination or by using one hand with the thumb in front of the abdomen and the fingers behind the loin (Fig. 4.4).

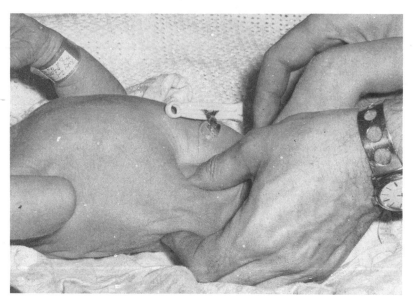

Fig. 4.4 Palpating the right kidney

Umbilicus

Even though the cord has been clamped at birth, it is possible to see whether there are three vessels in the cord. It is common for the skin of the abdomen to encroach on the base of the cord and this may suggest that an umbilical hernia will develop later. The base of the cord should be examined carefully for minor degrees of exomphalos which are easily missed; this is a hernia containing gut with a transparent membrane. Inflammation of the umbilicus is unusual in the first 24 hours.

Femoral pulses

The hips should be abducted into a frog position; the femoral pulses can be felt in the midpoint of the groin. They are sometimes rather difficult to find; it is important to wait for the baby to stop crying. If the pulses cannot be found, coarctation of the aorta may be present; but the usual reason is that they were not very obvious and they are easily palpable later in the first week. Coarctation may be present with normal femoral pulses because the ductus arteriosus can supply the aorta. It is, therefore, possible to find them on the first day, but they then disappear several days later when the ductus closes. Any baby with a suspected cardiac abnormality should have the femoral pulses examined repeatedly.

Hips

A careful examination for congenital dislocation of the hips is essential; it is described in detail on p. 190. The important findings are limited abduction and the sudden jump when the hip is dislocated or reduced.

Genitalia

Boys

The first week of life is the most important time to establish whether the testes have descended. A careful record that the testes have descended ensures that there is no later worry about whether testes are undescended

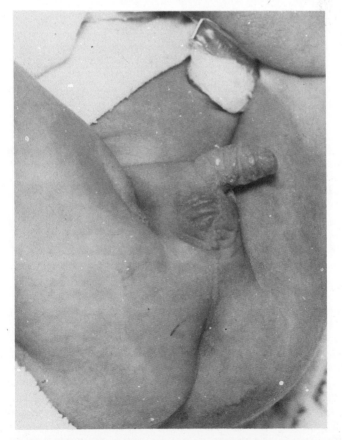

Fig. 4.5 Undescended testes in a baby of 35 weeks gestation

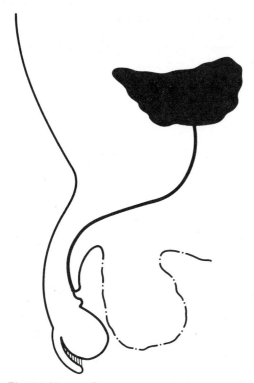

Fig. 4.6 Hypospadias

or merely retractile. Each of the testes should be present in the scrotum after 36 weeks gestation (Fig. 4.5). If the testes have not descended, an appointment should be made to see the baby in six weeks time because they often descend meanwhile. After six weeks the testes are unlikely to descend, unless the baby was very premature.

The penis should be examined carefully. The foreskin cannot be retracted at birth and the meatus may look very small, but this is not an indication for circumcision. Some boys have hypospadias: the urethral meatus is not on the tip of the penis but on the ventral surface somewhere between the tip and the scrotum. In this condition the foreskin is cleft on the ventral surface (Fig. 4.6) and is often called hooded. The baby looks as if he has been circumcised naturally. A careful search for the meatus should be made, as there is often a small dimple on the tip of the penis which is thought to be the meatus when in fact the urine emerges further down the penis. If there is any doubt, a nurse or the mother should be asked to watch micturition to see where the urine emerges and that the baby produces a good stream. A dribble rather than a good stream is an important physical sign and should always be recorded because a block in the urethra may be present which could lead to permanent renal damage unless it is relieved (see Chapter 9). A boy with hypospadias should not be circumcised because some of the skin may be needed for repair of the urethra. If circumcision is needed for religious reasons, it is possible to take a tiny piece of skin and leave plenty for the plastic surgeon.

A very small penis (micropenis) may be a sign of hypopituitarism, particularly if there is associated hypoglycaemia.

The scrotum is often pigmented and the usual reason for this is racial. However, do not forget adrenal hyperplasia which can produce the same appearance (see p. 197).

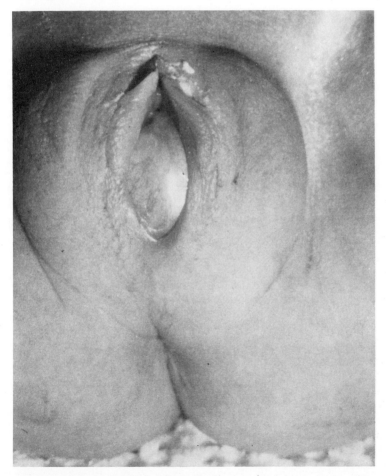

Fig. 4.7 Hydrocolpos (imperforate hymen)

Girls

The labia minora and the clitoris look surprisingly large in the newborn baby, particularly if the baby was preterm. If there is any doubt about the size of the clitoris a senior opinion should be obtained because some forms of adrenal hyperplasia may cause masculinization and need urgent treatment. Separate the labia majora; the vaginal opening should be obvious. If it is not, probe very gently because it is important not to miss an absent vagina. Discharge of meconium through the vagina is very suspicious because it suggests a fistula from the bowel.

There are often small tags around the vagina or even small cysts. Most of these disappear as the child gets older. If the hymen is completely sealed over it may be bulging from retained secretions and will need operation by a paediatric gynaecologist (Fig. 4.7).

Anus

The baby's bottom is often covered with meconium. Be careful to wipe it all away because a number of minor abnormalities of the anus still allow the baby to pass meconium. There should be a reasonable gap between the posterior part of the scrotum or vulva and the anus. Meconium may not be passed for the first 24 hours after birth. If there is any further delay, a gentle rectal examination should be done. If any obstruction is found, no force should be used otherwise the rectum could be ruptured. The commonest abnormality is atresia of the anus, but it is sometimes merely covered by a triangular flap of skin.

Legs

Straighten the legs to see if they are the same length. The are normally bowed outwards. The knees occasionally show dislocation with the tibia dislocated forwards on the femur.

Feet

Abnormalities of the feet are very common; the parents are often worried about clubbed feet. The commonest variety is talipes equinovarus (TEV) in which the foot is adducted and plantar flexed. This is described in the section on congenitial abnormalities. The most important procedure during examination is to see how far one can reduce the abnormality by pressure on the sole of the foot; TEV which is completely reducible is often called positional talipes and has an excellent prognosis (Fig. 4.8). Talipes calcaneovalgus is shown by a foot in eversion and dorsiflexion; this also has a good prognosis if the deformity can be completely reduced. Count the toes to look for any abnormalities such as extra toes or syndactyly.

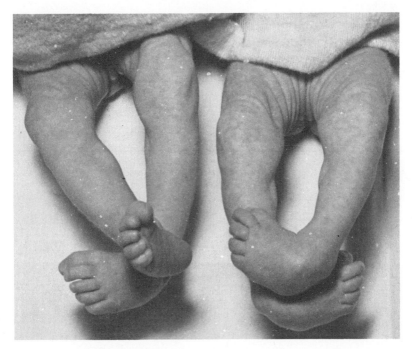

Fig. 4.8 Twins with talipes equinovarus. The one on the right has severe irreducible talipes and that on the left reducible (positional) talipes

The back

There is sometimes a pit in the lumbosacral region. If it is possible to see the bottom of the pit, no action need be taken, but if there seems to be a track passing inwards, the baby should be referred to a paediatric neurosurgeon as infection may spread to the central nervous system causing meningitis. Run a finger up the back to ensure that there are no swellings. It is particularly easy to miss a small encephalocele covered by skin and hair on the back of the head (Fig. 4.9). Mongolian blue spots are large areas, usually over the sacrum or buttocks which look rather like bruises. They are found in black or oriental babies and it is important that they are not confused with bruising due to non-accidental injury (Fig. 4.10). A simple capillary naevus is very common over the cervical and lower lumbar spine.

Neurological examination

During the examination, it should be possible to test the baby's responses.

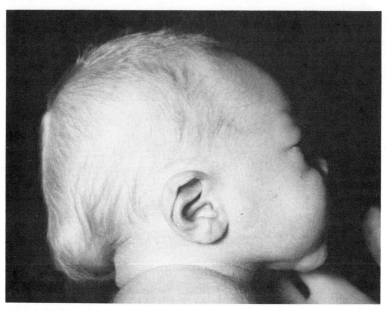

Fig. 4.9 A cervical encephalocele

A normal newborn baby has a number of simple reflexes which show that his skin is sensitive and that the central nervous system, nerves and muscles are working. The grasp reflexes are the easiest to demonstrate; a baby will clench his hand or foot in response to pressure on the palm or sole. When doing the palmar grasp it is usual to pull the baby forward to see whether he will respond by lifting his head slightly or pulling with his arms. A baby whose head flops helplessly backwards has abnormally low tone. The Galant reflex is shown when the baby has been turned over: a finger touches the loin and the baby swings his bottom over to that side.

The Moro response is the most famous primitive response; if the cot is slapped on either side of the baby, or the baby's bottom is lifted and allowed to fall gently onto the cot, or if the baby's head is lifted off the cot and allowed to fall back a few degrees onto the hand, a characteristic response follows — the baby flings his arms sideways, spreads his fingers and then adducts the arms as if in an embrace. During this the legs also extend. The baby looks startled and often cries. If it is felt necessary to elicit this response, it should be done very gently indeed as babies do not like it. It can, however, be useful when looking for a difference between the two sides in a baby who has brachial plexus palsy or a fractured clavicle. It is possible to make a formal score from the neurological examination but this is not necessary for a routine examination.

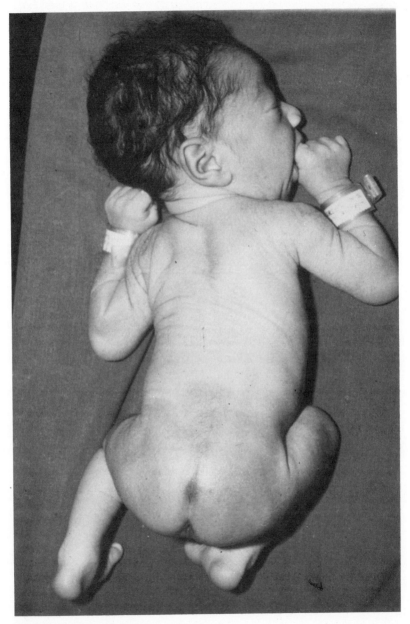

Fig. 4.10 Mongolian blue spot

The primitive responses which are usually described might suggest that the newborn baby is only capable of very simple neurological responses. In fact, he is much more alert to his surroundings than we used to think. There is a period of an hour or two shortly after birth when the baby is particularly alert and looks around. He will usually look at a face intently and is not so interested in non-human objects. He will also respond to being talked to. It is often important to explain this to the parents who may have been told by others that the baby cannot see or hear at birth.

Babies do seem to be sensitive. It is a misconception to think that they do not feel pain. Studies have shown that their palms sweat when a heel prick is done; a circumcision without an anaesthetic must be extremely painful.

At the end of the examination, it is nice to place the baby in the arms of one of the parents, so that they can explore his body fully and get to know their child. They may need encouragement to undress the baby and to look at him all over. The room should be kept reasonably warm so that the cold does not inhibit getting to know one another. It is also a nice time to put the baby to the breast.

The Discharge Examination

A baby needs several examinations during the first week if there are any worrying signs. However, every baby should be examined again before going home, although this is hardly necessary in those going home at 48 hours or sooner. This is just one of the regular examinations which should be done throughout childhood to ensure that an infant is progressing steadily and normally. The purpose of the discharge examination is to make sure that a baby has not developed an infection or other serious condition, which could not be managed at home, and has no congenital abnormality which has been missed. It is common for cardiac abnormalities to show no abnormal signs during the newborn period, but a murmur may appear later. The examination can follow the same plan but there are a number of specific checks to be made.

1 *Jaundice.* A baby who is still jaundiced at discharge needs another examination to make certain that the jaundice fades normally. The alternative is for the health visitor or general practitioner to check whether the jaundice has disappeared by two weeks of age. Prolonged jaundice has many causes (see Chapter 12).

2 *Heart.* Another complete examination of the cardiovascular system is needed in case any physical signs have appeared during the first week.

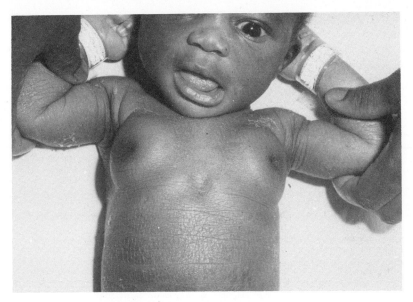

Fig. 4.11 Breast engorgement

3 *Hips.* The hips need rechecking since it is very easy to miss a congenital dislocation.

4 *Umbilicus.* This is a common site of infection. A note should be made about whether the umbilical cord has separated. The mother can be given simple information about cord care, for example applying powder containing an antiseptic such as chlorhexidine.

5 *Breast engorgement.* (Fig. 4.11). This may occur around seven to ten days of age in both sexes due to withdrawal of maternal oestrogens and normally subsides without treatment. Warn the mother not to try and express milk from them as this may lead to infection. Rarely, breast abscess may result (see Chapter 16).

Follow-Up

When a baby is discharged from hospital it is common to give the parents an appointment to come back to the follow-up clinic. However, it is important not to duplicate services which are available in the community since this may give the parents many unnecessary journeys to the hospital and it is likely that this will be much less convenient for them than calling at the local clinic to see the health visitor and the clinical medical officer.

It is extremely important to communicate information about the baby to them and the general practitioner. Modern methods of communication will make this easier. Electronic mail and computer networking will become increasingly important.

In general, there are two good reasons for follow-up. The first is that the baby has a high risk of disability, because of the birth history or other abnormalities. Follow-up is necessary for coordination of care and for detection of other developmental abnormalities. The second is that every neonatal unit running a special or intensive care service should monitor the number and types of abnormalities in the babies who have passed through the unit. Constructive changes in neonatal paediatrics can be made only by finding out whether babies survive and whether they survive without abnormalities. The following are suggested reasons for follow-up at the hospital:

1 *Birth weight under 1500 g*
2 *Major congenital abnormalities* (although it may be better to refer the baby to an appropriate specialist and to leave the coordination of care to the general practitioner and consultant paediatrician with a special interest in community child health)
3 *Urinary tract infections*, because of the risk of ureteric reflux and other abnormalities of the urinary tract
4 *Jaundice* with a peak bilirubin over 380 μmol/l in term babies, but lower in those of low birth weight
5 *Severe asphyxia*. We suggest that an Apgar score of less than 4 at five minutes would be a reasonable criterion
6 *Major neurological abnormality* in the neonatal period such as convulsions during the first 48 hours of life, or definite subarachnoid haemorrhage
7 *Symptomatic hypoglycaemia*
8 *Neonatal abnormalities* such as Erb's palsy which are likely to resolve fairly quickly and which are therefore more easily managed by a few visits to the outpatient department than by referral to another centre. Any long-lasting problems are not best managed from a maternity hospital.

This list, of course, does not include particular problems which are the special interest of an individual hospital.

Intermediate or Transitional Care Unit

To some extent the criteria for admission to special care nurseries have varied with the availability of paediatric and nursing expertise in the postnatal wards. In many units, babies who have been born by forceps delivery, for example, have been routinely admitted to a special care nursery, often even without consultation with the paediatric staff. The percentage of babies admitted to special care baby units has often fluctuated. Recently it became popular to admit many babies for observation and to receive the skilled attention of the doctors and nurses in the unit. In some units this even reached 40% of all births, whereas an admission rate of 6% was common in the early 1960s. We now think that it is a mistake to have a high admission rate because many babies would be separated from the mothers unnecessarily; it also reduces the skills of the nurses in the postnatal wards. The dangers of admitting well babies to special care nurseries are now appreciated: separation from the mother produces anxiety which may lead to impaired lactation or even cessation of breast feeding and a disordered relationship between the mother and her baby, sometimes called poor bonding. In addition there will clearly be an increased risk of healthy babies acquiring an infection if they are transferred to a unit in which there are already ill babies. There is good evidence that pathogenic and resistant bacterial strains are commoner in a special care nursery. The easy availability of phototherapy or a lower threshold for the use of antibiotics and other drugs may increase the risk of iatrogenic illness in such units.

As a result, it is becoming more common for a maternity hospital to have an intermediate or transitional care unit. This can be a section of a postnatal ward where babies needing special care can be nursed with their mother. The nursing staff in this area need special training and there should be a higher ratio of staff to babies than in an ordinary postnatal ward, because the babies need frequent attention, including feeding, daily weighing and four-hourly observations. The babies can be assessed by a paediatrician in the labour ward. The following are suggestions for an admissions policy:

1 Well babies of *low birth weight* but not less than 1700 g

2 *Rhesus disease* which does not require an immediate exchange transfusion

3 *Infants of insulin-dependent diabetics*. These have usually been observed in the special care baby unit for 24 hours, but in well-staffed hospitals they could easily be managed on a postnatal ward. Large babies or babies of mothers who have had an abnormal glucose tolerance test in pregnancy should be on a postnatal ward

4 Babies requiring *short-term tube feeding* before discharge

5 Suspected *meconium aspiration* with no respiratory problems

6 *Phototherapy* if it cannot be done on an ordinary postnatal ward.

Such a unit is not suitable for infected babies.

Transfer to Special Care Unit

The following are reasonable indications justifying transfer to a special care baby unit:

1 *Birth weight* under 1700 g or gestational age less than 32 weeks

2 *Birth asphyxia* with persistent central nervous system or respiratory signs or symptoms. Mild birth asphyxia (Apgar 5 or more at five minutes) with no subsequent problems is not an indication for transfer

3 *Aspiration* including meconium aspiration with respiratory symptoms and signs. Meconium staining of the skin with no evidence of aspiration is not an indication for transfer

4 *Rhesus haemolytic disease.* A rhesus-negative mother or a rhesus-positive mother with antibodies is not an indication for transfer; some mild cases do not need admission if they can be carefully observed on a postnatal ward or in intermediate care

5 *Respiratory* signs such as transient tachypnoea or respiratory distress syndrome. This would include such complications as pneumothorax or recurrent apnoeic attacks, as well as other causes of respiratory distress

6 *Congenital malformation* with symptoms such as congenital heart diseases

7 *Convulsions*

8 *Major infection,* for example meningitis, pneumonia or septicaemia. Minor infections such as those of the urinary tract or skin do not indicate a need for transfer, but some may need isolation only

9 *Persistent vomiting.* This does not include minor feeding problems, 'mucusy' babies or babies with regurgitations or occasional vomits. A baby who is persistently feeding poorly may need transfer

10 *Jaundice* requiring exchange transfusion. Phototherapy for full-term well babies should be given at the mother's bedside on the postnatal ward

11 *Fetal haemorrhage* or haemorrhage from the cord.

It is worth re-emphasizing those circumstances in which babies should *not* be routinely transferred. In addition to those already mentioned these include:

1 *Abnormal delivery* including forceps, ventouse and caesarean section

2 *Malpresentation*

3 *Mild hypothermia*

4 The babies of a *multiple pregnancy*

5 *Previous adverse history* for example, obstetric, neonatal death or stillbirth

6 The *jittery baby*

7 *Maternal illness* or therapy

8 *Traumatic cyanosis*

9 *Malformations* which do not threaten life such as Down's syndrome, cleft lip or talipes equinovarus
10 *Infant of a mother with well-controlled diabetes mellitus.*

Reasons for Isolating Babies

The usual reason that a baby needs isolation is that he is actually, or potentially, infected and is a source of infection to other infants:

1 Admission from outside the hospital
2 Staphylococcal skin lesions
3 Gastroenteritis
4 Severe ophthalmia
5 Group B β-haemolytic streptococcal infection
6 Mothers positive for hepatitis B surface antigen
7 Necrotizing enterocolitis
8 Colonization with a potentially dangerous organism.

There is a need for an isolation unit for infected term babies and also for a small isolation area within the neonatal intensive care unit because some of these babies are very ill.

Quite often the baby needs isolation because his mother is infected. An example is maternal tuberculosis but a more common problem is genital herpes.

Rooming-In

This means that the mother has her baby in the cot beside her for most of the 24 hours. The advantages are that mother and baby are able to get to know one another earlier. Unfortunately it is only really possible in single rooms or in units containing up to four beds. Otherwise there may be too much disturbance to mothers from babies other than their own. Nonetheless, even in many larger wards, rooming-in has been satisfactorily established.

Weighing

A normal newborn baby may lose up to 10% of his birth weight during the first week and not regain it until two weeks of age. Babies normally gain weight thereafter at the rate of some 200 g per week. There is no question that adequate gain in weight and length are crucial during the early months of life. This is the time when brain growth is at its greatest and any shortfall during this time may not be made up afterwards. Mothers, nurses and doctors make something of a fetish of daily weighing. It is perfectly adequate to weigh a well newborn baby on alternate days. In this way, day-to-day variation due to such things as an extra bowel action will not give rise to needless anxiety on the part of the mother or attendants. An ill or small baby, of course, requires more frequent weighing. Routine test weighing of breast-fed babies should not be done because it reduces the chance of successful breast feeding by making the mother worry about how much she should be producing. Weight is best plotted graphically, as inadequate weight gain is then more obvious.

Temperature

The baby's temperature is taken on admission and at 24 hours. Many check the temperature daily thereafter, but this is probably unnecessary in a well baby. Routine taking of the temperature rectally is undesirable as it may rarely cause rectal perforation. Axillary temperatures are quite satisfactory, but a figure below 36°C should be checked with a rectal reading. A low-reading thermometer should always be used.

Passage of Meconium and Urine

Failure to pass either meconium or urine within the first 24 hours should be reported to the paediatrician who should examine the baby carefully. Remember that less than one in a hundred babies will not have passed urine by 48 hours of age. Check for abdominal or bladder distension which might suggest urethral obstruction (much commoner in males and due to urethral valves; Fig. 9.25). Check for the position of the urethral orifice but do not attempt to retract the foreskin or to probe with a catheter. Check that the external genitalia are normal.

It is important to have noted the passage of meconium during delivery, as not doing so is a common reason for believing that the baby has not passed meconium in the first 24 hours. Low birth weight, preterm or ill babies may have delay in the passage of meconium, but always check for abdominal distension or vomiting indicating intestinal obstruction (see Chapter 10). If in doubt take an erect plain abdominal radiograph.

Baths

In the past, too much was made of the necessity for early and frequent bathing of newborn babies. This is not only unnecessary, but also leads to the real danger of the baby becoming cold. A full bath should never be done in the first 24 hours. This still leaves plenty of time for the first-time mother to be shown how to do it before she goes home. The baby's face can be cleaned shortly after birth to make him look nice and any very soiled areas can be cleaned. One unit in India greatly reduced the neonatal mortality rate by cutting out a bath shortly after birth. The use of antiseptic soaps for washing babies is discussed in Chapter 16.

BCG

Tuberculosis still occurs in Britain. It has a high prevalence among immigrants from outside Europe, North America and Australasia; it is therefore common in certain inner-city areas. In such areas, it is safest to immunize all babies against the disease shortly after birth. This is done by giving an injection of BCG before the baby leaves the maternity unit; 0.05 ml is given intradermally. There is a problem about giving it over the deltoid because of keloid formation. Some use the scapula or the upper buttock. BCG usually provides long-lasting protection against contracting tuberculosis.

If the mother is being treated for tuberculosis there is no longer any need to separate her from the baby or stop her breast feeding. The baby can be immunized with special isoniazid-resistant BCG and treated with a course of isoniazid. In this way one can be doubly sure that the baby does not get tuberculosis.

Guthrie Test

The Guthrie test is a simple blood test for abnormal amounts of phenylalanine, an essential amino acid converted in the liver to tyrosine. In those suffering from phenylketonuria (PKU), there is a lack of the liver enzyme which carries out this conversion. The enzyme is known as phenylalanine hydroxylase. In such babies the blood phenylalanine level becomes very high and causes brain damage, leading to severe mental retardation. The condition can be successfully treated from birth with a low phenylalanine diet.

Before birth, phenylalanine does not accumulate in the fetus because it

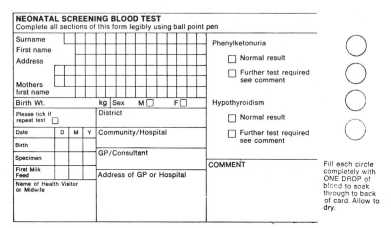

Fig. 4.12 The Guthrie test card

can pass across the placenta into the mother. After birth, the newborn baby with PKU has a steadily rising phenylalanine level after he starts to drink milk. Thus infants with PKU are not brain damaged at birth; they only become so once they have started ingesting phenylalanine in milk. The disease is uncommon; it occurs in about one in 7000 births in this country. However, once the parents have had one affected baby, there is a one in four chance of their having another infant with PKU because it is inherited as an autosomal recessive disorder. It is therefore sensible to have a universal screening test which can be used to detect the condition.

The test is carried out as follows: on about the sixth day of life the baby has a simple blood test. This is done by pricking the baby's heel and collecting four drops of blood on a piece of absorbent paper (Fig. 4.12). The test cannot be carried out earlier, because there has to be time for phenylalanine to be taken in by the baby as milk before abnormally large amounts can be detected in his blood. The paper is sent to a laboratory, where the blood spots are punched out and placed on an agar plate. This contains the phenylalanine antagonist beta-thionylalanine which inhibits the growth of a phenylalanine-dependent strain of *Bacillus subtilis*. If the level of phenylalanine in the blood sample is high, this inhibition is overcome and the bacteria are able to grow. This provides a simple and semiquantitative screen for raised levels of phenylalanine. Thus if, following overnight incubation, a turbid zone of growth is found around the test disc, this indicates a positive result. A rough serum phenylalanine level is determined by comparison with control discs. A value of 4 mg/100 ml (240 μmol/l) or more is presumed to be positive for phenylketonuria, but before diagnosis is firmly established a full investigation must be carried out.

The test should be explained to mothers before it is done and they must be warned that it is occasionally necessary to repeat the test, without this necessarily implying there is anything wrong with the baby. The commonest reason for repeating the test is that there was not enough blood to cover the circled areas on the card completely. The repeat test is nearly always satisfactory.

Modifications of the Guthrie test using agar media impregnated with other *B. subtilis* inhibitors can be used to detect a variety of other inborn errors of metabolism. Some centres do the screening by a plasma amino acid chromatogram. Thyroid-stimulating hormone (TSH) is now measured universally in the United Kingdom using blood spots on the Guthrie test card (see below).

Tests for Cystic Fibrosis

Screening tests for this disease are important because it is common: it affects about 1 in 2000 English babies. One test is the BM meconium test which estimates the amount of albumin in the first specimen of meconium that is passed. In cystic fibrosis the lack of pancreatic secretions produces an increase in albumin in meconium because it is not digested in the gut. The test is not very satisfactory and produces both false-positives and false-negatives. The false-positives are often seen in pre-term babies. A positive test was regarded only as a reason for sending the meconium to a laboratory for an accurate estimation of albumin. The test is probably being superseded by the use of blood immunoreactive trypsin. Any positive test is a reason for a definitive sweat test. It is still not certain that very early diagnosis of cystic fibrosis improves the prognosis but it does allow early genetic counselling.

The only effective way of reducing the birth prevalence of cystic fibrosis will be by *prenatal* screening. Progress is being made with an enzyme-based test (alkaline phosphatase) and gene marker identification. Neither test can be used to screen the population at large.

Screening Tests for Hypothyroidism

Congenital hypothryoidism is commoner than PKU as it affects about 1 in 4000 infants. If it is detected early it can be treated with thyroxine, so preventing mental handicap and ensuring normal growth. The gross physical signs—including prolonged jaundice, cretinous facies, big tongue, course cry and umbilical hernia—are often not present in affected babies and, therefore, a screening test is particularly useful. It is now carried out on all babies born in the United Kingdom, using blood from the Guthrie test card. It is possible to measure either T_4 or TSH. Ideally both should be measured, if no cases are to be missed, but TSH alone seems to be satisfactory and it is TSH that is measured in the UK. The rare pituitary and hypothalamic causes of congenital hypothyroidism will then be missed. This is not a major disadvantage as the hypothyroidism in these circumstances is less severe (so treatment is less urgent) and is usually part of a broader spectrum of hypothalamopituitary disease (so the problem may be suspected for other reasons).

Perhaps as many as one in eight to ten thousand babies will have TSH levels which are only temporarily raised. It is very important to check thyroid function fully before treatment with thyroxine is started to ensure that the problem is persisting. If it is not, treatment should be stopped as soon as the definitive results become available.

The presence or absence of any functioning thyroid tissue should be assessed by scanning following the injection of radioactive iodide (^{123}I) or technetium-99m pertechnetate. This will help to identify some inborn errors of thyroxine metabolism which run in families (autosomal recessive inheritance). Their final identification may require further special diagnostic procedures.

The initial dose of thyroxine replacement is around 10 µg/kg/day. The dose per kilogram falls with increasing age but remains around 100 µg/m²/day. The aim of treatment is to achieve normal growth and development. TSH levels may take many weeks to fall on treatment and provided T_4 levels are in the upper half of the normal range and growth is normal this is not an indication for increasing the dose of thyroxine.

Vision and Hearing Tests

Parents often ask if their babies can see and hear normally. It is easy to know that a baby can see something as he will blink in response to a bright light. It is also possible to show the parents that the baby will gaze at a smiling face with great interest. More sophisticated tests will be done during developmental checks later in the first year.

Tests of hearing are becoming more sophisticated. A baby will quieten at the ring of a bell in the first week and most parents will be certain in the first few months that their baby can hear something. All babies should be tested at eight months using a very soft rattle and other sounds at no more than 40 decibels. The baby turns his head towards the sound. Hearing tests for screening the newborn are being developed. A baby can be put into a cradle which analyses the startle response after a sound (Fig. 4.13).

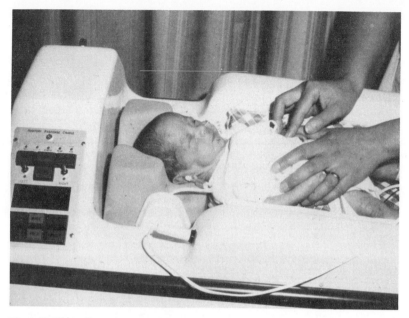

Fig. 4.13 The auditory response cradle

Tests for brain stem evoked responses are also becoming more widely available and can be used to evaluate the hearing of even very preterm infants.

Further Reading

See Further Reading to Chapter 1.

5

Care of Low Birth Weight Babies

Babies may be small at birth for two main reasons: because they are born early (preterm babies), or because they have not grown adequately in utero (small-for-dates babies). It is important to decide to which category a baby belongs, as each group has particular problems in the perinatal period. Some babies who weigh less than they should for their gestational age *and* are born early are doubly at risk.

It is best not to use the term 'premature' because it was used in the past for babies of 2500 g or less. A preterm baby is born before the end of the 37th week from the beginning of the last menstrual period; a small-for-dates baby weighs less than would be predicted from his gestational age, either two standard deviations below the mean (defining some 3.5% of all babies), or below the 10th centile. It is more useful to use the tenth centile as it will identify all babies who may be at risk of hypoglycaemia (see below). It does mean, however, that 1 in 10 babies is classed as small-for-dates.

To assess a baby's growth, intrauterine growth charts are used. These are derived by plotting the birth weights of a large population of newborn babies against their gestational ages. Lines are drawn which divide that population into centiles: 10th, 50th, 90th etc. A baby whose weight is just above the 90th centile for his gestational age is heavier than 90 out of every 100 babies in that normal population. A chart is reproduced in Chapter 4.

Before a baby's weight can be plotted on the graph, his gestational age must be known (see Chapter 2). After birth the gestational age may be estimated by observing a number of physical characteristics and neurological responses. The baby is scored on certain key features and the score enables the baby's gestational age to be read from a chart. The score is probably accurate within two weeks either way (see Appendix under Gestational Assessment). The baby's gestational age may then be plotted against the birth weight and the infant defined as large-for-dates, appropriate-for-dates or small-for-dates.

An appropriate-for-dates infant has probably grown at a normal rate in utero; he may be born before term, at term or after term. A small-for-dates baby has grown at a slower rate in utero, whether he is born before, at or after term. The commonest infant to be large-for-dates is the baby of a diabetic or pre-diabetic mother; those babies have their own special problems (see Chapter 15).

If the baby is small-for-dates, this may be because his growth rate was slow throughout pregnancy, or growth may have slowed only late in

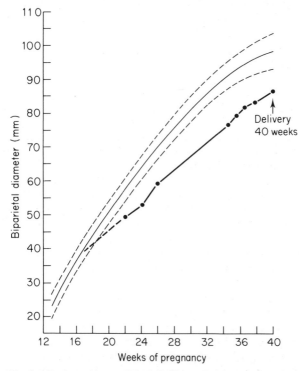

Fig. 5.1 Prolonged intrauterine growth retardation

pregnancy (Fig. 5.1; and see Fig. 2.8). These types may be distinguished by serial ultrasound measurements of biparietal diameter and lower thoracic circumference during pregnancy. The prognosis for growth and development varies with the time of the start of slow growth. Prolonged slow growth in utero produces long-term effects and may even affect mental development. Thus malnutrition during the period of most rapid brain growth (the middle and third trimesters of intrauterine life and the early months after birth) may reduce the number of brain cells produced and may permanently impair the baby's future intellectual development potential. Babies who grow slowly before about the 37th week may be short and light at birth, feed poorly as infants and show a number of dysmorphic features in childhood, such as asymmetry between the sides of the body, clinodactyly (short incurving little fingers) and short stature—the Russell–Silver syndrome. Some small-for-dates babies have an obvious reason for slow growth in utero; these include those with congenital rubella, chromosome disorders or major congenital abnormalities. Many such pregnancies end in spontaneous miscarriage. Only the unfortunate ones are born alive.

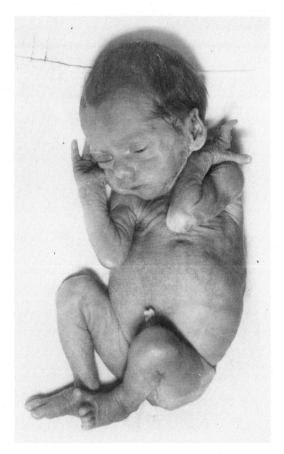

Fig. 5.2 A preterm baby born in 1954 at 28 weeks gestation and weighing 2 lb 7 oz (1.1 kg). He was discharged in good health after 11 weeks in hosptial

The Preterm Baby (Fig. 5.2)

If premature labour could be prevented, the perinatal mortality would fall considerably. This is because preterm babies are particularly at risk in the perinatal period. Unfortunately, except in certain specific cases (for example, mid-trimester abortions which may be prevented by cervical suturing), premature delivery cannot be reliably predicted or prevented in an individual patient.

There are a number of predisposing factors (risk factors). They are discussed fully in Chapter 2. Many women suffer from a combination of risk factors. For instance, there is an association between low social class, short stature, non-attendance for antenatal care, malnutrition, previous termination and so on. It is to these women that resources of money and manpower must be preferentially directed if perinatal mortality is to be further reduced.

Some immigrant groups have a particularly high perinatal mortality rate and the women may not attend for antenatal care. The Asian Mother and Baby Campaign is an example of the sort of action that needs to be taken. There should be literature in the appropriate language and interpreters to give health education.

The lower the gestational age, the greater the risk of perinatal problems: less mature lungs cause hyaline membrane disease, fragile capillaries in the brain rupture easily following trauma or hypoxia, infections are poorly resisted and anaemia may develop. These are the common and important problems of the preterm baby.

Feeding

The preterm baby of less than about 34 weeks gestation often has physical difficulty in taking, digesting and absorbing his feed. Sucking, swallowing and cough reflexes are particularly poorly developed before 34 weeks so that feeds may be taken slowly or go into the trachea. Aspiration into the lungs may occur if the baby should regurgitate or vomit because of slow stomach emptying. For these reasons, early feeds may have to be given through a tube passed into the stomach (nasogastric tube), or occasionally the duodenum. In the smallest babies (usually less than 32 weeks gestation), feeds are often given intravenously using a combination of special preparations (for details see Chapter 7). Preterm babies require a high energy intake (120–150 kcal/kg/day or about 500 kJ/kg/day) (or even higher) to grow adequately.

There is no ideal milk for very immature babies; expressed mature breast milk is not entirely satisfactory because of its low protein and fat content. Freshly expressed breast milk is still superior to any currently available artificial milk in preventing infection. New artificial milks have now been developed for low birth weight babies; they contain more protein and sodium than the ordinary baby milks. When enteral feeding is possible, feeds should be started early so as to avoid hypoglycaemia and this is one reason for putting the baby to the breast in the labour ward when possible. A 2 kg infant at 35 weeks gestation may not even need special care and might be completely breast-fed fairly quickly even though he is theoretically preterm and low birth weight. Many preterm babies require more than 200 ml/kg/day to grow adequately. Babies weighing less than 1300 g need sodium supplements (3 mmol/kg/day) (see Chapter 7 for details).

Jaundice

Neonatal jaundice has many causes and is discussed in Chapter 12. Preterm babies are particularly at risk of developing jaundice leading to bilirubin encephalopathy (kernicterus). There are several reasons for this:

1 their immature enzyme systems (especially liver glucuronyl transferase)
2 the low blood levels of 'Y' and 'Z' carrier proteins which facilitate entry of bilirubin into liver cells
3 relative hypoalbuminaemia (bilirubin is bound to albumin in the blood during transport to the liver for conjugation)
4 the greater risk of hypoxia and hypoglycaemia

A high unconjugated bilirubin level is dangerous, whatever the cause, because of the risk of kernicterus. Preterm babies may be damaged at lower bilirubin levels than mature babies, and this should always be remembered when assessing the significance of a bilirubin estimation.

Jaundice appearing within the first 24 hours of life needs immediate investigation and is never physiological or due to prematurity alone.

Hyaline membrane disease

This very important disorder is discussed in Chapter 6.

Hypothermia

The preterm baby has difficulty maintaining his body temperature and easily becomes cold. He is small and therefore has a high surface-area to body weight ratio, so that heat is lost rapidly. He is unable to produce heat by shivering. His deposits of brown fat are also smaller. Brown fat is situated in the neck and abdomen (Fig. 5.3); it has warm blood flowing through it and enables a mature infant to resist, to some degree, the stress of a low environmental temperature. The smaller preterm babies can lose a lot of water through the skin and therefore lose heat by evaporation.

Labour rooms are frequently too cold, providing comfort for mother, midwife and obstetrician but danger for the baby. A small, naked wet baby loses heat very rapidly so the resuscitation table heater must be switched on before delivery. The baby should be dried quickly. Warm towels and silver swaddlers are also valuable. Special care must be taken during baths, radiographic procedures, clinical examinations or surgery and when babies are naked in incubators. Hypothermic babies are more likely to die or to develop a serious illness, such as hyaline membrane disease. This has been known since the end of the nineteenth century (Fig. 5.4).

For each baby there is an ideal range of environmental temperature. If

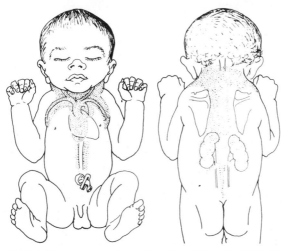

Fig. 5.3 The areas where brown fat is found. From S. Wallis & D. Harvey (1979) *Nursing Times*, by permission of the authors and editor

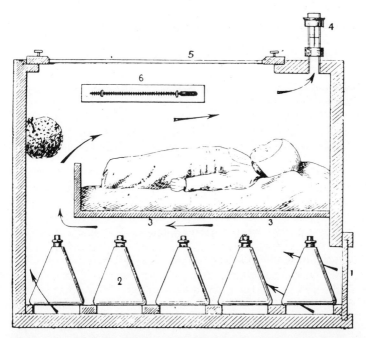

Fig. 5.4 An incubator used in Paris at the end of the nineteenth century. At the time it was shown clearly that cold babies were more likely to die

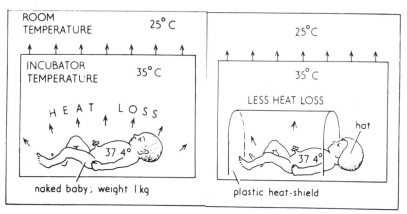

Fig. 5.5 How heat loss can be reduced by dressing the baby and using a plastic heat shield. From S. Wallis & D. Harvey (1979) *Nursing Times*, by permission of the authors and editor

nursed within this range he uses the least possible oxygen and energy to keep his body temperature normal. This temperature range is known as the neutral thermal environment and for a small naked baby is very narrow. In practice, special care nursery temperatures should be maintained between 26°C and 28°C, and incubator temperatures between 34°C and 37°C (Table 5.1). Perspex heat shields (simply and cheaply made in most workshops) are useful for reducing radiant heat loss without impeding a clear view of the baby (Fig. 5.5). One end of the Perspex shield should be closed to prevent its acting as a wind tunnel and cooling the baby. The head accounts for a large proportion of the preterm baby's total surface area; a scalp cap lined with gamgee will cut down heat loss significantly and clothes are often advisable, even when the baby is in an incubator. The aim should be to maintain the skin at 36.5 ± 0.3°C (Table 5.2). The probe is often placed on the proximal part of a limb and it is sometimes useful to connect it to the servocontrol of the incubator. In this way the incubator heater automatically increases or

Table 5.1 Suggested initial temperatures for nursing babies.

Weight	Incubator*	Cot†
1 kg	36°C	31°C
2 kg	35°C	28°C
3 kg	34°C	26°C

* Baby nursed naked with a Perspex heat shield
† Baby dressed

Table 5.2 Normal temperature ranges.

Rectal	36.6–37.5°C
Axillary	36.5–37°C
Anterior abdominal wall skin	36.2–36.8°C

reduces the heat produced to maintain the baby's temperature. This is convenient, but a disadvantage is that pyrexia may pass unnoticed and there may be swings of temperature in the incubator. When the servo-control is not in use the baby's axillary temperature should be taken regularly and checked by rectal temperature when necessary. Low-reading thermometers are essential.

Infections

Newborn babies have a number of specific and non-specific mechanisms for dealing with infection. In the preterm baby many of them are less well developed. In particular, IgG levels are low because less has been transferred from the mother across the placenta, making him vulnerable to many common bacterial and viral infections. His ability to produce IgM is low, leading to particular susceptibility to Gram-negative infections. Cellular immunity is also poorly developed. For a general discussion of infection in the newborn see Chapter 16.

Neurological disability

The preterm baby has a soft brain with fragile vessels. Damage, with tearing of blood vessels and of supporting structures such as the falx cerebri or tentorium cerebelli, is easily caused by trauma during delivery, but this is now less common. Until about 1960 the incidence of mental retardation, cerebral palsy (Fig. 5.6), convulsions, deafness and blindness was very high in these babies; but now, in the best centres, the incidence of mental retardation or major handicap has dropped to less than 10%, even though many more are surviving. Now that babies weighing less than 750 g are surviving there is some evidence that the number of survivors with neurological disabilities may be rising a little.

The improved outlook is associated not only with good paediatric care, but also with active obstetric intervention to prevent perinatal asphyxia, the gentle delivery of preterm babies with generous episiotomies or even less traumatically by lower-segment caesarean section. The elective use of caesarian section in the preterm baby is therefore becoming commoner and is being encouraged, especially for breech presentation.

Many preterm babies under 34 weeks have periventricular haemor-

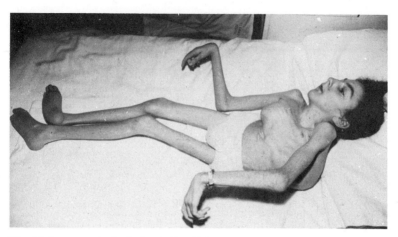

Fig. 5.6 Severe cerebral palsy in an older child

rhages which usually begin in the anterolateral walls of the lateral ventricles of the brain. Up to 30% of preterm babies have been shown by ultrasound (Fig 5.7) to have such haemorrhages. The technique of real-time ultrasound has shown other abnormalities in the brain, including cysts and ventricular dilatation, both of which are associated with a poorer outcome (see Chapter 14).

Sudden infant death syndrome (SIDS)

This condition occurs in 0.2–0.3% of live births but low birth weight infants are probably at much greater risk—perhaps 10 times as great. One study showed that 10% of postneonatal deaths (between 28 days and 1 year) in infants nursed initially on a neonatal unit were due to SIDS. Near miss SIDS also occurs more frequently in low birth weight survivors (see also p. 140).

Anaemias

Milk is a poor source of iron. The full-term baby has sufficient iron stores acquired in utero to last him about four to six months. A reason for introducing mixed feeding at about this time is to provide an increased dietary intake of this essential element. Preterm babies do not gain much of the iron which they would have stored if they had not been born too soon. Thus unless prophylactic iron supplements are given these babies will develop an *iron-deficiency (hypochromic) anaemia*. This anaemia, which would develop at around the age of six months, should be prevented by giving iron. Many centres give ferrous sulphate 30 mg twice daily from the third week of life. There are, however, certain

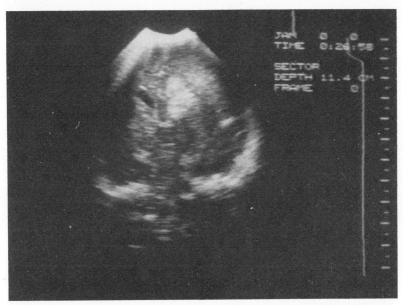

Fig. 5.7 Severe periventricular haemorrhage with blood in the ventricle and in the parenchyma of the brain.

worries about giving iron early with these babies: first, the iron may interfere with vitamin E absorption (see below) and second, evidence is accumulating that the availability of iron in the gut may encourage the growth of *E.coli*. On the other hand, there is now evidence that neurological development is delayed in iron deficiency.

Anaemia after six months should be contrasted with the *early anaemia of prematurity*. There are several reasons for the early drop in haemoglobin:

1 For adequate tissue oxygenation the fetus and neonate require about 11 g/dl of haemoglobin (Hb). As the placenta is only about 65% efficient at oxygenating haemoglobin, the total haemoglobin level in utero must be about 19 g/dl which is the level at birth. After birth the more efficient lungs oxygenate haemoglobin about 96% effectively and therefore the total haemoglobin can be allowed to fall to about 12 g/dl; the bone marrow goes into a resting phase and is restimulated as the level of oxyhaemoglobin tends to fall below 11 g/dl. The preterm baby' bone marrow is often slow to respond to such stimulation and thus an overshoot may take place, with anaemia developing during the second month of life.

2 At the same time, there is an extremely rapid rate of growth in the preterm baby leading to a rapid increase in circulating blood volume; the bone marrow is unable to respond adequately.

This early anaemia is normochromic and, if treatment is necessary, it should be by simple top-up transfusion. Transfusion is not indicated in most preterm babies because it tends to suppress bone marrow haemopoiesis further. Clear indications for transfusion are signs or symptoms of cardiac failure (such as shortness of breath on feeding, tachycardia or hepatomegaly). In addition, it is probably wise to transfuse those babies with a haemoglobin below 8 g/dl even if they appear well. The aim is to raise the haemoglobin level to about 12 g/dl. It is, however, common practice to transfuse any ill newborn baby with a haemoglobin below 10 g/dl, particularly if there is a respiratory disorder. Blood is best given slowly and partially packed so as to reduce risks of circulatory overload. It is useful to remember that a transfusion of 20 ml/kg (equivalent to 16 ml/kg of packed cells) raises the haemoglobin level by 25%. Alternatively, the volume required may be calculated from the formula:

$$V = W \times \text{number of g/dl by which the haemoglobin is to be raised} \times 6$$

where V is the volume of whole blood to be transfused (ml), and W is the baby's weight (kg).

A very few preterm babies (less than 1500 g birth weight) may show peripheral oedema due to a third and distinct type of anaemia. The blood film shows *haemolysis* with a high reticulocyte and platelet count and low packed cell volume. Vitamin E levels are low and the anaemia responds to treatment with this vitamin (15 mg/day). Some even doubt the existence of such a condition—certainly the cause is not fully understood—but giving iron supplements in the newborn period has been shown to interfere with vitamin E absorption.

Vitamins

Recommended vitamin intakes for newborn babies are:
Vitamin A   1500 units daily
Vitamin C   15–30 mg daily
Vitamin D   400 international units daily

Supplements are usually recommended for breast-fed babies in the form of proprietary vitamin drops. Artificial milks have added vitamins, but in inadequate amounts, so that drops are still necessary, although in smaller doses.

The enteral vitamin needs for preterm infants may not be satisfied by human milk (see also Chapter 7). The vitamin intakes from commercial formulae specifically designed for preterm infants by and large meet the minimum requirements for ascorbic acid, B_1, B_2, B_6 and niacin but there is considerable variation between different formulae. Folate supplements should be given (50–100 µg/day) to all babies under 1500 g birth weight.

In our present state of knowledge it is reasonable to suggest a vitamin B_{12} intake of 0.15 mg/100 kcal per day in formula-fed preterm infants. Infants born of vegetarian mothers should be particularly carefully monitored with regard to their vitamin B_{12} metabolism.

Early hypocalcaemia

Some preterm babies are found to have low levels of calcium and sometimes magnesium during the first three days of life. They respond to calcium or magnesium supplements or both (calcium gluconate 10% 0.5–1 ml orally with each feed, or magnesium sulphate 50% 0.5 ml orally with each feed). The mechanism of the hypocalcaemia may simply be immaturity of the parathyroid glands (magnesium is necessary for parathyroid hormone release). In many hospitals serving immigrant populations, however, a common cause of neonatal hypocalcaemia is osteomalacia (vitamin D deficiency) in the mother, who should be investigated.

Rickets

Rickets seems to be common in very immature infants, whether they are breast or artificially fed. Even large doses of vitamin D (up to 2000 units per day) will not prevent it. Babies of birth weight less than 1500 g should be regularly monitored for rickets with alkaline phosphatase measurements. If confirmed on X-ray, it should be treated with alfacalcidol 0.1 µg/kg/day.

Persistent ductus arteriosus

This is discussed in connection with hyaline membrane disease (Chapters 6 and 10).

Hypertyrosinaemia

Immaturity of liver enzymes causes hypertyrosinaemia in about one in 10 preterm babies, particularly those having a high protein intake or vitamin C deficiency. Blood levels of phenylalanine also rise and therefore these babies may have false-positive Guthrie tests (see Chapter 4). Normal tyrosine levels in neonatal blood are between 0.7 and 5.6 mg/dl (40–310 µmol/litre). The condition probably has no long-term effects and plasma levels usually return to normal by three months. It can be corrected by lowering the protein intake or giving a course of vitamin C (100 mg daily for several days).

The Small-for-Dates (SFD) Baby

Small-for-dates babies (Fig. 5.8) show the results of their impaired intrauterine growth: there is little subcutaneous fat, loose dry skin, muscle wasting, especially over buttocks and cheeks, scaphoid abdomen and thin umbilical cord. Scalp hair is sparse. They are often long and thin, as longitudinal growth is not as retarded as subcutaneous fat is diminished; only the most chronically and severely affected babies have head circumference and length, as well as weight, below the 10th centile. The babies are usually active and vigorous, but they are vulnerable to particular illnesses in the newborn period and differ in their susceptibilities from the preterm baby who may weigh the same at birth.

Perinatal asphyxia

SFD babies are frequently chronically hypoxic during the last part of pregnancy. Not surprisingly they are poor at withstanding the stresses of normal labour and may require active resuscitation. They need very careful monitoring in labour. Their chronic intrauterine distress may cause the passage of meconium into the amniotic fluid with gasping in utero. Thus before and during delivery these babies may aspirate meconium-stained liquor into the oropharynx, trachea and large bronchi. The first few breaths suck the meconium into the terminal bronchioles and alveoli (Fig. 5.9). If a SFD baby is expected because of the presence of any predisposing factors (listed in Chapter 2) or there is evidence of poor fetal growth (from serial ultrasound measurements or falling maternal urinary oestriols), a paediatrician should be present at the delivery. He should also be present if meconium-stained liquor is found when membranes rupture or are ruptured. The management of these babies is urgent and is described in Chapter 3.

Hypoglycaemia

Hypoglycaemia is common among SFD babies because of their large, metabolically active brains which need a lot of glucose and their small livers with poor glycogen stores. There is controversy as to whether asymptomatic hypoglycaemia causes brain damage in newborn babies. It is possible that the newborn's brain can utilize other substances, such as lactic acid, as energy sources. There is no doubt that symptomatic hypoglycaemia can cause brain damage and levels below 1.4 mmol/l (25 mg/dl) are undesirable. Symptoms are largely non-specific—limpness, apathy, poor feeding, apnoeic attacks—and therefore all babies at risk (those below the 10th centile for weight for their gestational age) should be screened routinely and regularly using blood glucose monitor-

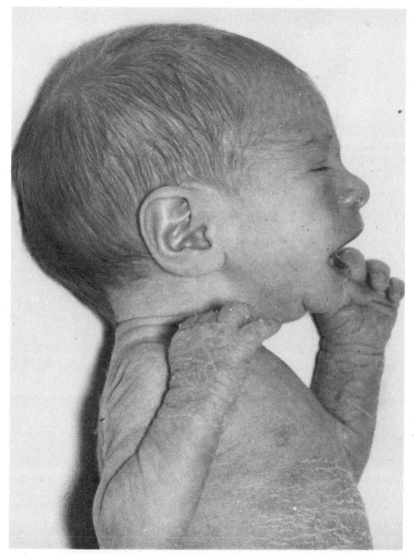

Fig. 5.8 The small-for-dates (SFD or dysmature) baby

ing strips. Estimations should be done four-hourly for 24 hours unless there are low levels, when they should be done more often. They may subsequently be checked less frequently. A reading below 1.4 mmol/l should be checked by blood glucose estimation (although this should not

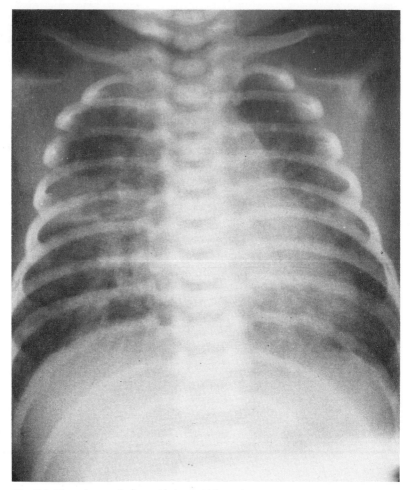

Fig. 5.9 Meconium aspiration with interstitial emphysema

delay treatment if the baby has symptoms). Asymptomatic hypoglycaemia should be treated (and can almost always be prevented) by early
and frequent feeding. If symptoms are present, glucose (dextrose) must
be given intravenously; 10 ml of 20% glucose can be used as an emergency
measure followed by 5% or 10% dextrose by intravenous infusion. Large
amounts of dextrose or continuous dextrose infusions should be avoided,
if possible, as they stimulate the baby's own insulin production and may
lead to sudden hypoglycaemia when treatment is stopped.

Heat loss

Like the preterm baby, the SFD baby easily becomes cold because of his high surface area and poor supply of subcutaneous fat.

Pulmonary haemorrhage

Pulmonary haemorrhage is an uncommon complication in SFD babies and its aetiology is not fully understood, but it is thought to be haemorrhagic pulmonary oedema from heart failure. It develops suddenly in the first few days of life and presents with blood welling up the trachea. It is commoner in babies who are also ill (for example hypoglycaemic or hypothermic). Some babies do survive and require mechanical ventilation. It may now be much less common because SFD babies are fed much earlier, kept warmer and are not allowed to become or remain hypoglycaemic.

Transient neonatal diabetes mellitus

This is a rare complication. The babies present with rapid weight loss and severe dehydration. They also have thirst and polyuria but for obvious reasons these are not usually noticed in a newborn baby. They look pale and lively in contrast to babies unwell with most other causes of dehydration, for example gastroenteritis. On testing, the urine contains sugar but no ketones, while despite high blood sugar levels they are not acidotic. Insulin levels are usually in the high normal range. On diagnosis babies should be treated with insulin to which they are very sensitive. For this reason it is best to start with 0.1 unit/kg/h as a continuous infusion. Normal saline is used initially and changed to a glucose solution when the blood glucose falls below 10 mmol/l. Potassium supplements are needed, so long as the baby is passing urine. Careful monitoring of ECG, blood glucose and plasma potassium is essential to prevent complications. This condition emphasizes the importance of screening SFD babies with blood glucose monitoring strips and testing their urine for glucose.

Skin infections

The dry, cracked, peeling skin provides a ready port of entry for organisms such as staphylococci which are widely present on attendants, linen and in dust. The ways in which such infections can be largely prevented are discussed in Chapter 16. In general, babies with infective skin lesions should be isolated and topical treatment is usually adequate. The main dangers are either that the infection will spread systemically (when systemic antibiotics should be given) or that other babies will be infected, with potentially serious results.

Poor feeding and poor growth

As indicated at the beginning of this chapter, some SFD babies have grown slowly throughout pregnancy while in others there is slow growth only at the end of pregnancy (see Figs 2.6 and 5.1). The latter group feed avidly from the first days after birth. Instead of losing weight initially and regaining their birth weight only by about the tenth day, they immediately gain weight and grow rapidly as if making up for lost time. In contrast, those babies who have grown slowly throughout pregnancy seem programmed for extrauterine slow growth also, however intensively they are fed. They have a retarded bone-age and, therefore, their epiphyses fuse late so that some catch-up growth may take place, but short stature may persist into adult life. The possible dangers of malnutrition during the period of most rapid brain growth have already been mentioned.

High packed cell volume with increased blood viscosity

Many SFD babies have haemoglobin levels over 20 g/dl and correspondingly high packed cell volumes (PCV, also called haematocrit) which is the proportion of the baby's blood volume made up of red cells. As the PCV increases above 65% the blood viscosity increases very rapidly and this leads to a number of complications. These babies look plethoric and lethargic and are cyanosed because there is more than 5 g of reduced haemoglobin present even with normal amounts of oxyhaemoglobin. They may become jaundiced, hyperexcitable or even develop respiratory distress or convulsions. It is customary to give additional fluid, orally if feeds are being absorbed, but this is not of proven benefit. If symptoms develop, exchange transfusion with 20–30 ml/kg plasma may be necessary. In practice this is rarely required.

The fetal alcohol syndrome

At one time, alcohol was felt to be safe in pregnancy. There is now increasing evidence that the drug has a serious effect on the growing fetus. The fetal alcohol syndrome was first recognized in the babies of chronic alcoholic mothers. It now seems that even a moderate intake may inhibit intrauterine growth. Quantities greater than two glasses of wine per day (or two other drinks) are thought to be deleterious.

Affected babies are small for dates and may have a number of dysmorphic features: microcephaly, a long phittrum to the upper lip, short palpebral fissures, maxillary hypoplasia and abnormal palmar creases. Ultimately, they may show developmental delay and mental retardation.

It is often useful to have problem sheets or even problem-orientated case notes for small and sick, or potentially sick babies. Their management may be made easier because problems are less likely to be overlooked.

Further Reading

Cole, T.J., Donnet, M.L. & Stanfield, J.P. (1983) Unemployment, birthweight and growth in the first year. *Archives of Disease in Childhood, 58*, 717–721.

Holland, B.M. & Wardrop, C. (1983) Anaemia in premature babies. *Maternal and Child Health, 8*, 44–49.

Illsley, R. & Mitchell, R.G. (ed) (1984) *Low Birth Weight: a Medical Psychological and Social Study*. Chichester: Wiley.

Stewart, A.L. (1985) Assessment of the Preterm Infant and Prognosis. In *Preterm Labour and its Consequences*, eds R.W. Beard & F. Sharp. London: Royal College of Obstetricians and Gynaecologists.

Stewart, A.L., Reynolds, E.O. & Lispscomb, A.P. (1981) Outcome for infants of very low birth weight: survey of world literature. *Lancet, i*, 1038–1040.

Wigglesworth, J.S. (1985) Perinatal Pathology of the Preterm Infant. In *Preterm Labour and its Consequences*, eds R.W. Beard & F. Sharp. London: Royal College of Obstetricians and Gynaecologists.

6

Respiratory Problems

Breathing difficulties are the most common problems of newborn babies. For example, hyaline membrane disease (HMD), due to lack of surfactant in the lungs, is common in babies born early, but it can be confused with a large number of other problems in the first few days of life. It is often very difficult to make a clear diagnosis even after examining the baby and having seen the chest radiograph. It is also difficult to exclude infection and this means that a number of babies have to be treated with antibiotics initially until the results of cultures are known.

A clue to diagnosis is the time of onset of the respiratory problem. *Hyaline membrane disease* and *transient tachypnoea of the newborn* begin during the first four hours of life. *Pneumonia* can occur at any time during the newborn period. *Pneumothorax* often causes a sudden deterioration in a baby who has had a respiratory problem. The *Wilson–Mikity syndrome* and *bronchopulmonary dysplasia* appear insidiously after the first week or two and are often complications in a baby who has required long ventilation for respiratory problems such as HMD or recurrent apnoeic attacks. *Apnoeic attacks* can occur as part of any respiratory problem but are particularly common in babies born at less than 32 weeks gestation and who may be otherwise completely well, or in those with an intraventricular haemorrhage. *Meconium aspiration* is an important cause of respiratory distress in small-for-dates babies or if there has been intrapartum asphyxia. One of the most difficult problems may be the differential diagnosis of cyanosis, which may be due to any of a number of respiratory problems or to some forms of congenital heart disease (see Table 10.2 p 225).

Hyaline Membrane Disease (HMD)

Hyaline membrane disease is thought to occur in 10% of all preterm deliveries, but it is a diagnosis usually made only at post-mortem. The clinical syndrome is called *respiratory distress syndrome* or RDS. It is very rare after 37 weeks gestation and is commonest in the very preterm baby. In the Perinatal Mortality Survey of 1970, it was still the largest single cause of death in babies born alive without major congenital defects.

Clinical features

Affected babies may be almost normal at birth with high Apgar scores. However, asphyxia during birth or a delayed onset of breathing makes the condition more severe. Gradually, over the next few hours, such babies become increasingly tachypnoeic with increased respiratory effort and expiratory grunting. Conventionally, the diagnosis is restricted to those infants who show two of three signs (tachypnoea greater than 60/min, expiratory grunting and chest wall recession) within four hours of birth, and when the illness lasts for more than 24 hours (Fig. 6.1).

The smallest and illest babies may not show all these signs and may be

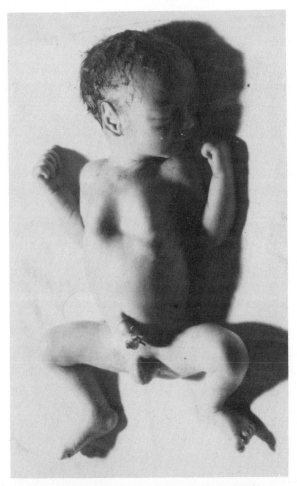

Fig. 6.1 A baby with respiratory distress syndrome (RDS)

Table 6.1 Plasma changes in blood gas and acid–base disturbances.

	Partial pressure of CO₂ (PaCO₂)	Blood pH	Plasma bicarbonate (HCO₃)
Respiratory acidosis (impaired CO_2 excretion)	↑	↓	Normal or ↑
Respiratory alkalosis (excessive CO_2 excretion)	↓	↑	↓
Metabolic acidosis (acid retention or alkali loss)	Normal or ↓	↓	↓
Metabolic alkalosis (alkali retention or acid loss)	Normal	↑	↑

deeply cyanosed with gasping or absent respirations. Since many babies are put straight onto a ventilator following resuscitation they do not show the classical earliest signs.

Over the following few hours, the baby needs a greater concentration of oxygen to prevent cyanosis. An arterial sample of blood shows hypoxaemia (low PaO_2). On listening to the chest there is diminished air entry, and there is also usually oedema and oliguria. The problems are greatest at 48–72 hours of age when, if death has not occurred, gradual recovery starts.

The cyanosis is caused by shunting of blood in the lung itself, past collapsed air spaces, with the result that reduced amounts of oxygen are carried in the blood. A shunt also occurs through a re-opened foramen ovale or patent ductus arteriosus. Besides hypoxaemia, other biochemical changes include acidaemia (low pH), high PCO_2 (Table 6.1), hypoglycaemia and hypocalcaemia.

A typical chest radiograph shows a ground-glass appearance of the lungs with an ill-defined heart border and an air bronchogram (air visible in the larger airways against the shadowing of collapsed small airways). In the most severe cases the lung fields appear virtually opaque (Fig. 6.2).

The diagnosis is often clear, but differential diagnoses include meconium aspiration, pneumonia, pneumothorax, pulmonary haemorrhage, cyanotic congenital heart disease, oesophageal atresia and diaphragmatic hernia. The immotile cilia (Kartagener) syndrome may cause prolonged tachypnoea in the newborn. Dextrocardia is the clue to this diagnosis in a proportion of cases.

An autopsy shows that the infant's lungs are collapsed and contain no air. The 'hyaline membrane' consists of fibrin with entrapped red cells, protein and necrotic alveolar epithelium.

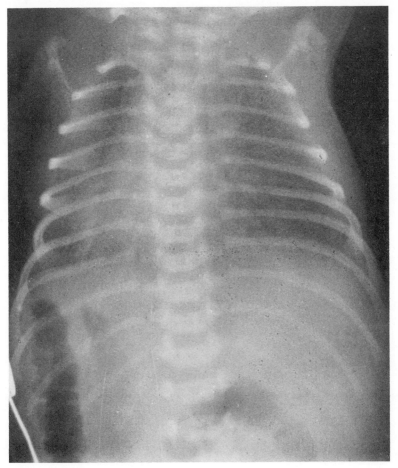

Fig. 6.2 The chest X-ray in respiratory distress syndrome

Aetiology and prevention

The anatomy of the normal lung provides a large surface area for gaseous exchange so that breathing air provides effective oxygenation of blood. The lungs of the fetus are filled with fluid; at birth, the first breath fills the lungs with air and the production of lung liquid ceases.

Surface tension in the fluid-filled lungs would be very high if a substance were not present to reduce surface tension and to allow the lungs to expand with air. *Surfactant* performs this task and is secreted by the lung from about 22 weeks gestation. It increases in quantity thereafter with surges at about 33–35 weeks and also at birth. Thus preterm infants are at risk because they have less surfactant present in their lungs.

Susceptibility therefore depends more on lung maturation than on gestational age. Babies who are especially at risk include those born before 37 weeks gestation, boys, second twins and babies of diabetic mothers. After birth the high surface tension causes alveoli to collapse at the end of expiration; this is the basis of RDS. Recovery is associated with increased surfactant production. Surfactant is a collection of fatty substances, which include large amounts of surface-active lecithins. Trials are in progress on the use of surfactant introduced into the trachea for the prevention and treatment of RDS. The first studies in humans used animal surfactant. This had major disadvantages in that it could produce immunological reactions in the lungs. Recently, artificial surfactant has been used; the ideal composition has not been determined but phosphatidyl glycerol seems an important component as it is always absent from the lungs of babies with RDS.

The concentration of human surfactant from amniotic fluid is being attempted. Preliminary work with artificial surfactant suggests that its use at birth, with a subsequent dose, improves the chances of a preterm baby's survival equivalently to the advantage of being a girl rather than a boy, or by about a one week increase in gestation.

Some events affect the rate of surfactant production in the fetus. Sudden intrapartum asphyxia resulting from antepartum haemorrhage, maternal hypotension or over-sedation impairs the ability to produce surfactant. Some chronic problems seem to increase lung surfactant: for example, retroplacental bleeding, ruptured membranes for more than 24 hours, placental infarction and pre-eclampsia or hypertension with intrauterine growth retardation. This may be because stress to the fetus causes glucocorticoids to be released from the adrenal glands and these steroids are thought to stimulate surfactant release. This now has clinical application; several trials indicate that treatment of a mother in premature labour with betamethasone (a steroid) may decrease the incidence of RDS and its mortality.

In utero, lung fluid containing surfactant flows up the trachea, out of the mouth and into the amniotic fluid. It is possible to measure the concentration of surfactant in amniotic fluid. Amniocentesis thus provides a clinical measure of fetal lung maturity before birth. This is expressed as the ratio of surface-active agents to sphingomyelin (a substance in lung secretions which remains relatively constant in concentration in the third trimester of pregnancy). This is known as the lecithin : sphingomyelin (L:S) ratio. A ratio greater than 2 indicates a low risk of RDS; under 2% of babies develop RDS with a ratio above 2. Over 75% develop RDS when the ratio is below 1.5; therefore a ratio of less than 1.5 indicates a high risk (Table 6.2). The obstetrician may therefore with more accuracy weigh the risk of the baby developing RDS after early delivery against the dangers of non-delivery. This is particu-

Table 6.2 The L/S ratio and the risk of RDS.

L/S ratio	Incidence of RDS (%)	Mortality from RDS (%)
>2.5	0.9 (0.7 diabetes)	nil
>2.0	2.2	0.1
1.5–2.0	40	4
<1.5	75	14

larly useful in such situations as intrauterine growth retardation and rhesus disease.

Very often spontaneous premature delivery cannot be prevented. Sometimes a cervical suture, or intravenous salbutamol, ritodrine or alcohol which inhibit uterine contractions, may delay birth to allow steroids to be given or the baby to become more mature.

Management

After birth, prompt resuscitation with early endotracheal intubation reduces anoxia, acidaemia and therefore the incidence and severity of RDS. Hypoxia immediately after birth must be avoided since hypoxia will reduce surfactant levels. Every baby of 30 weeks or less, and any baby of less than 35 weeks who has respiratory difficulty, should be intubated.

Supportive measures

General supportive measures should include the following:

1 *Adequate warmth.* In practice abdominal skin temperature should be maintained between 36.2°C and 36.8°C.

2 *Feeding.* Feeds given by mouth may well be aspirated into the lungs with lethal consequences. It is therefore usual to avoid nasogastric feeds. Adequate calories and fluid should be given via a peripheral vein or through a nasojejunal tube. It is possible to use an umbilical arterial catheter for 5% dextrose infusion in the first few days. A prolonged illness must be managed with total intravenous nutrition or nasojejunal feeding (see Chapter 7).

3 *Minimal disturbance or handling.* Feeding and crying have been shown to cause a fall in arterial Po_2, as does any handling. Manoeuvres such as taking rectal temperatures, over-vigorous sucking-out, frequent cleaning, nappy changing or repositioning should be avoided. Temperature, heart and respiratory rates, inspired oxygen concentration, arterial Po_2 and blood pressure should be monitored continuously without disturbance.

4 *Prevention of infection.* Scrupulous nursing care with due attention to asepsis in such procedures as tracheal toilet is of vital importance (see below). It is now usual to give antibiotics to any baby with a respiratory problem just after birth because it could be due to a group B β-haemolytic streptococcal pneumonia. High-dose parenteral penicillin should be used (150 mg/kg/day in six divided doses, intravenously or intramuscularly) and gentamicin appears to have a synergistic effect with it. The newer cephalosporins are also proving useful antibiotics in this situation (see Chapter 16).

5 *Parental visiting.* It is important for nurses and doctors to explain to parents what the extensive and frightening-looking supportive and monitoring equipment is, what it does and why it is being used.

Oxygen therapy

The temperature, humidity, flow rate and concentration of inspired oxygen must be adequately controlled and monitored. Oxygen concentrations above 30% cannot be effectively maintained in an incubator without the use of a headbox because the oxygen concentration drops when the doors are opened. It is convenient to use piped air and oxygen. The flow rate should be between 3 and 7 l/min, sufficient to prevent CO_2 accumulation in the headbox. Headbox oxygen should be used in conjunction with a humidifier so as not to chill the infant.

The inspired oxygen concentration is adjusted to maintain the Pao_2 in the normal range. The satisfactory levels of a baby's arterial blood gases are: pH 7.3–7.4; oxygen (Pao_2) 7–10 kPa (50–75 mmHg); carbon dioxide ($Paco_2$) 4.5–6 kPa (35–45 mmHg). They are best checked by continuous monitoring, using umbilical arterial catheters with oxygen electrodes at their tips, or transcutaneously. When the infant is shocked, intra-arterial monitoring is more satisfactory than transcutaneous monitoring. Less ideally, intermittent samples can be taken four-hourly (but more frequently when the infant's condition is changing rapidly or adjustments are made to therapy) from indwelling umbilical catheters or a radial artery. A small cannula can be placed in the radial artery by percutaneous insertion to monitor oxygen levels.

The umbilical catheter is inserted with full aseptic precautions so that the lip lies approximately at the level of the fourth lumbar vertebra. It should be tied in position and taped to the abdominal wall away from the perineum to minimize risks of contamination. The position must be checked by radiography. There is a characteristic downward loop on the X-ray as the catheter passes down into the pelvis via the umbilical artery into the common iliac artery. The catheter in the umbilical vein passes directly upwards.

As many as 10% may have a complication from the arterial catheter. Nurses should look particularly for disconnected tubing, through which the baby may bleed to death. Black or blue toes are an initial and commonly noticed sign of obstructed blood flow with insertion of umbilical artery catheters. White leg is associated with arterial spasm at the time of insertion or with a catheter which has passed down into the femoral artery so obstructing blood flow to the leg. Other complications include infection and thrombosis. To reduce these risks catheters are best removed after three to four days and subsequent samples can be taken from other arteries, though this has the disadvantage that handling and crying reduce the accuracy of the estimation as well as making the baby temporarily hypoxaemic.

Transcutaneous monitoring is now in widespread use for oxygen but has not proved so valuable for CO_2. Readings must be checked regularly by measurement from arterial samples. The reading is accurate because local heating is applied which causes vasodilatation and thus, particularly during the recovery phase of RDS, a close approximation to true arterial P_{O_2} is obtained.

The danger of uncontrolled oxygen therapy with prolonged high arterial P_{O_2} levels is that retinopathy of prematurity (retrolental fibroplasia) will develop. In affected babies there is initial vasoconstriction of retinal arterioles which, after some hours of exposure, becomes irreversible. On returning to normal oxygen tensions, the vessels proliferate intensely with new capillary formation which may result in retinal detachment and blindness.

It is important to realize that it is not high inspired oxygen concentrations in themselves that are dangerous; it is inappropriately high concentrations leading to high $P_{a}O_2$ levels which cause the damage. Thus oxygen therapy must be closely controlled to prevent this serious complication on the one hand and death or brain damage from hypoxaemia on the other. It does seem to be getting commoner once again with the survival of very small babies. It is possible that there may be factors other than oxygen in its aetiology.

Continuous inflating pressure and mechanical ventilation

Up to 30% of babies with RDS will require further support by one or both of these techniques to prevent hypoxaemia, apnoeic attacks or rising P_{CO_2} levels. The expiratory grunt of the baby with RDS is his own attempt to prevent alveolar collapse; by breathing out against a partially closed glottis (vocal cords) he keeps his alveoli expanded for as long as possible during expiration. The asthmatic or chronic bronchitic patient who purses his lips and puffs out his cheeks during expiration is doing the same thing.

This effect may be obtained artificially by applying a continuous inflating pressure against which the baby spontaneously breathes. Many techniques have been used for applying a continuous inflating pressure,

Table 6.3 Methods of applying continuous inflating pressure.

Method	Advantages	Disadvantages
Continuous positive airway pressure (CPAP)		
Face mask	Easy to apply	Leaks may occur if mask does not fit well. Stomach may be distended
Nasal catheters	Easy to apply, free access to baby's mouth	Ulceration of nasal passages if catheters used for a long time. Air may escape from the mouth. Stomach may be distended
Endotracheal tube	Artificial ventilation can be proceeded to quickly if needed	Complications of endotracheal tubes, trauma and lung infection
Head box		Tight seal around neck may traumatize skin and obstruct venous return from the head, leading to cerebral haemorrhage and hydrocephalus
		Poor access to baby's head. High noise level in box. Stomach may be distended
Continuous negative airway pressure (CNP)		
Body box	Easy access to baby's head	Tight seal around neck may traumatize skin and obstruct venous return from head leading to cerebral haemorrhage and hydrocephalus. Air leak may cool the baby. Poor access to baby's body

either with continuous positive airways pressure (CPAP) by headbox with neck seal, intranasal catheters, face mask or by applying continuous negative pressure (CNP) with subatmospheric pressure around the chest by means of a negative pressure body box. These methods have largely been superseded by the use of endotracheal tubes to give CPAP, which allows the immediate start of ventilation should an apnoeic attack occur.

All studies confirm a significant increase in Po_2 with CPAP in spontaneously breathing infants. It was employed increasingly early as it may act by limiting surfactant destruction, thereby reducing the length of the illness but it is now common to use mechanical ventilation. CPAP is still commonly employed in weaning babies off the ventilator. Complications are common, some due to the technique itself, some to the method of administration (Table 6.3). They include pneumothorax, a fall in cardiac output and, particularly with the neck seal, an increased incidence of intraventricular haemorrhage (see below). Some indications for CPAP include:

1 recurrent apnoeic attacks

2 Pao_2 less than 6 kPa (45 mmHg) when the baby is breathing 40% oxygen

3 to assist in weaning babies from the ventilator

Complications and CO_2 retention are commoner above 5 cm of water and much commoner above 10 cm, and such pressures are no longer used.

It is important when using CPAP to have an open nasogastric tube in place to prevent gastric rupture if gas should be blown into the stomach and to reduce the likelihood of aspiration of stomach contents into the lungs. The high incidence of complications and of subsequent ventilation with CPAP means that it should be used only in units with enough equipment and trained staff.

Babies with severe RDS may need mechanical ventilation to prevent hypoxaemia. There are two main methods: intermittent positive-pressure ventilation (IPPV), which is commonly used, and negative-pressure ventilation using a negative-pressure body tank with neck seal (now rarely used). Indications are:

1 prolonged apnoea with bradycardia unresponsive to stimulation

2 frequent or recurrent apnoeic attacks unresponsive to theophylline or CPAP

3 Pao_2 less than 6 kPa (45 mmHg) in 70% oxygen with or without CPAP, indicating severe respiratory failure

4 $Paco_2$ greater than 9 kPa (70 mmHg).

The ventilator must be carefully adjusted so that the baby's blood gases are normal at the least possible pressure. Ventilators suitable for newborn babies allow independent adjustment of respiratory rate, the ratio of inspiration to expiration, peak inspiratory pressure and peak end expiratory pressure (PEEP). CPAP should be available at the turn of a switch. A slow rate gives longer for oxygen uptake by the blood but may also allow the amount of CO_2 in the blood to rise. The $Paco_2$ can be reduced by increasing the rate. Normal babies spend about half the expiratory cycle breathing in and half out (in adults it is about one-third in and two-thirds out). The stiff lungs of the baby with RDS mean that he may need longer for inspiration (an I:E ratio of 2 or 3 to 1) although this may also cause CO_2 to accumulate. The I:E ratio must be reduced towards unity as the baby improves or his blood pressure may fall and he may become shocked. The least peak inspiratory pressure necessary to produce good chest movement and breath sounds should be used. The smaller the baby, the lower the pressure necessary to inflate the lungs and pressures above 30 cm of water are seldom necessary.

It is becoming commoner to use a higher frequency of ventilation with rates over 60/min. In this situation an I : E ratio of 1 : 1.5 or 1 : 2 is required. Higher pressures can be used since they are only applied for a small proportion of the ventilatory cycle.

Such ventilation may prove to reduce the incidence of pneumothorax and bronchopulmonary dysplasia. It is thought that bronchopulmonary dysplasia (see below) is largely due to ventilation at high pressures, for a

Table 6.4 Suggested initial ventilator settings.

Rate	30 per min
I:E ratio	1:1
Peak pressure	15–20 cmH$_2$O
PEEP	3–4 cmH$_2$O

The initial oxygen concentration should be that which the baby is already receiving and the peak inspiratory pressure the minimum which gives adequate chest expansion and air entry, as assessed clinically.

Table 6.5 Action if the ventilated baby remains hypoxaemic.

1 Increase the inspired oxygen

2 Increase the peak pressure stepwise to a maximum of 30 cm of water until adequate air entry has been achieved

3 Increase the I:E ratio (up to 3:1 if required)

4 Increase PEEP to 5 cmH$_2$O

5 If the arterial Pco$_2$ is high, increase the rate to 40 per min. A continuing high Pco$_2$ and low Po$_2$ may respond to a faster rate (60 per min) with I:E ratio of 1:1.5 and higher peak pressures (even up to 50 cm of water)

6 If the Po$_2$ is persistently low, transilluminate the chest for pneumothorax. If in doubt, take another radiograph

(As the respiratory distress resolves, remember to reduce the peak pressure, the I:E ratio to 1:1 and PEEP to 3–4 cm of water.)

high proportion of the ventilatory cycle. The most satisfactory machines are the constant flow, pressure-limited, time-cycled ventilators developed especially for the newborn. Reasonable initial ventilator settings are summarized in Table 6.4.

Action to be taken if the baby remains hypoxic (Pao$_2$ less than 7 kPa) is summarized in Table 6.5.

It is important for the nurse to assess ventilation clinically (chest wall movement, auscultation, colour) and blood gases must be checked as well, at least four-hourly or within 15 minutes of any adjustments in ventilator settings (if electrodes for continuous monitoring are not in place). Necessary clinical observations are summarized in Table 6.6. It is important to monitor the baby's blood pressure. This is best done via an intra-arterial transducer, but it can be measured using a flush technique. A small blood transfusion (10 ml/kg) can be given if the blood pressure is low (systolic less than 30 mmHg).

At all times when the baby is on a ventilator his chest should move and the manometer needle should move with each respiration. Adequate humidification helps prevent the accumulation of sticky secretions. Tracheal toilet should be performed four-hourly. On each occasion the

Table 6.6 Clinical observations that should be made of a baby on a ventilator.

1 Temperature	9 General activity
2 Heart rate	10 Blood gases
3 Blood pressure	11 Tracheal aspirate
4 Respiratory rate	12 Urine passed
5 Colour	13 Bowel actions
6 Chest movement	14 Concentration of inspired oxygen
7 Breath sounds, whether equal both sides of the chest	15 Ventilator settings
	16 Physiotherapy
8 Peripheral circulation	17 Drugs

baby may become hypoxic as he must be disconnected from the ventilator, so give him plenty of oxygen beforehand. The risk of infection is reduced by careful aseptic technique. All babies on ventilators should be given regular physiotherapy, with frequent changes of position to assist drainage of secretions from the lungs, together with stimuli to dislodge secretions so that they can be coughed up or sucked up the endotracheal tube. We have used an electric toothbrush with the head wrapped in cotton wool to provide gentle chest vibration. Another useful method is using a Bennet face mask which gives a cupping action, which physiotherapists find is effective and comfortable for the baby.

It is difficult to fix orotracheal tubes securely for positive pressure ventilation. Two useful techniques are shown in Fig. 6.3. Complications of ventilation include:

1 Pneumothorax, in up to 20% of cases, especially if high pressures are used. Suspect this if there is sudden deterioration.

2 Pneumonia. The risks are reduced by careful nursing and ensuring that tracheal toilet is performed with scrupulous aseptic technique.

3 Bronchopulmonary dysplasia (see below).

4 Mechanical failure. This danger should be eliminated by alarm systems for the heart rate and ventilating pressure monitors and by the presence of skilled nursing personnel.

A summary of the action to take if a baby deteriorates while being ventilated is shown in Table 6.7

The baby should be weaned off the ventilator as soon as possible. A good time to start is when his oxygen requirements start falling or if he shows signs of breathing on his own when the ventilation is stopped. The simplest way is to gradually reduce the ventilatory pressure and then the respiratory rate settings on the ventilator or by intermittent mandatory ventilation (IMV). It is sometimes very difficult to ventilate a big baby who fights the ventilator. Sedation can be used. If this is not sufficient to allow adequate ventilation, paralyse the baby with a drug such as pancuronium (dose 0.02 mg/kg intravenously and repeat as necessary). This appears to reduce the incidence of pneumothorax. Hypoxaemia can occur when the drug is given so monitor the Po_2 closely. If the baby is

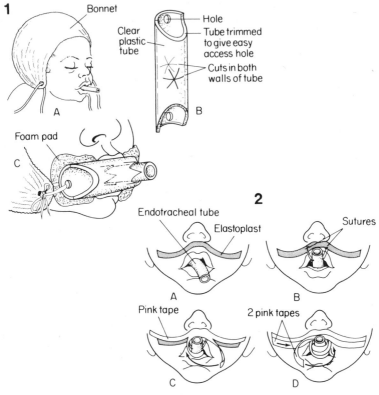

Fig. 6.3 Two methods of fixing orotracheal tubes in position. From S. Wallis & D. Harvey (1979) *Nursing Times*, by permission of the authors and editor

paralysed care should be taken by the nursing staff to change the position of the baby regularly to relieve pressure areas and also to perform passive limb exercises. Diazepam should never be given into an umbilical arterial catheter as fatal thrombosis has been reported.

Alkali therapy

The correction with alkali (e.g. 8.4% sodium bicarbonate) of the metabolic acidaemia associated with RDS was popular when there was no really effective treatment. Hypoxia causes lactic acidaemia and the best treatment is to improve tissue oxygenation or to allow the baby to correct his own pH. Respiratory acidosis can be corrected by ventilation; sodium bicarbonate may increase the $P\text{CO}_2$. It is possible that the over-enthusiastic

Table 6.7 Action to be taken if the baby deteriorates while being ventilated.

Chest moving	Chest not moving	
Always confirm breath sounds are present by listening to the chest	Listen to the chest	
	No breath sounds	Breath sounds one side only
? Insufficient oxygen. Increase inspired oxygen concentration to 100%, or until baby is pink. Increase inspiration/expiration ratio to 2:1	? ET tube blocked. Suck out the tube. It may be necessary to inject 0.5 ml normal saline down the tube to loosen sticky secretions	? ET tube slid down into right main bronchus. Try pulling it back a short distance ($\simeq$ 0.5 cm) and listen again
No change	No change	No change
? Blood bypassing parts of the lung that are being ventilated. Look for pneumonia producing lung collapse, pneumothorax, congenital cardiac anomaly	? ET tube displaced. Check position with laryngoscope and if in doubt change tube	? Secretions block bronchus beyond ET tube. Suck out the ET tube; it may be necessary to inject 0.5 ml of normal saline down tube to loosen sticky secretions
	No change	No change
None found	? Bilateral pneumothorax. Check position of heart beat. Has it changed, or is it difficult to feel? Confirm by transilluminating chest or with chest X-ray. If rapid deterioration insert chest drain immediately. Do *not* wait for X-ray to confirm diagnosis	? Pneumothorax. Check position of heart beat. Has it changed? Confirm by transilluminating chest or with a chest X-ray. If rapid deterioration insert chest drain immediately. Do *not* wait for X-ray to confirm diagnosis
? Illness causing circulatory failure. Consider septicaemia or intraventricular haemorrhage		

use of alkali therapy in the past was responsible for many deaths from intraventricular haemorrhage.

Intraventricular haemorrhage (IVH) is now probably the most frequent cause of death in babies with RDS (see Chapter 14). Careful resuscitation of all preterm babies at birth and the prevention of hypoxaemia and acidaemia almost certainly reduce the incidence of IVH and a reasonable indication for using alkali would be persistent acidaemia after attention to ventilation with a pH below 7.15 and base excess more than −7 mmol/l. Give sodium bicarbonate, 2–3 mmol/kg, slowly over about 30 minutes.

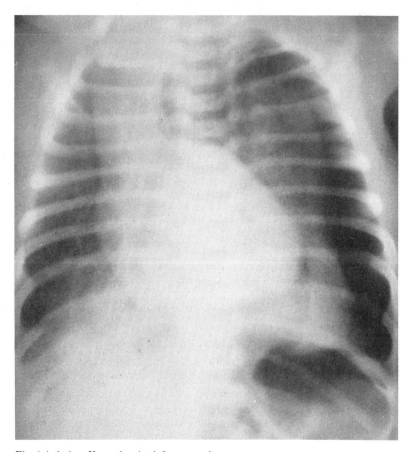

Fig. 6.4 A chest X-ray showing left pneumothorax

Pneumothorax

Pneumothorax can occur at any time during the newborn period but it usually appears as a complication of some other respiratory problem. For instance, it is common in babies who have been resuscitated at birth, especially if high pressures have been used to expand the lungs, and it often occurs as a result of ventilation or CPAP in a baby with hyaline membrane disease or after meconium aspiration. The usual presentation is sudden collapse and cyanosis. The classical physical signs found in adults are not always present in babies. It may be possible to find hyperresonance with absent breath sounds on the side of the chest where the pneumothorax has occurred. If the pneumothorax is under tension and is on only one side of the chest, there may be mediastinal shift to that the heart sounds are displaced, or it may even be possible to feel the displaced apex beat. Unfortunately, the diagnosis can often be difficult because these signs are not present. A major help in diagnosis is transillumination using a cold light source. Using this technique the chest will transilluminate brightly if there is a lot of air around the lung. It is only really satisfactory in very small babies (under 1300 g), although it can be useful in larger babies. In babies over about 2500 g the technique may not show any transillumination even though a large pneumothorax is present. If a pneumothorax can be found on transillumination, it is reasonable to drain the chest immediately if the baby is obviously very ill. Otherwise it is helpful to obtain a chest radiograph which usually makes the diagnosis quite clear (Fig. 6.4), although small pneumothoraces are sometimes difficult to diagnose because skin folds or items of clothing may give confusing shadows on a radiograph. In an emergency, when the baby has suddenly collapsed, it may be necessary to put a needle into the chest in order to see if a pneumothorax is present and to provide some instant relief. It is important to have an under-water seal and this is most easily done using a butterfly type of needle with the end of the plastic tubing under sterile distilled water. If a stream of bubbles appears, a chest drain can be inserted without radiographic confirmation because the baby may die without immediate treatment. Indiscriminate needling of the chest should not be done since it is very easy to damage the lung of a newborn baby and to *cause* a pneumothorax.

It is important to prevent pneumothoraces by avoiding pressures above 30 cm of water during resuscitation. One should choose the lowest pressure that will provide adequate mechanical ventilation of the lungs. It is common to see interstitial emphysema before the pneumothorax actually occurs. The radiographic picture is then very remarkable, with areas of translucency and collapse scattered through the lung so that it looks almost like a snowstorm. The air often escapes from the small alveoli into the substance of the lungs surrounding the bronchi; it then tracks up to the hilum of the lung and into the mediastinum. A lateral radiograph is essential whenever a pneumothorax is suspected because a pocket of air behind the sternum indicates that a pneumomediastinum is present. Sometimes radiographs show an even more dramatic picture with air in the pericardium or in the peritoneum (Fig. 6.5). When a very large amount of air has escaped into the mediastinum one may be able to feel the crackle of subcutaneous air around the neck or over the chest wall.

Careful thought should be given to the treatment of a pneumothorax. If the baby is in good condition, draining the air is not necessary. In a full-term baby, who is not at risk of retrolental fibroplasia, the use of high concentrations of oxygen will probably allow the pneumothorax to absorb more quickly. The baby's arterial oxygen tension should be

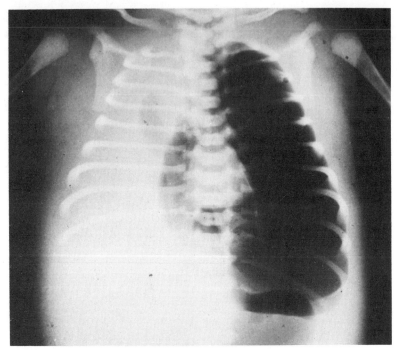

Fig. 6.5 Pneumopericardium with a large left pneumothorax

monitored and the pneumothorax is drained only if satisfactory Po_2 levels cannot be maintained. If the pneumothorax needs draining, it is important that a fairly large tube should be used. We suggest a proper chest drain; these are now available in pre-packed disposable units, with a metal stilette down the middle of the catheter. There are various sites where the drain can be inserted. It is commonest to use the front of the chest in the second or third interspace in the middle clavicular line. However, this has problems particularly in a girl; the hole produced by the chest drain will leave a scar which will be visible later and if the drain is inserted anywhere near the breast there is a danger that a part of the breast may not develop normally. It therefore seems reasonable to use the anterior axillary line in the fourth or fifth intercostal spaces. A small incision should be made through the skin, one intercostal space below the proposed site of insertion. The drain and stilette can then be passed through the skin and manoeuvred over the point of insertion through the intercostal space. It is wise to put artery forceps on the catheter as a guard, so that when the drain is pressed into the chest it does not suddenly go too far. When the chest has been entered, the stilette is withdrawn and the plastic catheter advanced upwards and anteriorly.

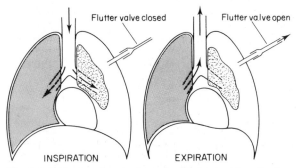

Fig. 6.6 A flutter valve. A piece of soft tubing with walls that collapse and lie closely opposed to one another, rather like an empty balloon. On inspiration the valve closes and prevents air entering the chest. During expiration the raised intrathoracic pressures force the walls of the valve apart and let the air out. From S. Wallis and D. Harvey (1979) *Nursing Times*, by permission of the authors and editor

The proximal end of the chest drain must be attached to some form of seal to prevent air entering the pleural space during inspiration. The most convenient seal is a Heimlich flutter valve (Fig. 6.6) which is available as a pre-packed disposable unit. An alternative is to use the simple under-water seal, but it is important to keep this below the level of the baby, otherwise water may enter the chest. We usually find that it is necessary to put a pump on the other end of the seal with a pressure of about 3–5 mmHg in order to drain the air satisfactorily. Fig. 6.7 shows a baby who has a right pneumothorax and is being artificially ventilated. A right intercostal drain has been inserted.

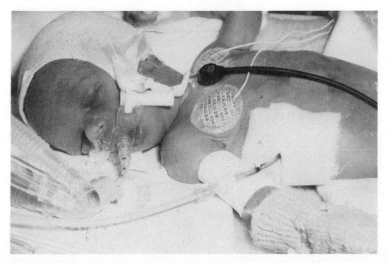

Fig. 6.7 Pneumothorax in a ventilated baby with respiratory distress syndrome

It is often difficult to decide when to remove the chest drain:

1 The chest radiograph should show that the pneumothorax has absorbed completely.

2 The drain should be clamped with artery forceps and the radiograph taken about six hours later.

3 If the pneumothorax has reformed, further drainage will be necessary but if there is no air in the chest it is reasonable to remove the drain.

If two pneumothoraces are present an attempt should be made to remove only one drain at a time. The second drain could be examined about 24 hours after the first.

Pneumopericardium is often lethal. If it is diagnosed during life, an attempt should be made to drain the air using a needle passed under the xiphisternum into the pericardium.

Meconium Aspiration

This subject is also discussed in Chapters 3 and 5. It can be a major problem and is particularly likely to occur in babies born at term and small-for-dates babies who have suffered from intrapartum asphyxia. When a baby does not have enough oxygen before birth he passes meconium into the amniotic fluid and makes gasping movements. Meconium is present in the liquor in about 10% of women at term, but a much smaller proportion of babies develop meconium aspiration. If meconium is present in the liquor, the anterior part of the mouth should be sucked out at delivery. It is best to clear the mouth completely as soon as the head is born so that it is done before the first breath when the chest is still in the birth canal. If the baby is covered with thick meconium, the larynx must be inspected so that any meconium on the vocal cords can be removed. If there is any suspicion that meconium has been aspirated into the trachea, the essential prophylactic measure is to pass an endotracheal tube and suck out the trachea. Some units perform tracheal lavage with 1–2 ml of normal saline but it does not seem to have any advantage over ordinary suction and may be hazardous.

If aspiration is suspected, it is important to observe the baby carefully for 12–24 hours as insidious deterioration may take place. The baby with severe aspiration usually shows an increase in respiratory rate and cyanosis. The chest radiograph is very variable but often shows large fluffy opacities in many parts of the lung field (see Fig. 5.9). The standard method of treating meconium aspiration is to give sufficient oxygen to keep the baby's arterial Po_2 between 7 and 10 kPa (50–75 mmHg). It is common to use antibiotics as pneumonia may follow. Pneumothorax is also a common complication.

In severe meconium aspiration, ventilation is often required but there is still doubt about the best way of ventilating the baby. It is common to use a rather higher rate than is usual for hyaline membrane disease (see above); we therefore suggest a rate of 35/min with pressure up to 25 cm of water. Some units use end-expiratory pressures of 4–5 cm of water since this has been shown to improve the oxygenation of the baby, but there is then a danger of over-expanding the normal parts of the lung. One of the major problems is a marked right-to-left shunt of blood as a result of persistent fetal circulation. This can be treated by over-ventilation to reduce the P_{CO_2} below normal or by use of a vasodilating drug such as tolazoline (dose 1–2 mg/kg bolus, then 1 mg/kg/h by intravenous infusion). Tolazoline is particularly used if the P_{O_2} remains low. It can produce a dramatic improvement in oxygenation, but it may cause hypotension.

The baby may remain ill for several days. The course of the illness is often complicated by pneumothorax, but if the baby survives the first few days, the tachypnoea will gradually reduce. The babies do not have any prolonged respiratory problems but lung function studies later in infancy have shown some abnormalities.

Pneumonia

Pneumonia is also discussed in Chapter 16. It may occur any time during the newborn period but is commonest shortly after birth, as a result of infection of the amniotic cavity. It should be suspected in any baby whose mother has had ruptured membranes for longer than 12 hours, is pyrexial or has had a long, difficult labour. Examination of gastric aspirate at birth gives a clue to the diagnosis since pus cells may be seen in large numbers in a baby who has pneumonia, but, since pus cells are often seen without infection, it may cause confusion. In addition a vaginal swab from the mother and a swab from the external ear of the baby may identify the causative organism. Babies with RDS or meconium aspiration may develop pneumonia, particularly if they are intubated or ventilated. The greatest danger is in babies with group B β-haemolytic streptococcal pneumonia and septicaemia. Babies are often rather larger than those who have hyaline membrane disease and they may be extremely ill and shocked. The chest radiograph may show patchy opacities but very often the picture is indistinguishable from hyaline membrane disease. If there is any suspicion that the baby might have pneumonia, it is important to start antibiotics very early. Penicillin is the most satisfactory drug. It should be given in high frequent dosage (150 mg/kg/day in six divided doses, intravenously or intramuscularly) usually in combination with gentamicin which seems to have a synergistic effect.

Transient Tachypnoea

This is an ill-defined and common syndrome. It is often diagnosed in babies who would not be expected to have hyaline membrane disease, for example a term baby who is breathing rapidly; the essential criterion for the diagnosis is a respiratory rate of more than 60/min. There may be recession, slight grunting or even cyanosis. The illness disappears by 24 hours and therefore does not fulfil the criteria for hyaline membrane disease. Some babies may have tachypnoea alone for longer than 24 hours but do not have the other criteria of grunting, recession, characteristic chest radiograph and cyanosis which would suggest a diagnosis of HMD. It may be that such babies have only mild surfactant deficiency and that this is the pathological mechanism underlying transient tachypnoea.

Another possible cause of transient tachypnoea is failure to absorb lung fluid satisfactorily after birth. Characteristic chest radiographs have been described; they show increased markings and opacification of the transverse fissure, suggesting oedema between the lobes of the lung on the right. Other characteristics are streaks which spread out from the hilum; it is suggested that these represent enlarged lymphatic vessels which are draining lung fluid. If the lungs were wetter than normal they would probably be stiffer and this could account for the fast breathing.

These babies need very little treatment apart from good standard incubator care and small and appropriate quantities of added oxygen to relieve cyanosis. If there are any opacities in the lung fields on the chest radiograph, it is wise to give antibiotics until the results of the cultures are known. Pneumonitis from chlamydial or cytomegalovirus infection has been described in newborn babies. These infections may be commoner than we suspect. Antibody tests should be done in any baby with an unusual respiratory illness.

Neonatal myasthenia gravis

This is a rare transient disorder which occurs in about 10–15% of babies born to mothers with myasthenia. Antibodies to striated muscle acetylcholine receptors cross the placenta and may cause muscle weakness, feeding difficulties and respiratory problems, usually in the first 24 hours of life. Intravenous edrophonium (1 mg) will confirm the diagnosis by leading to a marked improvement in respiratory effort and spontaneous limb movements, and less pooling of pharyngeal secretions. However, respiratory arrest may occasionally occur. Treatment with the anticholinesterase drug neostigmine is then necessary. This may be necessary for between a few days and several months.

The prognosis in terms of neuromuscular function is excellent. However, associated congenital deformities such as joint contractures may occur and require treatment in their own right with physiotherapy.

Bronchopulmonary Dysplasia

This condition has been seen more frequently in recent years as more small babies have been ventilated for long periods or have needed prolonged oxygen therapy.

The typical case is a baby under 1500 g who required prolonged ventilation for HMD and apnoeic attacks. He then remains dependent on oxygen and becomes cyanosed if no added oxygen is given. There is usually intercostal recession, a high respiratory rate and a very abnormal chest radiograph showing streaking of the lung fields alternating with translucent areas probably representing cystic or over-inflated parts of the lung. There is a high mortality and at post-mortem the histology of the lung shows focal areas of emphysematous alveoli, bronchiolar smooth muscle hypertrophy and perimucosal fibrosis.

There has been a lot of controversy about the cause of the condition. It occurs only in babies who have received prolonged oxygen therapy and ventilation and it is difficult to know whether it is the pressure effects of ventilation or the toxic effects of oxygen which cause injury to the lung. The evidence suggests that the pressure effects are more important since the syndrome has become much less common since low pressures have been used for ventilation. It is therefore wise to use the lowest pressure which will produce adequate ventilation of the chest. Reduction of ventilation pressures should be the first change in managing a baby who is improving. The oxygen concentration should also be reduced as soon as possible.

When a baby develops bronchopulmonary dysplasia it may be very difficult to wean him off the ventilator quickly. The illness may have a long course and the baby may need oxygen to prevent cyanosis for many months or even one or two years while he gradually improves. Theophylline and diuretics are often used. Steroids may sometimes lead to a dramatic improvement.

Wilson–Mikity Syndrome

This syndrome was described about 25 years ago as a characteristic illness of pulmonary insufficiency in very small babies. The chest radiograph shows streaking with cystic areas. The baby is cyanosed but does not always have very much tachypnoea. Rickets and rib fractures have been described as accompanying features. It is very doubtful whether this can be properly distinguished from bronchopulmonary dysplasia in most babies but it might be a reasonable diagnosis for chronic lung disease in a baby who has not received very much oxygen or ventilation therapy.

Apnoeic Attacks

The differentiation of primary and terminal apnoea is discussed in Chapter 3.

We define an apnoeic attack as a period of absent breathing lasting 10 seconds or more if accompanied by bradycardia or cyanosis, or lasting 20 seconds or more with no fall in heart rate or change in colour. An attack shorter than 20 seconds is not usually accompanied by cyanosis. In many preterm babies, periods of rapid breathing alternate with periods of slow breathing and this is a normal pattern.

Apnoeic attacks are common in otherwise normal babies born under 32 weeks gestation. They are a common complication of severe respiratory distress due to any cause; they may also complicate severe birth trauma, hypoglycaemia or maternal over-sedation. Severe and prolonged apnoeic attacks either in the normal preterm baby or, more commonly, in the baby with severe respiratory distress may be a sign of intraventricular haemorrhage and denote a poor prognosis (see above and p. 278). In the very preterm baby, the risk of apnoeic attacks is increased in certain circumstances: nasogastric tube feeds (with or without aspiration); excessive handling for nappy changing, temperature taking, or cleaning; too high an ambient temperature. The very immature infant often has phases of bradycardia which lead to apnoea if he is not stimulated.

In any baby, systemic infection must be excluded as a cause. Apnoeic attacks may also be the only presenting feature of neonatal fits (see Chapter 14). Some important causes of neonatal apnoea are summarized in Table 6.8.

Babies at risk should be nursed on apnoea mattresses which will automatically trigger an alarm after a predetermined period of absent breathing. In this way periods of prolonged apnoea with possible cerebral hypoxia are avoided and babies can be more easily resuscitated. The use of such monitors after the baby has left hospital is discussed on p. 316.

Treatment

Prevention

Apnoeic attacks are better prevented than treated:
1 Minimal handling. (If a baby has attacks, label the incubator **MINIMAL HANDLING**.)

Table 6.8 Some important causes of apnoeic attacks in the newborn.

Respiratory
Exhaustion (severe RDS, bronchopulmonary dysplasia)
Pneumonia—viral or bacterial; tracheo-oesphageal fistula
Pneumothorax—meconium aspiration; resuscitation; spontaneous; ventilation
Aspiration—blood; meconium; feed; vomitus
Vagal or pharyngeal stimulation (deep suction, passage of tubes)

Central
Apnoea of preterm infant (immature respiratory centre)
Seizures
Excess sedation with drugs (mother or baby)
Cerebral haemorrhage
Cerebral birth trauma
Kernicterus
Meningitis or other severe infections

Metabolic
Hypoglycaemia
Hypocalcaemia
Hypothermia
Acidosis, metabolic or respiratory
Hyponatraemia
Giving intravenous or intraarterial calcium or potassium too rapidly

Obstructive
Choanal or oesophageal atresia
Tongue (in Pierre Robin syndrome)
Mechanical (face covered by towels etc. during procedures)

2 An appropriate environmental temperature.

3 Nurse prone when possible.

4 Nurse on apnoea alarm set to a 10-second delay and use a heart rate monitor alarm set at 100 beats/min.

After the first attack consider nursing prone, removing nasal tubes and nursing on a sheepskin and adjust environmental temperature. A nasojejunal tube would also block the nose and should not be used. Intravenous alimentation may be necessary.

Do not give oxygen routinely: during an apnoeic attack the baby is not breathing so that it would have no effect. After the attack, breathing oxygen-enriched gases may be dangerous as the baby's Pa_{O_2} may rise to very high levels. However, it is possible for oxygen to be absorbed to some extent through mucous membranes, and the cold jet may make the baby gasp.

Physical stimulation can be obtained by stroking or patting the baby and changing his position. Suction of the posterior pharynx may provoke apnoea and clearing the airways should therefore involve suction only of the mouth. The baby can then be rapidly intubated if necessary.

If there is continued apnoea with bradycardia and physical stimulation fails, intubation and hand ventilation are needed (for technique see

Chapter 3). If regular spontaneous respirations with a normal heart rate return the baby can safely be extubated.

Recurrent apnoeic attacks

There is accumulating evidence that the use of the respiratory stimulant theophylline may prevent or greatly reduce the incidence of apnoeic attacks in preterm babies. The dose is still controversial. It is important to check blood levels regularly, so as to reduce the risks of toxicity—the most common of which are cardiac arrhythmias. A suitable loading dose is 6.2 mg/kg (Table 6.9). So far there have not been any reports of long-term side effects.

Continuous positive airways pressure (see earlier in this chapter for the possible techniques) can be used. There is good evidence that this method, however applied, prevents apnoeic attacks. The technique has its own dangers, however, and these are described above. There is some evidence that theophylline is more effective and is certainly easier to administer than CPAP. It is best employed in specialist units experienced in its use (Table 6.9).

Mechanical ventilation is indicated if adequate respiration is not maintained between attacks with or without the use of CPAP (for details, see Table 6.9).

Investigations

Any baby who needs treatment for apnoea should be investigated.

1 *Exclude infection* by blood culture, urine analysis and culture swabs from any obviously infected area and the external ear and white blood cell count. A lumbar puncture may often be indicated, but this may precipitate a further severe apnoeic attack. Be prepared for this.

Table 6.9 Management of recurrent apnoeic attacks.

Theophylline	Give the loading dose of 6.2 mg/kg either intravenously over 20 minutes or orally as choline theophylline. Then give maintenance dose of 4.4 mg/kg/day intravenously or Choledyl 1.5 mg/kg six-hourly. Plasma theophylline level should be checked the following day if possible.
CPAP	Administer via facemask, nasopharyngeal tube or endotracheal tube depending on infant's condition and size. Start at 2–4 cmH_2O and increase to a maximum of 4–6 cm. If response is poor, give theophylline or ventilate. If using a facemask, feeding should be intravenous. Pass nasogastric tube to aspirate stomach.
Ventilation	If apnoea is causing persistent acidosis (pH<7.2) and hypoxaemia (Pao_2<6 kPa) ventilate by endotracheal tube or facemask. Keep peak pressure low (<15 cmH_2O) or use IMV. Monitor response by blood gas analysis.

2 *Exclude hypoglycaemia* with glucose monitoring strips and a blood glucose estimation if the glucose monitoring strip result is low.
3 An *electroencephalogram* may reveal evidence that convulsions are presenting as apnoeic attacks.
4 *Ultrasound* or *computerized axial tomographic (CAT) scan* is useful to exclude subdural collections of blood or fluid and intraventricular haemorrhage.

Appropriate specific treatment (such as antibiotics, dextrose or anti-convulsants) may need to be given. If infection is suspected, do not await the culture results before starting treatment. Treatment should be started as soon as specimens have been obtained.

Diaphragmatic Hernia

This subject is discussed in Chapter 3 (p. 57).

Further Reading

Avery, M.E. & Fletcher, B.D. (1974) *The Lung and its Disorders in the Newborn Infant*, 3rd ed. Philadelphia: W.B. Saunders.

Gluck, L. & Kulovich, M. (1973) Lecithin–sphingomyelin ratios in amniotic fluid in normal and abnormal pregnancy. *American Journal of Obstetrics and Gynecology*, *115*, 539.

Gregory, C., Kitterman, J., Phibbs, R.M., Tooley, W.H. & Hamilton, W.K. (1971) Treatment of the idiopathic respiratory distress syndrome with continuous positive airway pressure. *New England Journal of Medicine*, *284*, 1333.

Kendig, Jr, E.L. & Chernick, V.C. (1983) *Disorders of the Respiratory Tract in Children*, 4th ed. Philadelphia: W.B. Saunders.

Liggins, G.C. & Howie, R.N. (1972) A controlled trial of antepartum glucocorticoid in premature infants. *Pediatrics, Springfield*, *50*, 515.

Strang, L.B. (1977) *Neonatal Respiration*. Oxford: Blackwell Scientific.

Wesenberg, R.L. (1973) *The Newborn Chest*. Hagerstown, MD: Harper & Row.

Roberton, N.R.C. (1977) Management of neonatal respiratory failure. *Journal of the Royal College of Physicians* (London), *11*, 389.

Tarnow-Mordi, W. & Wilkinson, A. (1986) Mechanical ventilation of the newborn. *British Medical Journal*, *292*, 575–6.

7

Nutrition

Breast Feeding

Breast feeding is the normal and natural way of feeding a newborn baby. It is only in very recent times, mainly during the last two centuries, that our industrial society has turned to the superficial attractions and convenience of bottle feeding. There are now a number of artificial milk preparations derived from cow's milk which are more or less adapted for human needs. Earlier in the century, bottle feeding was used largely by the upper social classes and women in the working class were more likely to breast feed. Until a few years ago there had been a continuing increase in the number of women who bottle fed their babies, but it is very interesting that more recently there has been a reversal of this trend and breast feeding is now much more popular than it was 15 years ago.

It seems likely that infant feeding habits have been largely socially determined. Unlike 50 years ago, breast feeding is now particularly popular amongst the higher social classes. It is the women in social classes IV and V who are less likely to breast feed now. In these days of smaller families, many young mothers have never even seen a baby being breast fed; they do not look upon it as natural. In addition, many mothers now wish or need to go out to work after the baby has been born in order to supplement the family's income. There is also no doubt that even the most friendly maternity ward is less relaxing for the new mother than her own familiar surroundings at home. Some of the suggestions made by maternity hospitals may seem more like rules to the young mother and may even hinder breast feeding; anxiety easily inhibits the natural development of lactation and can cause a woman to give up breast feeding. It takes at least two weeks to establish breast feeding properly and most mothers are discharged home long before this. Unfortunately some medical and midwifery advice has been to feed babies on a fixed routine of feeding schedules rather than to allow the mother to feed on demand, which is the natural way to breast feed a baby.

To encourage the spread of breast feeding in hospital, the attitude of midwives, obstetricians and paediatricians is of crucial importance. Women who have some doubt about the value of breast feeding should be encouraged to breast feed. Restricting the time of the baby on the breast by a schedule such as allowing the baby to feed only for three mintues the first day, five the second and seven the third has been shown to decrease the success rate of breast feeding when compared with a schedule that allows the mother to do what she and the baby want.

The time to teach the importance of breast feeding is in school. It could form part of the normal curriculum, like sex education, and both boys and girls should understand the vital importance of nutrition for a young baby. A breast-feeding mother could be invited to the school. Although it is less usual to persuade the mother to change her mind once the baby has been born, the advice and example of other mothers may be extremely helpful and breast-feeding mothers can be invited to antenatal classes. When there is a high rate of breast feeding within a maternity ward, undecided mothers are more likely to breast feed. The subject should be clearly discussed during the antenatal period, but one difficulty is that the mother who is less likely to breast feed is also less likely to attend for antenatal care.

The long-term establishment of breast feeding is greatly helped by putting the baby to the breast in the labour ward immediately after delivery. Recent trials have shown that more mothers continue to breast feed after discharge from hospital if this has been done. The establishment of breast feeding does take time and trouble, so a lactation midwife or infant-feeding sister, spending her entire day giving individual help to feeding mothers, is a great asset to a maternity department.

Newborn babies after the first 24 hours take many feeds each day. A baby who is allowed to feed as often and as much as he pleases may feed for only a minute or two and as often as twice an hour. The arbitrary stipulation that babies should be fed at regular intervals, and have a certain length of time on the breast, makes it very difficult to establish natural breast feeding. Babies should be fed on demand and, contrary to much popular belief, such babies have been shown to settle down to a routine more quickly than babies who are forced to fit into a rigid timetable. The practice of 'rooming in', where babies spend the night in cots by their mother's bedside, is also important for establishing breast feeding. It is otherwise only too easy for night nurses to give babies some milk complement; in some cases, the mother may not even be aware of this. It is thought that even one artificial feed may be sufficient to cause cow's milk allergy in a susceptible infant.

Advantages

It is worthwhile taking trouble to establish breast feeding because the breast-fed baby has a number of potential advantages over his bottle-fed peer. These advantages are worth considering in some detail:

Emotional relationships with the mother

Observation of infants in many different societies suggests that care of young infants is very different in modern industrialized societies from that in most parts of the world. In developing countries, and presumably in all countries in the past, a baby is carried around in close contact with his mother, is fed frequently on demand, is pacified immediately when miserable and sleeps in his parents' bed. In contrast, a baby in an industrial society is more likely to be fed less frequently, is allowed to cry when miserable, is rarely carried around and has much less bodily contact with an adult. The early part of infancy is a period of great need for emotional warmth and love manifested as close and regular body

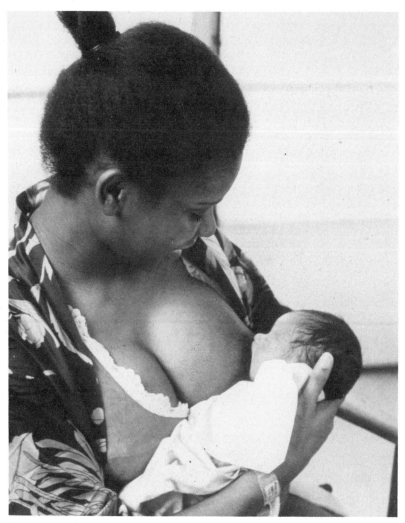

Fig. 7.1 Breast feeding

contact. Thus the baby who is breast fed is satisfying not only his nutritional needs but also his emotional needs (Fig. 7.1) There is good evidence that a baby at the breast takes in most of his fluid and energy requirements during the first few minutes of suckling. Much of the remainder of the time on the breast serves for oral pleasure and close body contact.

The bottle-fed baby is much more likely to be fed by other people than his mother. Feeding is more likely to be done in public and the baby may be deprived of the very close contact typical of breast feeding. Of course,

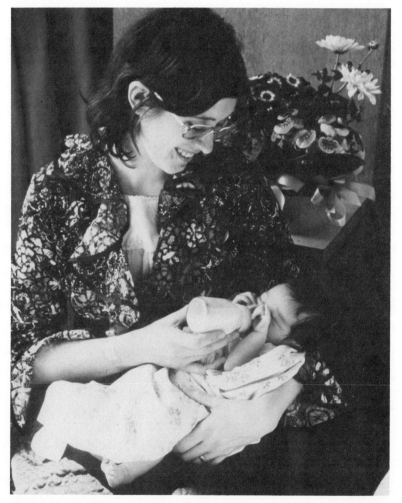

Fig. 7.2 Bottle feeding

many mothers who bottle feed their babies do establish a warm and loving relationship with them (Fig. 7.2) but one sometimes sees the baby being bottle fed at arm's length while the mother is engrossed in the television or her newspaper. A bottle-feeding mother may have to make a real effort to provide the emotional satisfaction that the breast-feeding mother does more naturally. We do not want this to sound too much like a sermon but there do seem to be very clear advantages to breast feeding.

Decreased likelihood of infection

The widespread morbidity and mortality among newborn babies in developing countries in recent years has partly stemmed from mothers' lack of knowledge of the rudiments of sterilization of bottles and feeds. Epidemics of infantile gastroenteritis have been the result. Even in the UK many mothers in socially deprived areas have neither the facilities nor the ability to produce properly sterilized artificial feeds. There are, however, specific factors present in breast milk, and not in artificially

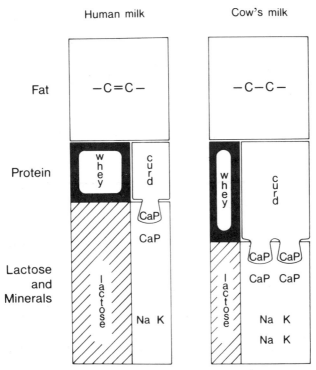

Fig. 7.3 The composition of human and cow's milk. From Wharton & Berger (1976), by permission of the author and editor

prepared cow's milk feeds, which protect the newborn baby from infection. An immunoglobulin, IgA, is secreted in high concentration in breast milk, and, more particularly, in colostrum during the first few days of life. This substance lines the breast-fed baby's gut and, in conjunction with lactoferrin also present in colostrum, helps establish a bacterial flora of non-pathogenic lactobacilli, while suppressing the growth of potentially pathogenic strains of *E. coli*. The bottle-fed baby's bowel flora is predominantly *E. coli*.

Reduced incidence of eczema and other forms of atopy

It is becoming clear that the incidence of eczema is much greater in babies who have had even one or two artificial feeds during the early weeks or months of life. There is a substance in the protein fraction of cow's milk which sensitizes many babies. This manifests itself as eczema during infancy and may be associated with the subsequent development of such diseases as asthma, urticaria, hay fever and allergic rhinitis. It is of particular importance that the breast-fed baby is not given any artificial cow's milk complement. In the early days of life, while mother's milk is still coming into the breasts, the newborn baby may be thirsty. He should be given feeds with clear fluids to satisfy this. If cow's milk complements are avoided, the risk of atopy is significantly reduced.

There has been a recent suggestion, based on epidemiological evidence, that breast feeding may help to protect an infant from the later development of diabetes mellitus. If this is true the mechanism would presumably be immunological.

Reduced likelihood of biochemical upset (including convulsions)

The composition of unmodified cow's milk and human milk is shown in Fig.7.3 and Table 7.4. The predominant protein in human milk (lactalbumin) is much more digestible than that in cow's milk (casein); there is more carbohydrate, but also the fat content, being much more evenly distributed throughout the milk, is much more easily digestible. In addition there are significant biochemical differences. For example, cow's milk contains some three to four times as much calcium as human milk but about seven times as much phosphate. It contains four times as much sodium and its osmolality is three times that of human milk. Until some years ago, the artificial milks available also contained too much phosphate. Many babies fed on these preparations developed hypocalcaemic fits during the second or third week of life. This is because there is an inverse relationship between calcium and phosphate in the body and ingesting too much phosphate tends to make the blood calcium levels low. In the last few years most available artificial milk preparations have reduced the phosphate load in the milk, thus making this problem much rarer.

An analogous problem has been the high sodium content of artificial milks. The newborn baby's kidney is not very efficient by adult standards. When a bottle-fed baby is well, there is just sufficient reserve to enable the kidney to fulfil the demands made on it. If such a baby develops diarrhoea, for example, this precarious balance is lost and severe biochemical disturbances can follow. Each baby milk preparation comes with its individual scoop. These are not interchangeable from make to make and failure to appreciate this may lead to feeds made up in the wrong strength. If baby milk powder is packed into the scoop or it is not levelled off, over-concentrated feeds are given to the baby. This may be very dangerous in itself, but if the baby is already unwell with gastroenteritis and crying for more feed because he is thirsty, he will be fed with an over-concentrated feed which will make his plight worse. It used to be common for such babies to be brought into hospital casualty departments dehydrated and with plasma sodium levels of over 160 mmol/l. There was considerable mortality amongst such babies and convulsions were common in those who survived.

Reduced incidence of cot deaths (sudden infant death syndrome, SIDS)

There is a much lower incidence of cot deaths amongst breast-fed babies. It does occur, but it is unusual. The reasons for this are not altogether clear; cot death is probably not one condition but has a multitude of different causes. Many of these deaths may be related to some of the factors already described, which are more likely in the bottle-fed baby. In addition, the bottle-feeding mother is less likely to have come for antenatal care and cot deaths amongst the infants of such mothers are commoner (see also p. 98).

Less likelihood of obesity

The fluid intake of the healthy baby amounts to 150–200 ml/kg/day. This is equivalent to 110–150 cal/kg daily (about 450–600 kJ); some preterm babies may need even more if they are to thrive. This is a rough guide as no two babies are alike. The natural way to allow a baby to feed is to let him take as much food as he likes as often as he likes. With rare exceptions, a healthy baby will regulate his own intake in a satisfactory manner. Attempting to fit him into an arbitrary feeding regimen may not be so satisfactory. There is a natural tendency among some bottle-feeding mothers to overfeed their babies. This is because of the mistaken idea that fat babies are healthy babies and because a baby who is feeding a lot and overweight tends to be a placid individual. There is evidence that the fat baby does not necessarily develop into the fat child and adult. Nevertheless, an obese baby is not a healthy one and is more susceptible to respiratory infection.

Contraindications

There are few contraindications to breast feeding. One recently recognized one is if the mother has acquired immune deficiency syndrome (AIDS). The reasons for preventing her from breast feeding are discussed in Chapter 16 (p. 308). The usual reason for not breast feeding is that a mother says she does not want to. It is not likely that you will succeed in persuading her once her mind is made up; to attempt to do so will only be counter-productive by suggesting that she is a less than adequate or conscientious mother for not wishing to breast feed.

Only rarely is breast feeding contraindicated because of drugs (e.g. lithium) that the mother is taking. In untreated tuberculosis, the mother who is already established on treatment may be allowed to breast feed her baby, who should, however, be protected with isoniazid-resistant BCG and also treated with isoniazid (10 mg/kg/day orally in three doses) for the first few months of life.

Breast feeding may be stopped temporarily because of breast engorgement or abscess, or psychosis; but many of the conventional contraindications such as maternal cardiac disease, diabetes or maternal renal disease should not prevent the baby being breast fed.

Some practical worries include temporary breast engorgement, which may be overcome by manual expression, and loose yellow frequent stools in the baby which are normal. You should explain to the mother that the baby does not chew on the nipple, but sucks it and the surrounding breast tissue into his mouth; he uses his gums to massage milk out of the breast.

The key to successful breast feeding is a relaxed mother. To achieve such relaxation in a hospital ward requires care, attention and patience from all those who attend her.

Breast milk drug excretion

Surprisingly little is known about the excretion of many drugs in breast milk. It seems likely that virtually all substances given to the mother will be excreted in some form, in greater or lesser concentration, in her breast milk. How much depends on the size of the drug molecule, its solubility in water and fat, its acidity and its degree of ionization at physiological pH. Excretory mechanisms are summarized in Table 7.1. As a general rule, the amounts are usually small, do not affect the baby clinically, and are not a contraindication to continuing breast feeding. The only important exceptions to this rule are mothers who have been given radioactive iodine for thyrotoxicosis and possibly other drugs affecting thyroid function, and those on cytotoxic drugs. It is commonly believed that breast feeding after eating a lot of fresh fruit or taking large amounts of purgatives can produce loose stools in the baby, but see Table 7.3. Such

Table 7.1 Excretion methods which allow drugs to appear in the milk.

1 Water-soluble substances with a molecular weight of 200 or less, e.g. ethanol or tetracycline, diffuse through pores and may achieve the same concentration in milk as in plasma

2 Active excretion, e.g. thiouracil

3 Most drugs are weak acids or weak bases and enter milk in their non-protein-bound, unionized forms to reach concentrations that depend on the pH difference between plasma (pH 7.4) and milk (pH 7.0), and on the degree of ionization of the drug at physiological pH, its protein-binding capacity and its lipid solubility. Weak acids reach *lower* concentrations in milk than in plasma, while weak bases reach concentrations in milk that are similar to, or *higher* than those in plasma

Table 7.2 Common drugs believed to have adverse effects in breast-fed babies when taken by the mother.

Drug	May cause
Sulphonamides	Neonatal jaundice Haemolysis in infants with glucose-6-phosphate dehydrogenase deficiency
Chloramphenicol	Possibility of grey baby syndrome
Phenindione	Increased prothrombin time
Barbiturates	Drowsiness
Thiouracil	Goitre Agranulocytosis
Radioactive iodine	Goitre Late risk of thyroid cancer
Cyclophosphamide and other anti-neoplastic drugs	Bone marrow depression
Propranolol	Cardiovascular and respiratory effects Hypoglycaemia
Ergot alkaloids	Ergotism
Diazepam	Sedation
Lithium	Hypotonia Hypothermia Cyanosis
Theophylline	Irritability

overindulgence in natural or artificial laxatives should clearly be avoided. The nurse and doctor should be particularly aware of possible complications when the drugs listed in Table 7.2 are being taken over a long period by the breast-feeding mother. Table 7.3 gives more information about the potential toxicity of a number of drugs now in common use or where information is available. Many nursing mothers receive drugs

Table 7.3 Potential toxicity to the baby of various drugs taken by breast-feeding mother.

Antibacterial drugs

Sulphonamides	Milk/plasma (M/P) ratios vary from 0.08 to 0.97 depending on ionization at plasma pH. Theoretical risk of neonatal jaundice by competition with bilirubin for hepatic sites. Haemolytic anaemia has been reported in a G-6-PD-deficient baby breast fed while the mother was taking sulphamethoxypyridazine
Penicillins	Amounts too small to have antimicrobial effect, but rarely may provoke antigenic response. Safe
Ampicillin	May cause diarrhoea and candidiasis
Isoniazid	High M/P ratio (too little information to be categoric about safety)
Tetracycline	High M/P ratio (too little information to be categoric about safety)
Streptomycin	Mother with normal renal function may take up to 1 g daily without causing ototoxicity in infant. Maternal renal failure increases milk concentrations up to 25-fold. Safe
Nalidixic acid	One report of haemolysis in infant with normal enzymes whose mother was uraemic
Chloramphenicol	M/P ratio is 0.5 but 50% in the form of an inactive metabolite. Not recommended
Oxacillin	Not found in breast milk
Nitrofurantoin	Not found in breast milk
Erythromycin	Occurs in small amounts in milk if taken orally by mother. Amounts increase ten-fold when it is given intravenously. Safe
Cephalexin/cephalothin	Trace amounts may occur in milk. Safe

Hormones

Insulin Adrenaline ACTH	Destroyed in infant's gut
Thyroxine Corticosteroids	If given in moderate amounts, are not found in the milk in significant quantities
Oral contraceptives	Male babies may develop gynaecomastia; females may show proliferation of vaginal epithelium. Infant is unlikely to be affected provided (*a*) drug is withheld until third or fourth week post partum; (*b*) daily dose does not exceed 50 μg ethinyloestradiol, or 100 μg mestranol + 2.5 mg 19-nortestosterone derivative

Anticoagulants

Heparin	Destroyed in gut. Safe
Ethyl biscoumacetate	Small amounts in milk

Table 7.3 Potential toxicity to the baby of various drugs taken by breast-feeding mother.

Anticoagulants	
Warfarin	Not detected in milk; baby's prothrombin time remains normal. Anticoagulant of choice in breast-feeding mothers
Phenindione	Increased prothrombin time reported; also large postoperative haematoma. Not recommended
Anticonvulsants	
Phenobarbitone	Probably no adverse effects
Phenytoin	No ill-effects. Insignificant amounts excreted. One child developed methaemoglobinaemia while mother was taking large doses of phenytoin and phenobarbitone
Psychotherapeutic drugs	
Diazepam	Diazepam and its active metabolite found in milk and in infant's serum and urine. Infants' EEGs show changes characteristic of sedative medication. Sedation and lethargy. Not recommended
Chlordiazepoxide	Minimal amounts in milk. Not harmful
Chloral hydrate Dichloralphenazone	Enter in sufficient amounts to cause minimal sedation after larger feeds
Imipramine	Not found in milk. Safe
Chlorpromazine	Evidence conflicting. Probably best to limit maternal dose to less than 100 mg/day
Lithium	Concentration in milk about one-half to one-third that in plasma. Complete absorption from gastrointestinal tract. Hypotonia and cyanosis observed in the baby of a mother taking lithium during pregnancy. Breast feeding is contraindicated if treatment is essential
Haloperidol	No reports of ill-effects
Narcotics	
Heroin Methadone	Enter milk, and infant probably already tolerant in utero. Nevertheless withdrawal symptoms common even if breast-fed
Morphine	Traces only. Safe, if indicated
Codeine	Not detected
Analgesics	
Salicylates	Small doses are harmless. Evidence of impaired platelet function in mothers taking large doses. ? similar effect in breast feeding. However, widely used and probably harmless
Phenylbutazone	Not detected. Safe
Iodides and thiouracil	
Thiouracil	M/P ratio is 3. Mothers who have to take this drug should probably not breast feed, but the thyroid function should be monitored

Table 7.3 Potential toxicity to the baby of various drugs taken by breast-feeding mother.

Iodides	Actively transported and goitrogenic. Sensitize infant's thyroid to co-goitrogens such as chlorpromazine, lithium and methylxanthines
Radioactive iodine	28% of dose may enter milk and be completely absorbed by baby. Stop breast feeding for 10 days after use. Also increases risk of later thyroid cancer
Technetium	Stop breast feeding for 48 hours
Alkylating agents	
Cyclophosphamide	Do not breast feed
Methotrexate	Weak organic acid with low M/P ratio but possible long-term effects on baby unknown
Miscellaneous	
Digoxin	Safe
Propranolol	Found in significant quantity in milk. Infants should be assessed regularly for cerebrovascular and respiratory effects and hypoglycaemia
25-Hydroxychole-calciferol	Large doses cause hypercalcaemia in baby. Monitor calcium levels
Antihistamines	Low levels. Unlikely to be significant
Tolbutamide	Found in milk. Could cause hypoglycaemia but seems safe
Metronidazole	High concentrations in milk and plasma. No harmful effect when mother receives 200 mg three times a day for seven days, but avoid high dosages; metallic taste may put baby off breast feeding
Ergot alkaloids	Avoid. May produce symptoms in suckling infants
Fluoride	Accepted daily dose for optimal tooth development under two years is 0.25 mg. This is provided in breast milk if local water supply provides 1 part per million. London water is not flouridated. Mottling of the teeth may occur if extra fluoride is taken or if local water concentration exceeds this level
Laxatives	Do not cause purgation except, possibly, for anthraquinone derivatives, e.g. cascara, senna, rhubarb, danthrone and aloes. In fact anthraquinone has not been shown to have any definite effect on the infant's bowel
Alcohol Nicotine	Probably not harmful in moderate amounts
Caffeine	Not enough occurs in milk to affect infant
Fava beans	Haemolysis reported in G-6-PD-deficient infants
Gold	Trace amounts in infant's serum
Thiazides	Small amounts; not harmful

without particular justification. Paracetamol and nitrazepam should not be routinely prescribed to all post-partum obstetric patients.

Expressed breast milk and milk banks

Since breast feeding improves the survival of preterm babies it is important to encourage it whenever possible. Many units give expressed breast milk (EBM), either from the mother or a bank, to babies who are not yet able to suckle at the breast. When a mother is expressing milk herself, by hand or pump, it is common practice to give this immediately to the baby. This 'raw' milk has all the immunological properties of milk obtained by suckling. In some developing countries such milk, given via nasogastric tube, has greatly reduced the incidence of infection in preterm infants.

It is important to keep a very strict control over milk which has been expressed but will not be given immediately to a baby. Specimens must be taken to ensure that the mother is not producing infected milk and it is wise to treat the milk with heat to reduce the risk of bacterial contamination. Milk can be pasteurized, by holding at 60°C for 30 minutes, and then deep frozen. Heating does reduce the immunological properties of the milk although it does not alter the mineral content. Pasteurization does not destroy so much IgA as older and fiercer methods, such as boiling. The establishment of a breast milk bank is important in emphasizing the importance of breast feeding for the preterm and encouraging mothers to express milk for their own babies. Unfortunately EBM may not contain sufficient calories or protein for adequate nutrition in a small baby. Attempts have been made to boost the nutritional content of banked breast milk with protein, fat or carbohydrate but we are still uncertain about exactly what needs to be added. It is fairly common practice to add carbohydrate as Caloreen (up to 5 g/kg) to EBM given to a small baby who is not gaining weight satisfactorily.

Milk that has been collected by allowing it to drip from a breast while the baby sucks the opposite breast has, unfortunately, a very low fat content. Expressed milk is the only satisfactory milk for a bank at present. Technological advances in the future should allow the fractionation of human milk into components containing protein, carbohydrate and fat. In this way a human milk product with more protein and energy than in the current banked milk could be produced.

At present, if a mother is intending to breast feed her preterm baby, we use banked EBM—boosting the energy content if necessary, depending on the baby's progress. When a baby is not going to be breast fed we use a formula feed designed for low birth-weight babies (there is rarely sufficient EBM in the bank to meet the needs of every small baby on the unit).

The disadvantage of currently available formula feeds for low birth-

weight babies is their high sodium content. Despite their high energy
and protein content this limits their usefulness as volumes need to be
restricted to less than 150 ml/kg/24 hours.

Feeding Techniques

Breast feeding

From what has been said already, it should be clear one must not
interfere with the mother's ability to breast feed. The baby should be
offered the breast in the labour ward and fed very frequently during the
newborn period for as long as the mother and the baby wish. The baby
should suck well from the nipple; inverted nipples can be corrected, to
some extent, by wearing a nipple shield (Woolwich shell) inside the bra.
The nipple usually becomes long and erect during the early part of
suckling; it reaches as far as possible into the baby's mouth so that he can
suck on the areola. The midwife should help the mother to get comfortable, as it must be miserable to breast feed in a cramped or difficult
position.

Bottle feeding

If the mother has decided to bottle feed, it is usually possible to establish
bottle feeding in a term baby without much difficulty. The occasional
baby needs a change of teat to provide one that he can suck on more
easily; preterm babies born at less than 34 weeks gestational age usually
need special techniques of tube feeding before progressing to bottle
feeding. The choice of milk needs a little thought; in general, it seems
reasonable to choose a milk that is chemically similar to breast milk.
Table 7.4 shows the composition of breast milk. The figures refer to
pooled mature breast milk and there is, in fact, a lot more variation than

Table 7.4 Composition of breast milk, and artificial powdered milk and cow's milk.

Composition	Breast milk	SMA (S26)	Cow's milk
Carbohydrate*	6.8	7.2	4.9
Fat*	4.5	3.6	3.7
Protein*	1.1	1.5	3.5
Sodium (mmol/l)	7	7	22
Phosphorus (mg/l)	140	330·	920
Calcium (mg/l)	340	445	1170

* grams per 100 ml of formula.

is suggested by average figures. One example of artificial milk is also shown in the table. The concentration of chemicals looks very similar in some artificial baby milks and breast milk but there are still important differences, particularly in immunoglobulins and, of course, in the live cells which breast milk contains. It is important that the amount of sodium should be very little higher than in breast milk since hypernatraemia used to be a common complication of gastroenteritis in the early months of life before milks were modified to contain less sodium. However, very small newborn babies may develop hyponatraemia and could need sodium supplements (3 mmol/kg/day).

Special feeds have been developed in recent years which are thought to be appropriate to the special needs of the preterm baby (but see above).

Nasogastric feeding

Indications for nasogastric feeding include any baby who has considerable difficulty in sucking or is unable to suck. This commonly means the preterm baby, generally less than about 34 weeks gestation, an ill baby of any size or maturity and babies with difficulty in breathing such as babies with heart failure. Such infants may be gradually introduced to breast or bottle feeding at the appropriate time with the number of (intermittent) nasogastric feeds gradually reduced. The aim is to achieve a weight gain of about 200 g/week.

Technique A tube is inserted through the baby's nostril and passed down the oesophagus into the stomach. Different size tubes are now available for babies of different weights: FG4 for babies of less than 1.2 kg, FG5 for 1.2–1.7 kg and FG6 for greater than 1.7 kg. FG8 gastric tubes are used for orogastric feeding only. The nose–umbilicus length is a good guide to how far to insert the tube. It is wise to choose the smaller nostril so as to leave the larger one for the baby to breathe through. There may be a case for passing the tube through the mouth. There is usually very little difficulty in passing the tube. When the tube is thought to be in the stomach, a syringe is attached and an attempt made to aspirate stomach contents. The liquid from the stomach is acid and will turn blue litmus paper red. If there is any doubt about the position of the tube, air can be gently blown down the tube while listening with a stethoscope over the upper abdomen. Once the position of the tube has been confirmed, it can be fixed in position by strapping on the baby's cheek.

Amounts of feed for the preterm baby (usually full-strength expressed breast milk):

60 ml/kg/24 hours on Day 1
90 ml/kg/24 hours on Day 2

120 ml/kg/24 hours on Day 3
150 ml/kg/24 hours on Day 4

These amounts should be increased as shown and then gradually every day. The intake may need to exceed about 200 ml/kg/day before the very tiny baby will grow adequately.

Very preterm babies of less than about 1.3 kg need oral sodium supplements (3 mmol/kg/day) after the first week. Babies of less than 1 kg or in whom the plasma sodium is less than 125 mmol/l need about 6 mmol/kg/day of extra sodium. The plasma sodium should be measured at least every day.

Feeds can be given as often as hourly to reduce the risk of aspiration. For similar reasons, the baby may be nursed prone.

Expressed breast milk should be used when available. There seems to be no ideal milk for very preterm babies because they need the anti-infection qualities of fresh breast milk but with a higher energy and protein content for growth (see above).

Dangers. There is some evidence that a baby who is tube fed for a long time may be slow to learn sucking. For this reason, it is useful to allow even a very small baby a little time for sucking at the mother's breast or on a dummy well before this is likely to be his normal means of feeding.

Trauma from the tube is uncommon if the tube is passed gently. If resistance is met, the tube should be withdrawn slightly and a further attempt made at re-insertion.

Airway obstruction may occur in the smallest babies, as the diameter of the tube may approach that of the nasal passages. As the young baby is an obligatory nose breather, care must be taken to ensure that a small enough tube is used, and that the opposite (larger) nostril is never allowed to block.

Aspiration of feeds should largely be prevented if babies are fed upright, prone or on their sides. In addition, particular care should be taken when passing the tube that it has actually reached the stomach. The risks of aspiration into the lungs of feed from a tube which is coiled up in the oropharynx are considerable. Nasogastric feeding is not suitable for babies with respiratory problems; it should certainly not be used for 24 hours after endotracheal extubation or when giving CPAP (see Chapter 6).

Continuous intragastric feeding

This method has proved extremely useful for the small preterm baby. It may well be more physiological than the large bolus feeds described above as such babies would normally take very small amounts of feed at very frequent intervals. The overall amounts given are similar to those given by intermittent feeding. Because the baby is handled less, he is less likely to become infected. A constant infusion pump may be used to regulate the rate that the milk is given. It is vital that babies fed in this way are nursed prone, otherwise the risk of aspiration of feed into the lungs is very high. Once again, care must be taken that the nasogastric tube is in the stomach and not coiled up in the oropharynx. If these precautions are taken, this is an extremely simple and safe technique to use in small babies. It may be wise to aspirate every three hours to ensure that milk is not collecting in the stomach. Agitate the bottle or syringe fairly often to keep the fat mixed with the rest of the milk and keep the pump below the level of the baby or most of the fat (and therefore the calories) will be left in the syringe. Alternatively place the barrel exit uppermost.

Nasojejunal (NJ) feeding

Indications. Nasojejunal feeding is used to maintain full nutrition in small babies who are ill, not receiving sufficient energy or being ventilated or receiving CPAP by mask or nasal tube because there would be a serious risk of aspiration with gastric feeds. Sometimes, also in very small babies, it may offer an alternative to intravenous feeding. Therefore consider it in babies weighing less than 1.25 kg, respiratory distress syndromes, congenital heart disease, septicaemia, surgical conditions, seizure disorders and sedated babies.

The method of passing the tube is as follows:
1 A 125 cm French gauge silicone coated Vygon tube is selected.
2 The baby's nose-to-pubis (gastric mark) and chin-to-heel lengths (jejunal mark) are measured and the tube is marked with pen and black thread respectively at these distances from the tip.
3 The infant is turned onto his right side and the attendant's hand is placed in his left hypochondrium to compress his stomach gently.
4 The nasojejunal tube is passed through the smaller nostril and into the stomach until resistance is felt at the nose-to-pubis length.
5 The tube is aspirated to see whether acid gastric juice or bile is obtained. If bile is obtained the tube is advanced to the chin-to-heel mark over five minutes, aspirating occasionally. Once the tube has reached the stomach it can be flushed with 1 ml of 4% dextrose/0.18% saline to help keep the tube patent and, by stimulating peristalsis, helping the tube to advance further.
6 If bile is not obtained, the infant is left on his right side. Every 15 minutes a further attempt is made to advance the tube.
7 When bile is obtained and the tube is advanced to the second mark, a supine radiograph is taken of the baby's abdomen. Successful passage of the tube is indicated by (a) the tube crossing the mid-line and traversing

the duodenal loop into the proximal jejunum; (b) aspiration of bile; and (c) aspiration of a nasogastric tube (see below) before feeding shows no residual volume present on successive occasions.

8 A little air should then be blown in to clear the end of the tube.

9 Pass a nasogastric tube through the same nostril (so as not to produce respiratory obstruction). This tube should be tied to the nasojejunal tube.

10 A radiograph of the abdomen should be taken after two hours.

It is important that a silicone-coated or silastic tube is used. Polyvinyl-chloride tubes, which were used for this purpose, became rigid within a few days of being passed and led to a real risk of bowel perforation. Silastic or silicone tubes should probably be changed about every 10–14 days.

Most nasojejunal tubes pass within eight hours. The best feed for the baby is expressed breast milk which may conveniently be given by infusion pump. The baby's total fluid requirements should not be given immediately. The feed should be increased by 1–2 ml per hour until the baby's calculated requirement is reached within 12–24 hours.

Precautions. A number of precautions should be taken with the baby being fed nasojejunally:

1 The nasogastric tube should be aspirated between two- and four-hourly. If there is no aspirate, blow 0.5 ml of air to clear the tube, and re-aspirate. If the aspirate is less than 5 ml, replace it down the tube. If it is more than 5 ml, discard it, but remember to include it as fluid deficit. If milk is aspirated through the nasogastric tube check to see if the aspirate is acid in case the nasojejunal tube has slipped into the stomach.

2 The girth should be measured eight-hourly. Mild distension is fairly common. If it becomes progressive or marked, nasojejunal feeding may have to be discontinued for 8–12 hours. An abdominal radiograph may be necessary if there is any suspicion of necrotizing enterocolitis (see p. 296).

3 Record the size and frequency of any vomit and whether the fluid vomited has been replaced. If vomiting is excessive in frequency or quantity the position of the tube should be checked.

4 The frequency and characteristics of the stools passed should be checked and recorded. Test them daily for blood.

5 Blood for electrolytes and calcium should be checked twice weekly, or if the volume of aspirate is particularly large.

Nasojejunal feeding is a useful way of giving feeds to small, sick babies over long periods of time. In most units it is less risky than intravenous alimentation and, if the precautions described above are taken, it is a relatively safe procedure. However, the following complications have been reported: abdominal distension, altered gut flora, gastric reflux, frequent loose stools, disturbance of peristalsis, bowel perforation and peritonitis, necrotizing enterocolitis and intussusception.

Intravenous feeding

Indications

You should balance the possibility of serious complications against the need for improved nutrition to avoid severe weight loss and maintain growth. Parenteral nutrition is most often indicated when oral nutrition cannot be maintained for a prolonged period. Thus common indications are:

1 Extreme prematurity, with failure to establish feeding by means of a nasojejunal tube or when a nasojejunal tube blocks the nostrils of a very small preterm infant and if nasogastric feeding is also contraindicated.
2 Respiratory disorders lasting longer than four or five days.
3 Necrotizing enterocolitis.
4 Prolonged diarrhoea or malabsorption.
5 After serious neonatal surgery, particularly intestinal operations.
6 Seriously ill term or preterm infants.

Before instituting this type of feeding it is essential to ensure the ability to maintain strict aseptic techniques. Skilled nursing care is required, with frequent biochemical monitoring using microtechniques. Any acidosis and dehydration must be corrected. Do not use fat emulsions if there is hyperlipidaemia, impaired bone marrow function or jaundice.

Before starting, remember to explain to the parents what is being done and why.

Required constituents

The solution used must supply adequate energy, water, nitrogen, vitamins, electrolytes and trace metals. The constituents of some of the solutions available are shown in Tables 7.5 to 7.9.

1 *Aminoacid solutions.* Vamin is the solution of choice, as it contains glucose. It may produce acidaemia if given too rapidly.
2 *Fat emulsions.* Intralipid is the solution of choice. It has no serious side-effects, apart from the possibility that it unhooks bilirubin from albumin. It may, however, interfere with blood tests, and the laboratory should be informed when it is being used.
3 *Glucose.* Other possible energy sources such as sorbitol have not been fully evaluated in infants. Fructose should not be used as it can produce profound metabolic acidaemia.
4 *Vitamin supplements.* We use Solivito and Vitlipid Infant (KabiVitrum). Solivito is a yellow mixture of water-soluble vitamins (thiamine, riboflavine, pyridoxine, cyanocobalamin, nicotinamide, folic acid, biotin, pantothenic acid and ascorbic acid) and is added to glucose

Table 7.5 Ped-El: 1 ml contains:

Ca^{2+}	0.15 mmol
Mg^{2+}	25 µmol
Fe^{3+}	0.5 µmol
Zn^{2+}	0.15 µmol
Mn^{2+}	0.25 µmol
Cu^{2+}	0.075 µmol
F^{-}	0.75 µmol
I^{-}	0.01 µmol
$PO_4{}^{3-}$	75 µmol
Cl^{-}	0.35 mmol
K^{+}	<1.0 µmol
Na^{+}	<1.5 mmol

Table 7.6 Solivito: one reconstituted vial contains:

Vitamin B_1	1.2 mg
Vitamin B_2	1.8 mg
Nicotinamide	10 mg
Vitamin B_6	2 mg
Pantothenic acid	10 mg
Vitamin C	30 mg
Biotin	0.3 mg
Folic acid	0.2 mg
Vitamin B_{12}	2 µg

Table 7.7 Vitlipid Infant: one 10 ml vial contains:

Retinol palmitate corresponding to retinol	100 µg (333 IU)
Calciferol	2.5 µg (100 IU)
Phytomenadione	50 µg
Fractionated soya bean oil	100 mg
Fractionated egg phosphatides	12 mg
Glycerol	25 mg
Sodium hydroxide	to pH 8
Water for injection	to 1 ml

solutions (see below). Vitlipid is a white sterile emulsion containing the fat-soluble vitamins A, D_2 (calciferol) and K_1 (phytomenadione).

5 *Electrolyte and trace element supplements* must include sodium, potassium and magnesium. Very preterm babies are usually hypocalcaemic in the first 48 hours of life and therefore need calcium supplements. In practice many ill babies need repeated small blood transfusions which provide sufficient iron, so it is not now necessary to give iron by deep intramuscular injection. Trace metals are most conveniently given as weekly infusions of plasma (10 ml/kg) or as Ped-El which is intended to cover daily losses of electrolytes and trace metals. The Ped-El infusion should not be started before renal function is reasonably established, that

Table 7.8 Vamin-Glucose: 1 litre contains:

Alanine	3.0 g	Proline	8.1 g
Arginine	3.3 g	Serine	7.5 g
Aspartic acid	4.1 g	Threonine	3.0 g
Cysteine/cystine	1.4 g	Tryptophan	1.0 g
Glutamic acid	9.0 g	Tyrosine	0.5 g
Glycine	2.1 g	Valine	4.3 g
Histidine	2.4 g	Glucose	100.0 g
Isoleucine	3.9 g	Sodium	50 mmol
Leucine	5.3 g	Potassium	20 mmol
Lysine	3.9 g	Calcium	2.5 mmol
Methionine	1.9 g	Magnesium	1.5 mmol
Phenylalanine	5.5 g	Chloride	55 mmol

Table 7.9 Intralipid 20%: 1 litre contains:

Fractionated soya bean oil	200g
Fractionated egg lecithin	12 g
Glycerol	25 g
Water for injection	1000 ml
Phosphorus (organic)	15 mmol
Energy	2000 kcal (8.5 MJ)

is after the second day of life. In practice, it is often unnecessary to start vitamin and electrolyte supplements until full-strength intravenous feeding is established, say after the fourth day.

Fluid requirements

In the premature neonate, we give 60 ml/kg on the first day of life, 90 ml/kg on the second day, 120 ml/kg on the third day and 150 ml/kg on the fourth day and subsequently. Increased water loss, for example during phototherapy, means than an extra 30 ml/kg is required for each of these days.

Volumes of each nutrient solution are increased stepwise achieving maximum values after four or five days (Tables 7.10 and 7.11).

In practice four solutions are made up:
1 Vamin with glucose
2 10% dextrose
3 4% dextrose with 0.18% saline
4 20% Intralipid

One and a half times the required quantity is ordered to cover for priming the intravenous sets. The solutions and additives are conveniently made up under full aseptic conditions, ideally in the pharmacy (see Table 7.12).

Table 7.10 Incremental intravenous feeding schedule for low birth weight infants (ml/kg/24 hours)

	Vamin-Glucose	20% Intralipid	10% Dextrose	Energy kJ	cal
Day 1	18	2	30	126	30
Day 2	36	6	60	252	60
Day 3	50	12	105	412	98
Day 4 onwards	50	20	120	504	120

The balance of fluid requirements should be given as 4% dextrose with 0.18% saline.

The amount of 10% glucose may have to be decreased if the renal threshold is exceeded and glycosuria occurs, with the attendant problems of osmolar diuresis and hyperosmolar dehydration. Insulin may be needed to control hyperglycaemia—insulin dose 0.5 units/kg/dose intravenously and repeated three-hourly if necessary, or by continuous infusion of 0.1 unit/kg/hour. Calcium supplements will be required from the outset in most babies; phosphorus should be provided as soon as the serum calcium has stabilized. On day 4, calcium and phosphate supplements can be stopped and replaced with Ped-El at 4 ml/kg/day.

Vitamins may be started from day 4 onwards. Solivito (water-soluble vitamins) at 0.5 ml/kg/day. Vitlipid (fat-soluble vitamins) at 1 ml/kg/day. The total amount of Vitlipid should not exceed 4 ml/24 hours.

Intralipid 20% should be infused at 0.65–0.85 ml/kg/hour. Although it can be started on day 1, it often has to be postponed because of jaundice.

Table 7.11 Composition of fluids for complete intravenous feeding in small infants (values per kg/24 hours).

Solution	Volume (ml)	Energy (kJ)	Nitrogen content (amino acid) (g)	Na$^+$	K$^+$	Cl$^-$	Ca^{2+}	PO$_4^{2+}$	Mg^{2+}
Vamin/glucose	50	32.5	0.47	2.5	1.0	2.5	0.125		0.075
10% glucose	120	40							
4% glucose with 0.18% saline	10	1.5		0.308		0.308			
20% Intralipid	20	40						0.3	
8.7% K$_2$HPO$_4$ (1 mmol/ml)	0.5				0.5			0.5	
10% calcium gluconate	3.5						0.81		
Ped-El	4					2.1	0.9	0.45	0.15
Solivito	0.5								
Vitlipid Infant	1								

Table 7.12 Chart for daily prescription of intravenous alimentation solutions.

Name .... Weight............. Ward.......
　　　　　　　Requirement for Day ....

		kcal
Protein		
Vamin with glucose (providing 650 kcal/1000 ml)	. . .ml	. . .
Vamin N (providing 250 kcal/1000 ml)	. . .ml	. . .
Fat		
Intralipid 20% (providing 2000 kcal/1000 ml)	. . .ml	. . .
Vitlipid infant	. . .ml	
Carbohydrates		
10% Glucose (providing 375 kcal/1000 ml)	. . .ml	. . .
4% Glucose with 0.18% saline (providing 150 kcal/1000 ml)	. . .ml	. . .
Electrolytes and vitamin supplements		
Ped-El	. . .ml	
Solivito	. . .ml	
Calcium gluconate	. . .mmol	
K_2HPO_4	. . .mmol	

Total day's fluid intake of . . .ml/24 hours.

Notes from pharmacy
1 Intralipid with vitamin supplement (when required) will always obviously be supplied separately
2 If incompatibilities between electrolytes exist then the other alimentation would be supplied split between two containers
3 An extra volume will always be provided for manipulation but containers will be labelled to show the day's requirement

Methods of administration

Intravenous fluids may be given:
1 *Into peripheral veins* using short cannulae or butterly needles. Intravenous feeding may be continued in this way for several weeks, but the needle needs resiting at least every 48 hours. The greatest care should be taken to stop infusions promptly if the needle comes out of the vein as the hypertonic solutions cause severe tissue necrosis.
2 *Into a central vein.* This method of infusion has the advantage that the cannula does not need frequent resiting so there is less handling. The major disadvantage is serious infection, often with fungi or unusual bacteria resistant to the common antibiotics, so most units now favour the use of peripheral veins instead. It is important that umbilical vessels are not used because of the risk of portal vein or aortic thrombosis, necrotizing enterocolitis, and septicaemia.

The following techniques can be used for placing a catheter in a large vein or the right atrium:

1   Scrub up and wear mask, gown and gloves.

2   Open pack and assemble equipment: cut-down pack, 19 gauge butterfly needle, 25 gauge butterfly needle, syringe and needle, heparinized saline, chlorhexidine in spirit, pointed scalpel blade, antibiotic spray, sleek and micropore, splint and dressing, silastic catheter, sterile tape measure.

3   Measure the silastic catheter with sterile tape measure and note length.

4   Connect silastic catheter to 25 gauge needle and run through heparinized saline (0.5 u/ml). Thread the plastic needle cover back over the needle to protect it from cutting through the catheter.

5   Suitable veins in order of preference are antecubital, saphenous, scalp, external jugular.

6   Having chosen a vein in advance and prepared the skin, an assistant must apply a suitable tourniquet to fill the vein and hold the baby still.

7   Clean the skin carefully with chlorhexidine in spirit and allow to dry. Measure the distance from the chosen vein to the right atrium.

8   Make a small incision with a scalpel blade 0.5 cm away from the vein to facilitate manoeuvring of the 19 gauge butterfly needle.

9   Cut the tubing off the butterfly needle and pass it under the skin to enter the vein, taking care not to transfix the vein.

10   Blood will flow freely back out of the needle. Stem the flow by pressing with a finger on the skin over the tip of the needle. Thread the silastic catheter through the needle and into the vein.

11   At this stage blood should flow back into the catheter if the end is open.

12   Thread the catheter into the vein until sufficient has been passed to reach the right atrium (the length remaining can be measured with the sterile tape measure).

13   Spray the area with antibiotic spray and fix the catheter to the skin with tape leaving the entry point open. Apply a sterile dressing and splint as required.

14   Do not use the line for feeding until the position has been confirmed radiographically. This is done by injecting 0.7 ml of Conray 280 through the 25 gauge butterfly needle and silastic tube. Take a radiograph of the limb and chest just as the injection finishes.

15   If necessary withdraw the catheter until the position is correct. It is not usually possible at this stage to push the catheter in further, so it is important to be generous in the initial measurements; however, do not be too generous or you may knot the catheter in the right atrium.

Precautions and monitoring

A baby who is being fed intravenously must be carefully observed clinically for signs of complications (see below). The baby's growth should be checked by daily weight, weekly length and head circumference measurements. Fluid intake and output must be recorded scrupulously.

Intravenous drugs should not be infused into the central line. Penicillin, fusidic acid, adrenaline, papaverine and many other drugs are of low pH and may be unstable in infusates.

Urine is tested eight-hourly for sugar, and more frequently in tiny infants, as blood sugar may rise very rapidly. Blood sugar should be estimated (using testing-sticks) at least daily and if there is glycosuria. Electrolytes, calcium and acid–base status are estimated daily initially, but later every second day. Phosphorus and magnesium are estimated once weekly. Amino acids and albumin, total protein, bilirubin and transaminases are measured weekly. Chromatography of urinary amino acids may also be helpful for the detection of hyperaminoacidaemia, including tyrosinaemia which may respond to high doses of vitamin C. A Guthrie test should be performed weekly.

A full blood count, including packed cell volume, should be performed twice a week.

The complete intravenous tubing distal to the Millipore filters is changed every 24 hours.

Intralipid infusion is stopped every day at 5 a.m., so that one may be certain that the fat is being cleared. This is done at 8 a.m. by spinning a sample of blood in a centrifuge and examining the plasma. We do not use Intralipid while the baby is significantly jaundiced.

Bacteriological monitoring demands appropriate cultures from the intravenous site, blood and catheter if it appears infected. Blood culture should be done daily. Also urine for *Candida* is sent routinely. All babies on antibiotics are given oral nystatin in addition.

Complications

1 *Septicaemia* is usually caused by *Candida albicans*, staphylococci, *Pseudomonas aeruginosa*, *E. coli* or diphtheroids. It may follow contamination during insertion of the intravenous line but is more likely to occur if catheters are left in place for prolonged periods.

2 *Hypoglycaemia* can follow abrupt termination of intravenous feeding, possibly due to high levels of endogenous insulin. Therefore, reduce the intravenous input gradually whilst simultaneously increasing oral feeds. Do frequent blood glucose estimations during the transition.

3 *Hyperglycaemia* can cause osmolar diuresis and dehydration.

4 *Heart failure* may occur, since acid solutions contain relatively high sodium concentrations, as do several antibiotics such as ampicillin and cloxacillin.

5 *Hypophosphataemia* may occur even if phosphate is being given in theoretically adequate amounts. This problem may be associated with

Table 7.13 Representation of energy reserves in babies of different birth weights

Weight at birth of neonates	Carbohydrate (g)	Fat (g)	kcal	Reserves (calculated in days)
1000 g	0	10	90	1
2000 g	9	100	936	5
3000 g	34	560	5176	18

haemolytic anaemia, cerebral symptoms, muscle weakness, shock.

6 *Trace metal deficiencies* such as zinc.

7 *Mechanical complications* from catheter malpositioning or dislocation may include thromboembolism, thrombophlebitis, intracardiac curling or knotting of the catheter, arteriovenous fistula or pneumo- , haemo- , or hydrothorax.

Small babies have poor energy reserves (Table 7.13). Despite the risks intravenous alimentation may be life-saving and ensures optimal brain growth during a very important period.

Further Reading

Brooke, O.G. (1982) Low birthweight babies. Nutrition and feeding. *British Journal of Hospital Medicine*, *28*, 462–469.

Davies, D.P. (1978) The first feed of low birthweight infants: changing attitudes in the 20th century. *Archives of Disease in Childhood*, *53*, 187.

DHSS (1974) *Present Day Practice in Infant Feeding*. London: HMSO.

Ebrahim, G.J. (1978) *Breast Feeding: The Biological Option*. London: Macmillan.

Hyde, J. (1978) Transpyloric feeding in the newborn. *British Journal of Hospital Medicine*, *19*, 618.

Jeliffe, D.M. & Jeliffe, E.F.P. (1978) *Human Milk in the Modern World*. Oxford: Oxford University Press.

Lewis, P. (1978) Drugs and Breast Feeding. In *Clinical Pharmacology and Obstetrics*, pp 366–375. Bristol: John Wright.

Mackeith, R. & Wood, C. (1977) *Infant Feeding and Feeding Difficulties*, 5th ed. Edinburgh and London: Churchill Livingstone.

Martin, J. & Monk, J. (1983) Trends in breast feeding. *Maternal and Child Health*, *8*, 72–78.

Panter-Brick, M., Wagget, J. & Dale, G. (1978) *Intravenous Nutrition in Paediatrics*. Kent: Abbott Laboratories.

Shaw, J.C.L. (1973) Parenteral nutrition in the management of sick low birthweight infants. *Pediatric Clinics of North America*, *20*, 333.

Stanway, P & Stanway, A. (1970) *Breast is Best*. London: Pan.

Wharton, B.A. & Berger, H.M. (1976) Problems of childhood. Bottle feeding. *British Medical Journal*, *i*, 1326.

8

Congenital Disorders:
General Principles

Congenital malformations are common (Fig. 8.1) and are a major cause of death in the perinatal period. Some children who survive are left with very little handicap because the abnormality can be corrected, but many children have lasting problems. Congenital abnormalities seem to be a particular problem as a cause of perinatal death in the British Isles because of the high incidence of neural-tube defects. The overall incidence of congenital malformations is about 2%. The number of babies in whom congenital malformation was the primary finding at post mortem examination in the 1958 British Perinatal Mortality Survey was 5.8 per thousand. There appear to be major differences in the incidence of congenital malformations around the world and in different parts of the British Isles. In general, neural-tube defects, including anencephaly and myelomeningocele, are commoner in Western Europe; in the British Isles they are commoner in the North and West. There appear to be more neural-tube defects in cities where there is a large population of Irish descent and this has been shown in some of the large cities of North America. Cleft palate and cleft lip appear to be commoner in East Asia.

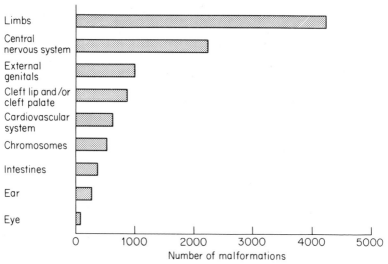

Fig. 8.1 Incidence of congenital malformation (England & Wales 1975). (OPCS)

Many surveys are difficult to interpret because one cannot establish the true incidence of congenital abnormalities at birth. Some abnormalities are immediately obvious, like anencephaly or cleft lip, whereas others are obvious only later, such as a ventricular septal defect which may not be accompanied by a murmur in the newborn period but only several weeks later. The prevalence of congenital abnormalities varies

Table 8.1 Approximate incidence of some important congenital abnormalities and inborn errors with multifactorial inheritance

Abnormality	Incidence (in total births)	Risk to siblings
Myelomeningocele		
South-east England	1/600	1/20 (5%) for either myelomeningocele or anencephaly, i.e. 1 in 40 for each
South Wales/Ireland	1/250	1/18 for either myelomeningocele or anencephaly, i.e. 1 in 35 for each
Anencephaly		
South-east England	1/800	1/20 for either myelomeningocele or anencephaly, i.e. 1 in 40 for each
South Wales/Ireland	1/300	1/18 for either myelomeningocele or anencephaly, i.e. 1 in 35 for each
Cleft lip and palate		
Whites	1/750	1/25 (4%)
Chinese	more common than in caucasian	
Blacks	1/2500	
Cleft palate only	1/2000	1/33 (3%)
Congenital heart disease		
Overall	1/150	
VSD	1/400	1/23 (4.4%)
ASD	1/1000	1/30 (3.3%)
PDA	1/2000	1/70 (1.4%)
Tetralogy of Fallot	1/3300	1/100 (1%)
Congenital dislocation of the hip		
Newborn (dislocatable or dislocated)	1/200	
Established (untreated)	1/1000	If ♀, risk for next ♀ 1/12 (8%), risk for next ♂ 1/60 (1.6%). If ♂, higher risks. Overall about 1/25 (4%)
Talipes equinovarus	1/1000	1/35 (2.9%)
Hirschsprung's disease	1/5000	If brother affected: 1/25 (4%)
		If sister affected: 1/8 (12.5%)
Hypospadias		
Whites	1/120	1/14 (7%)
Blacks	1/500	

Table 8.2 Approximate incidence of some important congenital abnormalities and inborn errors with inheritance by single mutant gene.

Abnormality	Incidence	Incidence of heterozygotes
Autosomal recessive (recurrent risk 1 in 4)		
Cystic fibrosis		
Whites	1/1500 to 1/7200	1/20 (5%)
Black Americans	1/17 000	
Africans	Rare	
Orientals	Rare	
Congenital adrenal hyperplasia		
(21 hydroxylase deficiency)		
Western Europe	1/5000	1/37 (2.7%)
	(50% are salt-losers, c.f. USA 30%; Alaska 100%)	
Autosomal dominant (recurrence risk 1 in 2)		
Achondroplasia	1/10 000	
X-linked recessive (if mother is a carrier 1/2 daughters is a carrier and 1/2 sons has the disease)		
Glucose-6-phosphate dehydrogenase deficiency		
African type		1/4 (25% of black
Black Americans	1/8	American ♀)
Whites	Rare	
Factor VIII deficiency (haemophilia)	1/4000 ♂	

according to the age at which a survey is taken because, for example, dislocation of the hips is relatively common at birth but becomes less common as the child grows older, particularly if treatment is used, and some congenital malformations correct themselves, for example, a ventricular septal defect which may close spontaneously.

The incidence of some important congenital malformations and inborn errors is shown in Tables 8.1 to 8.3. These figures, particularly the risk of a sibling being affected, are useful when counselling for future pregnancies. In most cases, however, it would be wise to seek the advice of a clinical geneticist, especially where there is some complication such as consanguinity, several cases of an abnormality within a family or several abnormalities in one baby.

Table 8.3 Incidence of some common chromosomal abnormalities.

	Incidence in total births (all conceptuses)	Incidence in total liveborn births	Risk if sibling affected (apparently normal parents)
Down's syndrome (trisomy 21) Overall	1/300	1/700	1/65
Regular (non-disjunction) depends on mother's age:			
<25 years	?	1/2000	1/90
25–34 years	?1/100	1/1300	1/50
35–44 years	?1/25	1/250	1/90
45 years +	?1/6	1/80	?
D/G translocation	?	about 4% of all babies with Down's syndrome	1/5 if maternal translocation
			1/20 if paternal translocation
Trisomy-18 (Trisomy E, Edwards' syndrome)	?1/2000	1/3000 increases with advancing maternal age	
Trisomy-13 (Trisomy D, Patau's syndrome)	?1/3000	1/5000 increases with advancing maternal age	low
Turner syndrome (females)	?1/500	1/10 000	Not increased

Aetiology

A few congenital abnormalities have a well-known aetiology:

Congenital rubella, particularly in the first trimester of pregnancy, usually produces abnormalities. The babies have microcephaly, retinal pigmentation, patent ductus arteriosus or other congenital heart anomalies, mental handicap and deafness and are small-for-dates at birth. It is interesting that the incidence of congenital abnormalities is less if the virus invades the fetus later in pregnancy.

A large dose of *radiation* in mid-trimester is well known to produce severe damage to the brain. Microcephaly was seen in the fetuses in the survivors of radiation from atomic bombs in Japan in 1945.

Some *drugs* produce congenital abnormalities but the list is relatively short. The most famous and disastrous example is thalidomide, which produced congenital limb deformities in the babies of women who took this sleeping tablet around 1960 (see Fig. 2.9). Other drugs which are known to cause congenital abnormalities are listed in Chapter 2. Thalidomide produced obvious and unusual abnormalities but it can be very difficult to know whether a drug causes abnormalities because the number produced could be very small and the abnormality is otherwise common. Thus very careful studies are needed before a drug can be used widely in pregnancy.

Diabetes mellitus appears to produce a higher incidence of congenital abnormality; several surveys have suggested 6% rather than 2% for the general population. It is not clear whether the illness in the mother produces the abnormalities or whether the cause is among the drugs she is using, such as insulin. It is also not yet clear whether careful control of diabetes very early in pregnancy would reduce the incidence of congenital malformations.

Some abnormalities appear to be commoner in one *social class* rather than another. The most well known example is anencephaly, which is commoner in social class V than in social class I.

A *mutant gene* can produce a congenital abnormality, such as achondroplasia, extra fingers or some types of hydrocephalus. Although single gene abnormalities such as these examples do occur, it is probable that many congenital abnormalities are produced by a number of genes acting together; this is polygenic inheritance. It is thought to be true of neural-tube defects.

There are many conditions with a rather more doubtful aetiology. Women anaesthetists are said to have babies with a higher incidence of congenital anomalies and this may be related to the anaesthetic gases which they accidentally inhale during induction of anaesthesia. Many hypotheses have been made about items of diet such as blighted potatoes, corned beef or even tea as an aetiological factor of neural-tube defects, but these have been disproved. Vitamin A depletion is, at present, being investigated. It is possible that some environmental factors such as an item of diet could act together with genetic factors. Vitamin supplements before conception probably reduce the incidence of neural tube defects.

Classification

There are many ways of classifying congenital malformations; the most usual is according to the part of the body where the anomaly occurs. A useful scheme for those looking after newborn babies is to divide the lesions into those which need immediate treatment, usually meaning an urgent referral to a neonatal surgical unit, and those requiring early treatment within the first week of life, compared with those where treatment can be left for some time or which may need no treatment at all.

Problems requiring immediate treatment

1 *Tracheo-oesophageal fistula with or without oesophageal atresia*. It is essential to avoid feeding the baby, who must be transferred rapidly to a surgical centre for closure of the fistula and repair of the oesophagus. The oesophagus should be drained during transfer. The operation is often done within the first 24 hours.

2 *Congenitial diaphragmatic hernia* produces a characteristic syndrome of cyanosis and dextrocardia immediately after birth. It requires immediate surgical attention; unfortunately, the results are often poor because of pulmonary hypoplasia underneath the herniated gut in the thorax (see p. 57).

3 *Pierre Robin anomaly*. Affected babies can easily die from asphyxia because the tongue falls back into the pharynx. The baby needs careful nursing in the prone position.

4 *Choanal atresia*. When this is complete and bilateral, the baby cannot breathe satisfactorily and an oral airway should be passed until an opening can be made in the nose (see p. 60).

5 *Gastroschisis and exomphalos* need urgent referral (see p. 60).

6 *Spina bifida*. A decision should have been made within 24 hours whether or not a surgeon is to be consulted about closing the lesion. A baby with meningocele should be referred immediately; in a baby with myelomeningocele, there should be careful discussion with the parents about possible treatment (see p. 186).

7 *Talipes equinovarus*. If the feet are not reducible, they require early strapping which, if started at birth, is thought to improve the prognosis (see p. 192).

Lesions requiring early treatment (within the first week)

1 *Imperforate anus*. Some would include this in the urgent group, but in fact one often waits for one to two days to allow air to reach the lower end of the rectum so that a radiograph can be taken to estimate the length of the atresia. Some babies have only a covered anus with a flap of skin over the anus, but even here operation is often delayed for one to two days.

2 *Abnormal external genitalia*. Only rarely is there a reason for operating on these babies but investigations should be started within the first few days and careful discussions held with the parents.

3 *Cleft palate or lip*. In some units the lip is closed during the first week and a dental prosthesis is fitted into the cleft.

4 *Teeth*. A natal tooth can often cause an ulcer on the tongue and therefore should be removed as soon as the baby is reasonably well.

5 *Congenital adrenal hyperplasia* in a girl can usually be suspected at birth but may present more difficulties in a boy. Investigations and treatment should be started in the first three to four days.

6 *Intestinal obstruction*. The higher the obstruction, the more likely that bilious vomiting will occur, unless the atresia is in the first part of the duodenum; the lower the obstruction the more likely that distension will occur. Any baby with definite intestinal obstruction should be referred for treatment at once. In some cases it is now possible to make the diagnosis even before birth by the use of ultrasound.

Lesions requiring treatment later or not at all

There are many congenital abnormalities that require very little attention. Some of those that will need attention but only after the first week, include:

1 *Cleft lip*, which is often closed within the first six months. Some surgeons will repair it even within the first few weeks.

2 *Hydrocephalus*. Where this is present at birth, the prognosis is often poor and no operation is done but hydrocephalus that develops in the first few weeks needs a shunt.

3 *Hypospadias*.

4 *Urethral valves* causing urinary obstruction in boys.

5 *Birth marks*

Most babies with a congenital malformation can be nursed at their mother's bedside. We think it is very important that a mother who gives birth to a baby with a congenital abnormality should have every opportunity to get to know her baby and learn how to look after him. The family is then in a better position to decide whether they will be able to cope with the baby at home. We separate mother and baby only if there is an abnormality that requires surgical or intensive care, in particular a condition where the baby's airway may suddenly become obstructed. It is important not to cause too much parental anxiety in cases of normal variations.

Surgery

Surgery on the newborn baby is technically extremely demanding, and the paediatric care must also be highly skilled. The baby is vulnerable to heat loss and, because of the baby's small blood volume, measurement of blood loss and total fluid and electrolyte replacement must be scrupulous. The baby is also at risk of picking up infection.

Many babies will require transfer to a regional neonatal surgical unit for operation. The greatest risks to such a baby are aspiration pneumonia and hypothermia. It is usually advisable to take time at the referring hospital to stabilize the baby by correcting hypoxaemia, acidosis or hypothermia. No baby requiring surgery should be transferred without a nasogastric tube in situ and without a normal body temperature (although the massive heat loss from a large gastroschisis makes the latter impossible—here, and with a diaphragmatic hernia, urgent transfer may be preferable).

Frequent oral and pharyngeal suction will be necessary. Vitamin K should be given (see below). Ensure that a specimen of maternal blood and a parental consent form accompany the baby. There must be a full referral letter with details of the obstetric history, delivery, birth weight and gestational age, nature and sequence of symptoms (When was meconium first passed? Has the vomitus contained bile?), family and social background, drugs given and investigations performed with their results.

The general principles of management prior to surgery involve two main areas:

(a) Explain to the parents what is involved. Tell them why the operation is necessary, what the risks are and what the prognosis is.

(b) Anticipate and prevent predictable complications. In particular:

1 Ensure that the baby's airway is clear and that he is adequately oxygenated.

2 Have cross-matched blood available by the time the baby goes to theatre. The newborn baby's blood volume is only 80 ml/kg (100 ml/kg in the preterm baby). It is easy, therefore, to underestimate the need for replacement.

3 Reduce the risk of bleeding from hypoprothrombinaemia by giving vitamin K (Phytomenadione): 0.5 mg should be given to all babies before operation.

4 Pay careful attention to reducing heat loss and keeping the room warm (see Chapter 5).

5 Replace fluid and electrolyte losses correctly. The baby's maintenance requirements are 60–80 ml/kg on Day 1, 80–100 ml/kg on Day 2 and 100–120 ml/kg on Day 3. About two-thirds of these totals should be given during the first 24 hours after operation. The baby will need 3 mmol/kg/day of sodium and 2 mmol/kg/day of potassium. Energy requirements (120 kcal/kg daily or more; about 450 kJ) are best given as 10% dextrose. Abnormal fluid losses (e.g. aspirate) will need to be added to these basic requirements when the total fluid volume required is calculated. If the bowels are not working (e.g. following a gastrointestinal resection), the fluid must be given intravenously. Once there is normal gastrointestinal function, fluid may be introduced orally starting with

30 ml/kg on Day 1 and increasing by 30 ml/kg per day until a total of 150 ml/kg/day is reached on Day 5. 150 ml of milk contains 110–120 kcal (about 450 kJ). The intravenous fluid should be reduced by an equivalent amount as the oral feed is increased.

6 Keep a careful watch for the metabolic abnormalities such as hypoglycaemia, hypocalcaemia, or acidosis. The specific treatment for each is discussed elsewhere.

7 Prevent infection first by aseptic theatre technique and postoperative care and secondly with early investigation by swabbing, blood culture and suprapubic aspiration of urine, and the use of appropriate antibiotics if there is any deterioration in the baby's condition.

Many young doctors and nurses find the management of families of infants with congenital abnormalities difficult. Some ways of helping the staff to help these families are described in Chapter 18.

Further Reading

Blyth, H. & Carter, C.O. (1969) *A Guide to Genetic Prognosis in Paediatrics.* London: Heinemann Medical.

Clayton, B. (1976) Screening and management of infants with amino acid disorders. In *Recent Advances in Paediatrics*, 5, ed. D. Hull, Edinburgh and London: Churchill Livingstone.

Fraser, G. & Mayo, O. (1975) *Textbook of Human Genetics.* Oxford: Blackwell Scientific.

Harper, P.S. (1984) Carrier detection in genetic disorders. In *Recent Advances in Paediatrics*, pp 1–16 ed. Meadow, R. Edinburgh: Churchill Livingstone.

Langman, J. (1969) *Medical Embryology*, 2nd ed. Baltimore: Williams and Wilkins.

Lorber, J. (1971) Results of treatment of meningomyelocele. *Developmental Medicine and Child Neurology*, *13*, 279.

McKusick, V.A. (1975) *Mendelian Inheritance in Man*, 5th ed. Baltimore: Johns Hopkins University Press.

Nixon, H.H. (1978) *Surgical Conditions in Paediatrics.* London: Butterworths.

Pembrey, M. (1984) The new genetics and prevention of disease. In *Recent Advances in Paediatrics*, pp 17–34, ed. Meadow, R. Edinburgh: Churchill Livingstone.

Phelan, P.D. (1984) Screening for cystic fibrosis. In *Recent Advances in Paediatrics*, pp 103–120, ed. Meadow, R. Edinburgh: Churchill Livingstone.

Rickham, I.P., Lister, J. & Irving, I.M. (1978) *Neonatal Surgery*, 2nd ed. London: Butterworths.

Smith, D.W. (1982) *Recognisable Patterns of Human Malformation*, 3rd ed. Philadelphia: W.B. Saunders.

Solomon, L.M. & Esterly, N.B. (1973) *Neonatal Dermatology*, Philadelphia: W.B. Saunders.

Weatherall, J. (1982) A review of some effects of recent medical practices in reducing the numbers of children born with congenital abnormalities. *Health Trends*, *14*, 85–88.

9

Congenital Disorders: Specific Conditions

Some individual congenital abnormalities are now discussed (for congenital heart disease see Chapter 10). Many of them require surgical intervention.

Alimentary System

Cleft lip and palate

Cleft lip, whether unilateral (Fig. 9.1) or bilateral (Fig. 9.2), is among the

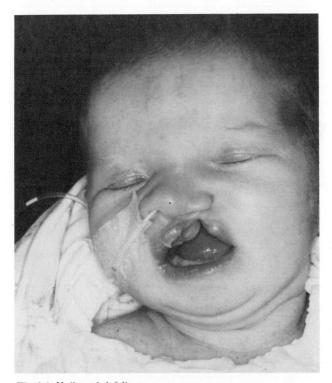

Fig. 9.1 Unilateral cleft lip

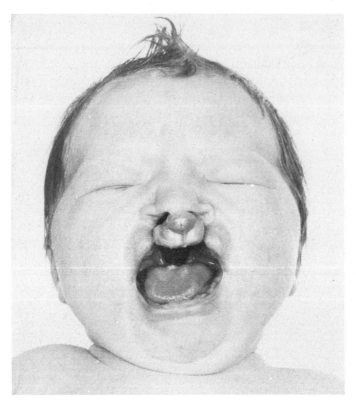

Fig. 9.2 Bilateral cleft lip and palate

most immediately obvious and distressing abnormalities to the new mother. It may occur on its own or associated with cleft palate. Cleft palate may itself occur alone and its detection at the first postnatal check is extremely important. The embryological development of the nose and mouth region is complex and specific causes for such defects are seldom present. Genetic factors clearly play a part; these defects are commoner in some families, and there is an increased risk of producing subsequent affected babies. Associated malformations are not uncommon, sometimes as part of a chromosomal disorder such as Patau's syndrome (trisomy D, see below).

Cleft lip, with or without cleft palate, occurs about once in every thousand births. Cleft palate alone occurs about once in 2000 births. The chance of having another baby with cleft lip is about 1 in 25 if both parents are normal, but 1 in 10 if one parent has a cleft lip. The chance of an affected parent having an affected child is about 1 in 50. With isolated cleft palate the recurrence risk is about 1 in 30 with normal parents, but as high as 1 in 6 if both parent and older child are affected (see Chapter 8). It is now thought that there is no evidence that barbiturates taken in the first trimester of pregnancy are associated with cleft palate.

Unilateral or bilateral cleft lip virtually never produces any feeding problems. It is very reassuring to the mother for the paediatric department to have photographs of previous babies, before and after surgical correction, so that the worried parents may see the excellent results that modern plastic surgery can produce. The timing of surgery is a matter for the individual surgeon. Bilateral defects are usually closed one side at a time.

The management of cleft palate is more difficult. Many mothers, given the proper encouragement, are able to breast feed, but some babies with large defects are unable to suck as they cannot create the negative pressure necessary because of the palatal defect. There is in addition an increased risk of aspiration of feeds. The baby must then be taught to swallow feeds delivered to the back of the tongue. This may be done either by bottle feeding with a specially large hole in the teat or by cup-and-spoon feeding.

Subsequent management requires a multidisciplinary approach. A plastic surgeon repairs the defect; this is often done at about the age of one year. An orthodontist makes sure that the alveolar arch develops normally with correct alignment of teeth; some recommend fitting dental plates soon after birth to stimulate forward growth of the upper jaw.

A speech therapist corrects defective speech which results from the inability to prevent air from escaping into the nose during phonation. An ENT surgeon will be required because of recurrent and frequent attacks of otitis media; these may be associated with high-frequency deafness. Adenoids should only very rarely be removed, as they help ensure an airtight fit between the posterior pharynx and palate. The paediatrician is responsible for explaining to the parents what is involved and coordinating the efforts of the other specialist members of the team. The parents may need considerable support throughout childhood.

Congenital teeth

Normally the first dentition begin to erupt at about the age of six months. From time to time, a baby has one or more lower incisors present at birth (Fig. 9.3). They are removed to prevent their being aspirated into the lungs or ulcerating the tongue.

Pierre Robin anomaly

This condition is discussed below under Respiratory system (p. 179)

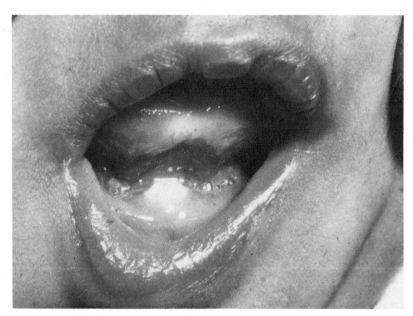

Fig. 9.3 Congenital teeth

Neonatal intestinal obstruction

There may be a block anywhere in the baby's bowel, from oesophagus to anus. Early diagnosis is important. The problem is best considered according to the region affected.

Oesophageal atresia

Babies with this abnormality commonly have an oesophagus with a blind end, usually with a fistula between the upper trachea and lower oesophagus. A number of variations may occur, however (Fig. 9.4).

It is important that the diagnosis is made before the first feed. If not, the feed will cause acute choking, coughing and cyanosis. If the diagnosis is still not made, dehydration, electrolyte disturbances and starvation will follow. Once lung complications have occurred, the baby's prognosis is much poorer and surgery is less successful.

Three clues should lead to the diagnosis before the first feed:
1 Maternal polyhydramnios, which is present in two-thirds of cases, sometimes predisposing to preterm delivery.
2 Noisy breathing after birth with bubbly or frothy mucus regurgitating from the mouth.
3 Frequent cyanotic attacks during the early minutes and hours of life.

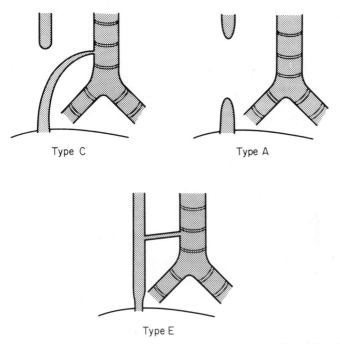

Type C

Type A

Type E

Fig. 9.4 Types of oesophageal atresia and tracheo-oesophageal fistula. Type C (85%): blind-ending upper oesophagus with fistula from trachea to lower oesophagus. Type A (9%): no fistula. Type E (4%): fistula with atresia. Types B and D together account for less than 2% of cases

If the diagnosis is suspected, it can be confirmed by passing a thick catheter down the oesophagus. It is important not to push too hard and also to use a catheter which is not so thin that it coils up, giving the erroneous impression that the tube has passed further than it has. In practice a size 12 French gauge catheter is best. In oesophageal atresia it will not pass more than 5–10 cm from the mouth. A radiograph will confirm that the tip is in the upper oesophagus. Confirmation may also be obtained by aspiration; the contents of the pouch contain no acid. Alternatively, a little air can be blown down the tube, and no sounds will be heard in the abdomen. The use of radio-opaque material should be avoided because of the risk of aspiration of oily material into the lungs with subsequent pneumonia.

If one congenital abnormality has been demonstrated, others are more likely to be present. In the case of oesophageal atresia associated abnormalities include those of the heart, lower bowel and skeleton.

Before surgery, the upper oesophageal segment should be sucked out regularly to prevent aspiration into the lungs; this is particularly important during transfer of the baby to a surgical unit. Antibiotic cover should be given. Full-term babies in whom the diagnosis is made early often have an operation within 24 hours. Usually the fistula is closed through a right thoracotomy and in the majority of cases an end-to-end anastomosis of the two oesophageal segments can be made. Postoperative feeding is initially by gastrostomy. Preterm babies, or those diagnosed late and showing lung complications, may need to be fed intravenously or by gastrostomy before surgery is feasible. The mortality among full-term babies diagnosed before the first feed is less than 2%; however, the overall survival rate is only 85%. This emphasizes the importance of early diagnosis before the first feed is given and also the worse prognosis in preterm babies.

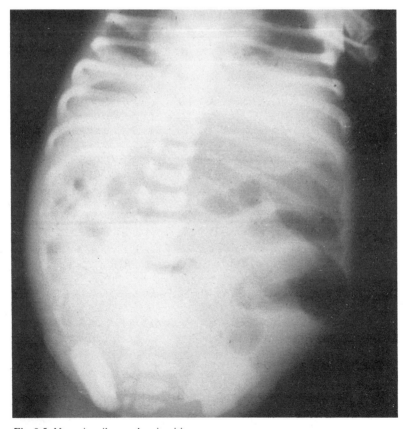

Fig. 9.5 Meconium ileus and peritonitis

Small and large bowel obstruction

These lesions may be considered in two groups—high and low obstruction—as the timing of onset of signs may differ in the two groups (see below). The obstruction may be within the lumen of the bowel (e.g. meconium ileus from cystic fibrosis) (Fig. 9.5), an abnormality of the bowel wall (e.g. duodenal atresia) or an extrinsic lesion constricting the bowel (e.g. peritoneal bands).

An early diagnosis is possible on the basis of findings on examination at birth or subsequently, and certain pointers in the maternal or family history. A maternal history of polyhydramnios suggests the possibility of intestinal obstruction; upper bowel distension in utero can even be seen by ultrasound. Ganglion-blocking agents or other drugs such as methyldopa given to the mother to treat hypertension cross the placenta and may cause paralytic ileus in the baby. A family history of gastrointestinal abnormalities or cystic fibrosis may be relevant.

Early symptoms and signs are:
1 *Vomiting.* Depending on the level of lesion, the vomitus may or may not contain bile. Bile is present if the obstruction is below the bile ducts
2 *Delayed or absent passage of meconium* (particularly in low lesions)
3 *Abdominal distension* (most noticeable with low lesions)
4 *Respiratory distress* following aspiration into the lungs (particularly with high lesions)
5 *Dehydration* with acid–base or electrolyte disturbances
6 *Septicaemia*; this may complicate distension and bowel perforation.
As the obstruction has often been present for some time by the time of birth, bowel perforation may well have taken place in utero. The most useful investigation is a plain erect abdominal radiograph. This may show either fluid levels due to obstruction or air under the diaphragm if perforation has taken place. The presence of grey, inspissated meconium containing air bubbles indicates the presence of meconium ileus (Fig. 9.5). Intraperitoneal calcification indicates previous perforation and meconium peritonitis.

In *duodenal atresia* the plain abdominal radiograph is characteristic, with a double bubble of gas visible in stomach and dilated duodenum but no air below this level (Fig. 9.6).

Imperforate anus (Fig. 9.7) must always be specifically excluded by testing the patency of the anus as part of the routine examination of every newborn baby. Thus delayed diagnosis should not occur. Should this happen, the baby will present with bile-stained vomiting and abdominal distension. Meconium is not passed. Occasionally the presence of a rectovaginal or rectourethral fistula causes meconium to be passed from vagina or urethra. Sometimes the anus is covered by a triangle of skin which allows meconium to be passed.

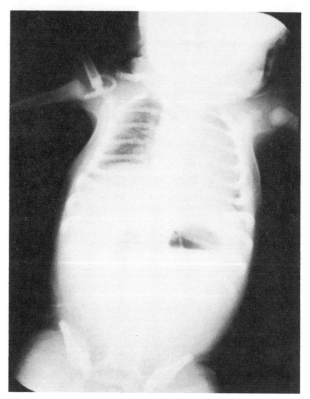

Fig. 9.6 Duodenal atresia

In all these conditions the key to a successful outcome is to make the diagnosis early. Babies who develop electrolyte abnormalities or an aspiration pneumonia are much less likely to survive. In the case of imperforate anus, it is useful to know the total length of terminal bowel which is absent. To demonstrate this, time must be allowed for air to reach the lower bowel (usually 24–48 hours). The infant is then suspended head downwards for several minutes and a lead marker (e.g. a coin) is placed on the perineum. A plain radiograph shows gas in the blind rectal pouch and the distance between the gas and the anal skin can be estimated. The scale of the operation will, of course, depend on the length of the gap demonstrated.

In *Hirschsprung's disease* the defect is a congenital absence of ganglion cells of the myenteric parasympathetic nerve plexus of Auerbach from a segment of colon. This extends from the internal anal sphincter for a variable distance up through the rectum and often lower colon. This aganglionic segment is narrow, but there is great hypertrophy and

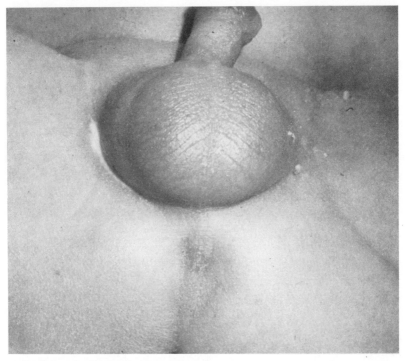

Fig. 9.7 Imperforate anus

distension of the normal colon above it. On rectal examination a tight sphincter is often found, but this is not an infallible sign. Passage of the finger often produces a rush of faeces and gas. The diagnosis is confirmed by rectal biopsy and balloon studies which show that the anal sphincter will not relax normally. With modern surgery these infants usually do extremely well, but a colostomy is often required to allow the abdominal distension to subside before a definitive procedure is undertaken. The most serious postoperative complications are necrotizing enterocolitis and incontinence of faeces. The characteristic presentation is delay in the first passage of meconium; a rectal examination should be done in any baby who has not passed meconium by 24 hours of age.

Diaphragmatic hernia

This condition is discussed in Chapter 3 (p. 57).

Exomphalos

This is a rare abnormality involving herniation of bowel and other viscera

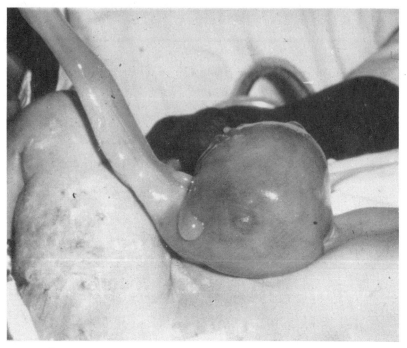

Fig. 9.8 Exomphalos

into the base of the umbilicus (Fig. 9.8). It is covered by fused layers of amnion and peritoneum, not skin. Rupture and evisceration can occur after birth with secondary infection. Associated abnormalities are present in three-quarters of the affected babies. Watch out for Beckwith's syndrome: exomphalos, large tongue and internal organs, plus severe hypoglycaemia (1 in 7 affected). Complete repair is possible when there is a small defect in an otherwise healthy baby. Larger lesions may be covered by skin to provide protection and definitive repair deferred until the peritoneal cavity is larger (by about one year of age). In the most unfavourable cases, painting the sac with 2% aqueous mercurochrome provides temporary protection by epithelialization. Alternatively a tent of inert material may be sewn over the lesion. There is a considerable mortality in those babies most severely affected. (For early management see Chapter 3.)

It is common to see babies of African descent with umbilical hernias, sometimes containing gut or omentum. The sac is completely covered by skin. No treatment is required because the hernias disappear spontaneously by about three to five years of age.

Gastroschisis

Gastroschisis is antenatal evisceration of abdominal contents through a defect to one side of a normally inserted umbilical cord. There is no covering membrane sac and the defect is usually small. Associated anomalies are much less frequent than with exomphalos, but resultant malrotation and intestinal atresia are common. Gastroschisis is particularly common among preterm babies, but in the best hands about three out of four babies survive surgical repair. The acute management of the condition in the labour ward is described in Chapter 3.

Respiratory system

Choanal atresia

This condition is discussed in Chapter 3.

Congenital laryngeal stridor

Some babies have a low-pitched stridor on inspiration. The common variety from a soft collapsing larynx is not usually noticed until after the first week of life. Many babies have a short-lived stridor after endotracheal intubation. Since there are some important, though rare, causes of stridor, such as laryngeal webs, polyps or haemangioma, direct laryngoscopy should be performed for any persistent stridor.

Pierre Robin anomaly

This consists of (Fig. 9.9):
1 Small lower jaw (micrognathia).
2 Midline cleft palate without cleft lip.
3 Glossoptosis (an abnormal attachment of the genioglossi muscles allows the normally sized tongue to fall back and block the airway, especially during feeding).

It is likely that the primary abnormality is hypoplasia of the mandibular area before the ninth week of intrauterine life. This allows the tongue to be pushed backwards and prevents the normal closure of the posterior palate.

Cyanotic and choking episodes with the risk of bronchopneumonia are prevented by nursing these babies in a prone position. The baby may be suspended using tube gauze stuck to the head. Anterior fixation of the tongue surgically may sometimes be necessary. Alternatively, in some centres a dental prosthesis is used to fill in the cleft and prevent the tongue falling into the nasopharynx. The Pierre Robin anomaly is most

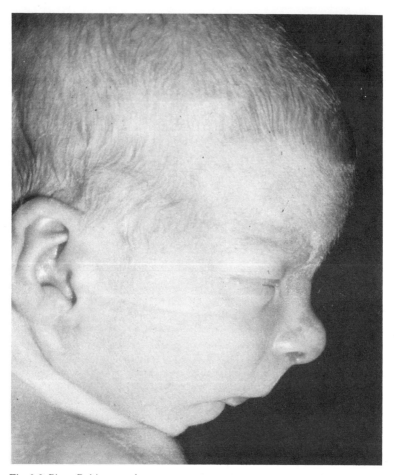

Fig. 9.9 Pierre Robin anomaly

commonly seen in otherwise normal babies. If they survive the neonatal period without episodes of hypoxia and aspiration pneumonia, the prognosis is extremely good. The retrognathia improves with time. Occasionally the anomaly is but one feature in a syndrome of multiple defects, for example, trisomy 18 (see below).

Congenital lobar emphysema

This results from a congenital abnormality of bronchial cartilage causing bronchomalacia and therefore air-trapping in the affected lobe (usually left upper lobe). The obstructive emphysema present with rapid breathing, cough, stridor, and shortness of breath during feeds. Sometimes

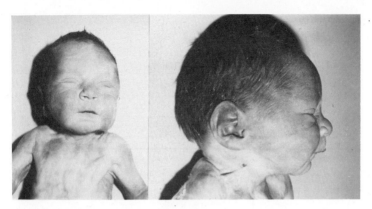

Fig. 9.10 Potter's syndrome (renal agenesis)

the significance of these symptoms is not realized for many weeks or even months. They may be attributed to recurrent chest infections if a careful history is not taken. On chest radiography there is distension of the affected lobe, with herniation across the midline and compression of remaining lung tissue. Treatment is by resection of the affected lobe.

Potter's syndrome

This name is used for babies whose mothers had oligohydramnios, usually because the baby had passed very little urine in utero, for example due to renal agenesis. There is amnion nodosum, small nodules of desquamated skin on the fetal surface of the placenta. The baby has a squashed face (Fig. 9.10) with a flattened nose and grooves below the eyes. Other compression effects are seen, such as talipes equinovarus and dislocation of the hips. The baby often dies immediately after birth because the lungs do not grow normally in such fetuses (pulmonary hypoplasia) and resuscitation is therefore impossible.

Central Nervous System

Neural tube defects

The nervous tissue in the embryo forms as a neural plate and then a tube which develops from the head downwards and is complete by the fourth week of intrauterine life (Fig. 9.11). The spinal cord is derived from the surface of the embryo (neuroectoderm). The meninges and vertebral column come from tissue below the surface (mesenchyme).

A bifid lumbosacral vertebra occurs in 10% of the normal population. There is no underlying abnormality of meninges or spinal cord and the

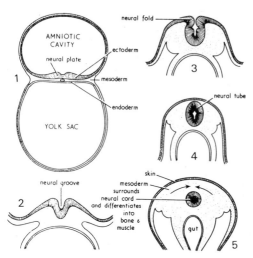

Fig. 9.11 Normal development of the spinal cord. From S. Wallis & D. Harvey (1979) *Nursing Times*, by permission of the authors and editor

condition is known as spina bifida occulta. Its presence may be marked by an overlying patch of hair, lipoma, naevus, dermal sinus or other abnormality, usually minor.

In contrast, spina bifida cystica occurs when there is protrusion and dysplasia of the meninges only (meningocele) (6%) or of meninges and spinal cord (myelomeningocele) (94%). These are much more serious conditions and are colloquially referred to as spina bifida (Fig. 9.12). A myelomeningocele is usually accompanied by neurological signs.

The incidence of the condition varies from country to country and regionally within countries (see also Chapter 8). For example, it is much commoner in Ireland and Wales than in south-east England. Both genetic and environmental factors are thought to play a part in its aetiology. The overall incidence in the UK is about 2 per 1000 live births. The risk increases when there is a family history of babies born with neural tube defects. When the parents have already had a child with a neural defect they have about a 1 in 20 chance of having another such baby and of these approximately half will have anencephaly and half spina bifida. The risk is higher in some areas. When the parents have had two affected children the risk is 1 in 8.

The defect is always in the midline. It may be anywhere from the head (encephalocele) to the sacrum (Fig. 9.13). Defects are commonest in the lumbosacral region. This is probably because it is this area which, embryologically, is the last to form the neural tube by fusion of the neural plate. A sac of variable size is then seen on the baby's back (Fig. 9.14). It is covered by a thin neuroepithelium (arachnoid membrane) rather than

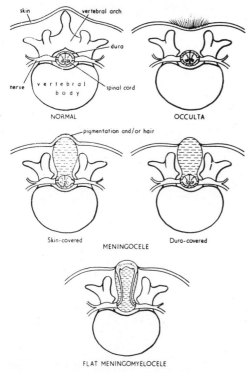

Fig. 9.12 Various forms of spina bifida. From S. Wallis & D. Harvey (1979) *Nursing Times*, by permission of the authors and editor

skin, with neural tissue on the surface. Many myelomeningoceles do not have a sac at all, so the spinal cord is exposed and only about 15% of spina bifida are closed by a membrane.

The natural history of such lesions is that the sac becomes infected within a few days or months of birth with meningitis and eventual death. Thus until about 25 years ago such lesions were almost always fatal. Only about 5% survived the first year, the lesion becoming covered by skin within the first few months. During the 1960s it was found that early closure of the defect surgically (within 24 hours of birth) would prevent the onset of meningitis and death.

Many of these surgically treated infants have considerable further problems:

1 there is often extensive flaccid paralysis, depending on the level of the lesion, with associated sensory loss. Such children are therefore often confined to wheelchairs.

2 There is commonly dribbling incontinence of urine without normal

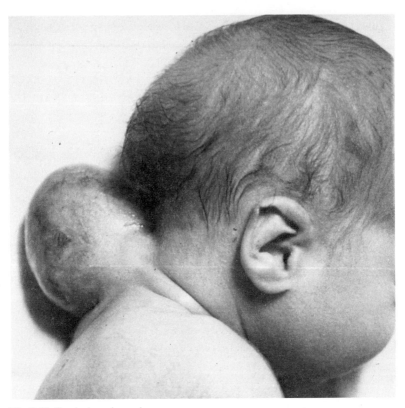

Fig. 9.13 Cervical meningocele

control due to loss of parasympathetic outflow to the bladder. The anal sphincters are similarly affected with resulting incontinence of faeces. There is a high incidence of ureteric reflex and ascending urinary tract infection with renal damage and eventual renal failure. To prevent this, many urological operations are necessary.

3 Hydrocephalus is commonly associated; it is due to the so-called Arnold–Chiari malformation which is a protrusion of the cerebellum through the foramen magnum at the base of the skull (Fig. 9.15). This causes obstruction to the downward flow of cerebrospinal fluid (CSF) so that its pressure rises within the head. To allow CSF to circulate freely, shunt operations were devised but they have a significant morbidity and mortality. Severe mental handicap is often present in addition.

4 Orthopaedic deformities, for example kyphoscoliosis, congenital dislocation of the hips and talipes equinovarus (Fig. 9.14), are common in this condition and may require many operations for their correction.

It is felt by many paediatricians that the quality of life enjoyed by many

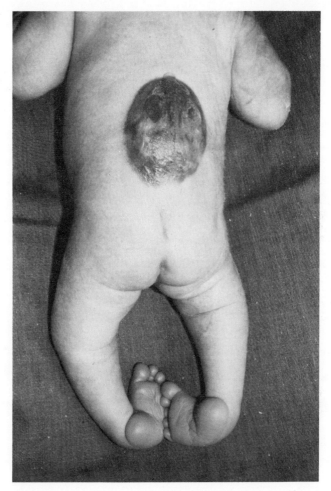

Fig. 9.14 Myelomeningocele with bilateral severe talipes

of these unfortunate children is extremely poor. For this reason the policy of automatic operation was reviewed.

A decision should be made at birth about the baby's prognosis. Criteria, following the work of Lorber in Sheffield, have now been developed to enable a more rational decision to be made. Meningocele has a very good prognosis. The presence of any of the following adverse factors increases the chance of early death or poor quality of life and would tend to make the paediatrician advise against surgery for a myelomeningocele:

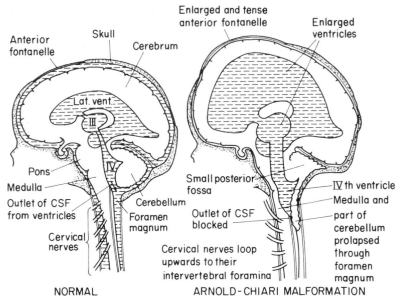

Fig. 9.15 Normal circulation of the cerebrospinal fluid and the development of hydrocephalus following obstruction of the circulation by the Arnold–Chiari malformation. From S. Wallis & D. Harvey (1979) *Nursing Times*, by permission of the authors and editor

1 flaccid paralysis of the lower limbs, often with urinary incontinence with dribbling and a patulous anus
2 hydrocephalus (defined as 2 cm above the 90th centile for the baby's gestational age)
3 other congenital abnormalities
4 kyphosis
5 large lesions (more than 5 cm in diameter)
6 high lesions (thoracolumbar or higher)
7 meningitis.
   It now seems that a very early decision regarding the need for surgery may not be as crucial as used to be thought. When a decision is made that immediate surgery is not indicated, it is usual to avoid other active treatment such as antibiotics. Such babies should be kept warm, fed and free from pain but they will probably die within days or weeks. It is kindest to feed the baby on demand and sedate him if he is uncomfortable. Strong analgesia may be required if the spinal cord is drying out. Some babies do not die; this must be explained to the parents before any decision is made. The baby may even need operation later, either to correct a very ugly hydrocephalus or to make nursing easier by closing the back.

The parents must be fully informed about the prognosis for their baby. It seems wrong, however, to expect them to make a decision for or against surgery. This is made by the paediatrician in consultation with the parents. He should give his decision which they are free to accept or reject, but in their emotional state of grief and anxiety the onus of treating or not treating should not be placed on their shoulders. In this way we hope the strength of parental guilt feelings when the baby does die may be much reduced.

Those children who are operated on will require prolonged follow-up by the paediatrician, neurosurgeon, urologist, orthopaedic surgeon and psychiatrist acting as a team.

It is likely that such agonizing decisions will have to be made less commonly in the future. Many cases of spina bifida can now be prevented provided the parents are willing to accept termination of pregnancy. The amniotic fluid surrounding babies with open spina bifida or anencephaly contains raised concentrations of alpha-fetoprotein (AFP). Clearly not every pregnant mother should have an amniocentesis, since the procedure carries at least a 1% risk of subsequent abortion and a small increased risk of respiratory distress and congenital abnormalities (congenital dislocation of the hips or talipes equinovarus), but where there is a family history of the condition it should be carried out. If amniotic fluid is obtained for another reason, for example to do a chromosome analysis, the AFP concentrations should always be measured. It is now possible to measure alpha-fetoprotein in maternal blood. This is done between 16 and 18 weeks gestation. This unfortunately means two visits to hospital early in pregnancy; the first (at about 12–14 weeks) is for blood group and Wassermann reaction (WR). If abnormally high levels of AFP are found the patient is examined by ultrasound to exclude wrong gestation, fetal death, twins or anencephaly. It is often possible to scan the back for spina bifida. An amniocentesis is performed for estimation of AFP when two samples suggest high plasma AFP concentration. Anticholinesterase levels are now also measured on amniotic fluid. Raised levels are found in open spina bifida. If AFP or anticholinesterase levels in the amniotic fluid are high, termination of pregnancy may be offered as the fetus is very likely to have a neural-tube defect. A few other conditions may give rise to high levels of alpha-fetoprotein in blood and amniotic fluid. As these are all extremely serious, there is little risk of terminating normal babies or babies with only minor abnormalities. Real-time ultrasound is proving increasingly useful in assessing movements of the legs and in allowing a lesion to be seen in utero.

It is likely that screening of the whole population will become possible in the future.

There is evidence from animal experiments that vitamin supplements taken during pregnancy by the mother might reduce the incidence of neural-tube defects. Unfortunately it is now ethically impossible to carry out properly controlled trials in women.

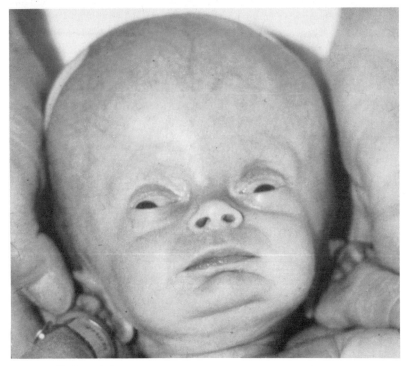

Fig. 9.16 Hydrocephalus

Hydrocephalus

Hydrocephalus (Fig. 9.16) has already been mentioned as a common association with myelomeningocele. It may also occur separately, due either to primary structural abnormalities (such as aqueduct atresia or stenosis) or to blockage secondary to infection (such as toxoplasmosis or meningitis) or intraventricular haemorrhage. The commonest way of detecting hydrocephalus is by measuring the head circumference regularly. Every baby in a special care baby unit should be measured once weekly and the result plotted on a head circumference against gestational age chart (see p. 64). If the baby's head is enlarging too rapidly, the plot will gradually cross the centiles for the normal population. It is the abnormally fast rate of rise that is crucial for the diagnosis. A large, but normal, baby may have a head circumference above the 90th centile for age, but the head should grow parallel to that centile.

The head enlarges too quickly because the CSF is accumulating under increased pressure. Associated findings therefore include palpable separation of the skull sutures, a bulging anterior fontanelle and prominent scalp veins. A confirmation of hydrocephalus can be obtained by

CAT scan or now more easily by real-time ultrasound scan by measuring the size of the lateral ventricles. If the ventricles continue to enlarge too rapidly, the brain substance will be stretched and damaged. To prevent this, a shunt operation is performed which allows the CSF under raised pressure to drain into the baby's right atrium or peritoneal cavity. A one-way valve prevents blood from entering the ventricle. Unfortunately, such shunts need revising as the baby grows or if they become blocked or infected. Low-grade infection by such organisms as *Staph. epidermidis* are common. For these reasons shunt operations should not be performed unless absolutely essential. Spontaneous arrest of hydrocephalus sometimes occurs, thus obviating the need for surgery.

Many babies, whether or not they have needed shunts, grow up with normal motor and intellectual function.

Microcephaly

A very small head circumference is associated with mental handicap. Antenatal ultrasound scanning may warn the paediatrician by showing a small and slowly growing fetal head. Some babies with perinatal or postnatal brain damage, due for example to asphyxia or cytomegalovirus infection, may have a normal head circumference at birth but the skull does not grow. A measurement of the occipitofrontal circumference during the first week of life is therefore essential to provide a base-line measurement and to identify babies whose heads are already small. A number of insults to the brain can cause microcephaly at birth, particularly a large dose of radiation in the second trimester or congenital rubella. A number of cases cannot be explained.

The floppy baby

This condition is discussed in Chapter 14.

Cardiovascular System

Congenital heart disease is discussed in Chapter 10.

Single umbilical artery

After delivery the cord vessels should be counted on the cut end of the cord. There are normally two small thick-walled arteries pouting above the cut surface and one large thin-walled vein. Sometimes (in about 0.5% of all deliveries) a single artery is present. About one-third of these babies have congenital malformations, especially of the gut (e.g. oesophageal atresia or imperforate anus), heart or kidneys. Such babies should therefore be examined carefully for detectable lesions and observed closely during the newborn period for signs such as heart murmurs or those of urinary tract infections. Some paediatricians do an intravenous urogram on all babies with a single umbilical artery, but most merely follow them up. An ultrasound scan of the abdomen is a useful non-invasive way of looking at the anatomy of the kidneys and urinary tract.

Skeletal System

Congenital dislocation of the hip

A check for dislocated hips is one of the most important parts of the routine examination of the newborn. Repeated checks are necessary, but even so it is likely that not every case can be diagnosed during the newborn period. Those not detected may not present until toddler age when the child will walk with a limp or may be diagnosed during later checks in infancy by finding limited abduction of the thigh. Treatment of those diagnosed late is much less satisfactory and involves orthopaedic operations. Diagnosis during the newborn period and treatment by splinting is often successful in saving the baby from surgery and a possibly permanent disability.

Congenital dislocation is commoner in girls, breech presentations, oligohydramnios, full-term babies and, for reasons that are unknown, the left hip. It seems that such things as the amount of liquor and intrauterine posture are relevant to the aetiology.

Diagnosis is made as follows (Fig. 9.17): the baby is laid on her back, feet facing the examiner on a flat surface. The legs are grasped with the thumbs along the inner side of the thigh and the middle fingers over the greater trochanters. The bent knees are held comfortably in the palm of the examiner's hands. Each hip is tested individually. The hip is gradually abducted while the middle finger presses upwards on the greater trochanter. If a hip is dislocated it will be felt to 'clunk'; this must not be confused with the much more commonly detected tendinous clicks which do not represent true dislocation. A further sign of true dislocation is that the dislocatable hip will not abduct fully; this sign is often absent in the newborn period. Radiographs are usually unhelpful in the newborn. Treatment sometimes advocated is placing the baby in a double thickness of terry towelling nappies to keep the hips abducted. This almost certainly has no beneficial effect in true dislocation and babies with tendinous clicks get better without treatment. We therefore do not recommend it. In all suspected cases an orthopaedic opinion should be sought early, and careful follow-up is necessary.

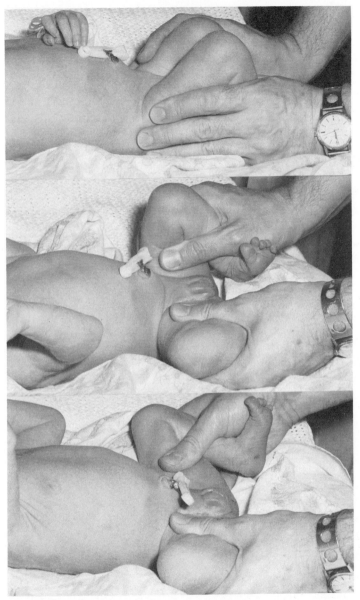

Fig. 9.17 Examination of the hips to exclude congenital dislocation

Talipes

This club foot defect (see Fig. 4.8) is found not uncommonly in newborn babies. Usually the foot is plantarflexed (equinus) and inverted (varus). Less commonly the foot is dorsiflexed (calcaneous) and everted (valgus). Both deformities probably derive from mechanical pressure in utero and if the foot can be over-corrected into the opposite position easily the defect is said to be 'positional' and will get better without treatment. If correction is not possible by manipulation a permanent deformity will result if treatment is not started as soon as possible. An orthopaedic opinion should be sought urgently. Initial treatment is usually by special strapping so that the kicking movements of the baby automatically help to correct the position. Often such strapping is all that is required, but careful follow-up will detect those babies who require operations to produce a satisfactory result.

It is often the mother who first notices the club foot defect and she will require considerable explanation and reassurance about the outcome.

Talipes is a common finding in severe myelomeningocele and a quick check of the back should always be made in case a cystic lesion there has been overlooked.

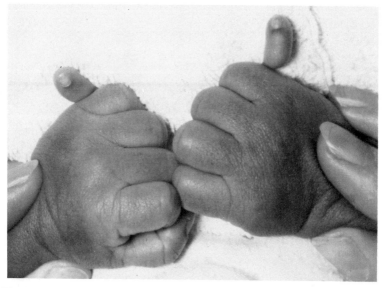

Fig. 9.18 Extra digits

Extra digits

Extra digits are quite common in babies whose parents come from the West Indies and they have an autosomal dominant inheritance. The fingers vary in size from tiny bumps to miniature fingers with a nail (Fig. 9.18). They are almost always attached to the ulnar side of the hand. If there is a tiny pedicle, the finger can be tied off with silk. The finger then becomes gangrenous and drops off. When there is a thick base, a proper removal by a surgeon is necessary. Analogous deformities may occur in the feet.

Syndactyly

Syndactly (Fig. 9.19) usually requires no treatment. Any webbing of the fingers will need attention by a plastic surgeon. In some cases, all, or almost all, of the digits are joined together. This may be associated with other congenital abnormalities, for example in Apert's syndrome, which includes cleft palate and craniofacial synostosis.

Skin

Birth marks

These are blemishes on the baby's skin and are present at birth or from a

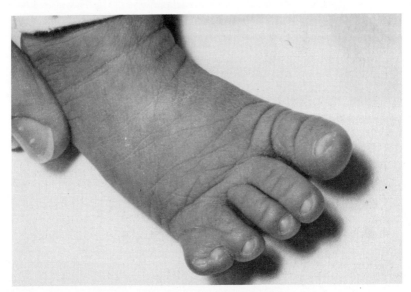

Fig. 9.19 An extra digit with syndactyly

few days afterwards. They are a common source of concern to the infant's mother.

Local blood vessel malformations. There are three types of abnormality involving localized malformation of blood vessels in the skin.

1 *Stork-bites (naevus simplex)* are so common that they could be considered normal. They consist of pink capillary haemangiomata on the upper eyelids, in a V shape on the forehead, on the nose and upper lip and often at the back of the head just above the hair-line. Their name obviously derives from the idea that the stork who brought the baby has carried him in these places and it may amuse the mother to be given this light-hearted information provided she is also reassured that the marks almost always disappear within the first year but, even if they do not, are nearly always practically invisible. Those on the nape of the neck do not go but are covered by hair.

2 *Port-wine stains* are very different from simple lesions in their poor prognosis. Although they are capillary haemangiomata, they are much denser and better defined, as well as being larger and blue or purple in appearance. Unfortunately they are permanent. Treatment in later life is usually by cosmetics to cover them up. Some extensive lesions on the trunk may be excised and grafted with skin from elsewhere on the body, but the scarring that is produced may not be a very great cosmetic improvement on the original. Port-wine stains of one side of the head and face (usually confined to one branch of the fifth cranial nerve) are particularly serious as they are often associated with a similar underlying abnormality of the meningeal coverings of the brain. These intracranial haemangiomata may give rise to fits on the opposite side of the body.

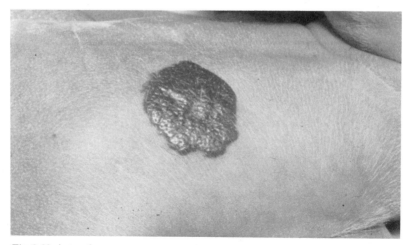

Fig. 9.20 A strawberry naevus

This combination of port-wine stain and fits is known as the Sturge–Weber syndrome.

3 *Strawberry naevi* are also capillary haemangiomata but, because they are more cavernous in nature, are usually raised above the level of the surrounding skin, looking like small strawberries (Fig. 9.20). They are not obvious at birth, but appear only during the early days or weeks of life. They start as tiny flattened lesions which escape notice. They can occur on any part of the body and there are often many lesions. They continue to grow during the early months of life, but gradually they begin to epithelialize from the middle, becoming bluer and then whiter, and gradually flatter and fading away altogether. As they nearly always disappear on their own without treatment before the age of about five years, they are best left untreated. Surgical excision always leaves a scar and may be hazardous as quite large feeding blood vessels are sometimes involved. The only indication for surgery is for those which press on vital organs such as the eye. Some are easily abraded and are commonly rubbed, causing bleeding and secondary infection. In other cases bleeding from lesions is uncommon and usually insignificant. Occasionally, it may be necessary to reduce the growth of the rapidly expanding lesion with topical steroids. Very rarely, in the case of enormous naevi, coagulation occurs in the naevus and thrombocytopenia may result.

Pigmented naevi (common brown moles) are less often a source of concern to the mother; she will often have many such small lesions herself. They usually grow with the infant and are permanent. Some hairy moles can be very big and ugly; they may look like a black pair of trousers. They are difficult to treat by surgeons when they are large, but abrasion produces impressive results. When they occur over the scalp there are sometimes lesions on the meninges.

'Mongolian' blue spot (see Fig. 4.10). These spots are found on babies of African or Asian descent. They appear as poorly defined blueish areas of pigmentation which are described as being confined to the sacral area. In practice they are often multiple and may extend well up the back or even on to the shoulders and limbs. It is important to recognize such lesions for what they are, as at first glance they look rather like areas of bruising. It has not been unknown for mothers to come under suspicion of having battered their infants when such lesions have been misdiagnosed at routine follow-up examinations. The lesions usually disappear as the babies grow. This may be because their own brown pigmentation becomes more prominent.

Remember that many mothers tend to brood about what, to the doctor, may seem to be trivial blemishes. These worries must be appreciated and full reassurance given. For advice on talking to the mother of the more severely handicapped or abnormal child, see Chapter 18.

Milia

These are small white sebaceous spots present on the nose, forehead or cheeks of practically every newborn baby. They are harmless and gradually disappear.

Toxic erythema (urticaria of the newborn)

This rash is common in babies after the first 48 hours of life. It usually disappears by seven to ten days. At first the lesions are white papules with a red flare, as if the baby has been stung by a nettle, but they then develop a central yellow vesicle like a pustule. They seem to be rare in the preterm baby. They are most frequent on the trunk, followed by the face. Occasionally severe examples may be confused with infected pustules, but the lesions characteristically change their position within a few hours and scrapings from the central spot show eosinophils rather than organisms or pus cells. No treatment, other than explanation, is necessary.

Genitourinary System

Hypospadias

In babies with hypospadias, the external urethral meatus opens on the ventral aspect of the penis (glans or shaft) or on the perineum (see Fig. 4.6). In the worst cases, the scrotum is bifid and the sex of the genitalia may look ambiguous. When necessary surgical repair is carried out in several stages during the second or third years of life. Such babies should not be circumcised as the surgeon requires the redundant foreskin to fashion a urethral passage.

At birth, some babies look as if they have been inexpertly circumcised. On closer inspection they are found to have a mild degree of glandular hypospadias. The penis may be bent (chordee) (Fig. 9.21), but do not make the diagnosis before an erection has been seen, as the penis may straighten properly. Some babies in this group may safely be left alone. Others, and some of those in the more severe groups, may require an operation soon after birth for correction of chordee and meatotomy for meatal stenosis.

Before surgery is contemplated for the perineoscrotal type of severe hypospadias, the baby's karyotype should be checked. In this way, the occasional girl virilized in utero due to congenital adrenal hyperplasia will not be misdiagnosed (see below).

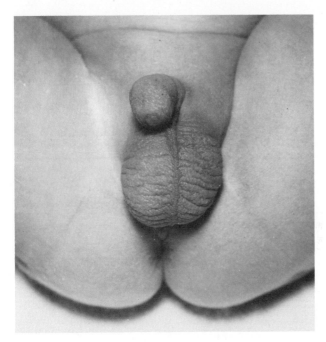

Fig. 9.21 Chordee

Congenital adrenal hyperplasia (CAH)

This is due to an enzyme defect which prevents the steroid cortisol being synthesized by the adrenal gland. This leads to overproduction of adrenocorticotrophic hormone (ACTH) by the pituitary gland because cortisol does not inhibit the hypothalamus or pituitary from producing it in excessive amounts. Abnormal steroids are formed by the uncontrolled stimulation of the gland by ACTH (Fig. 9.22). The commonest variety is 21-hydroxylase deficiency which occurs in about 1 in 5000 live births. The lack of the enzyme leads to hormones (androgens) being produced which masculinize the female fetus and infant (ambiguous genitalia) (Fig. 9.23). There is no obvious change in boys in the newborn period. Some of these infants cannot make the hormone aldosterone and there-fore cannot retain salt. They become dehydrated, hyponatraemic and hyperkalaemic within the first few weeks of life—the so-called salt-losing crisis. Two clues to the diagnosis are therefore ambiguous genita-lia in a female infant or a salt-losing crisis during the early weeks of life. A family history of CAH or of any unexplained neonatal death should also be sought. Most babies who present with dehydration will be losing fluid into the gut due, for example, to gastroenteritis. Sodium loss in the urine

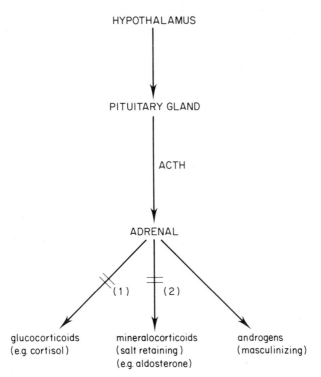

Fig. 9.22 Congenital adrenal hyperplasia. (1) A block in cortisol biosynthesis, often associated with (2) a block in aldosterone biosynthesis. Raised ACTH levels thus result in raised adrenal androgen levels (see text).

may be due to a kidney problem or to CAH. A useful distinction is that there is hyperkalaemia in CAH and aldosterone levels are low—they will be high in renal disease. Treatment of the salt-losing crisis is a matter of urgency; this is best done by simple salt replacement. Once this has been achieved a full investigation and diagnosis can be made. Long-term replacement steroid therapy is then necessary. In 21-hydroxylase deficiency a useful clue to the diagnosis is a very high plasma concentration of 17-hydroxyprogesterone. A male baby without the salt-losing tendency may not be diagnosed until later childhood when he is growing abnormally rapidly and showing signs of precocious sexual development. His ultimate height prognosis is, by then, very poor. It is possible to screen for the 21-hydroxylase deficient form of CAH by measuring 17-hydroxyprogesterone levels on the Guthrie test card blood spots. This would both prevent this problem and give advance warning of an affected male baby who might develop a salt-losing crisis. This test is being carried out in some centres but universal screening might not be cost-effective.

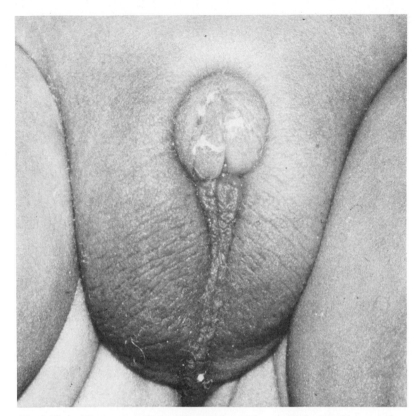

Fig. 9.23 Ambiguous genitalia in a female infant with congenital adrenal hyperplasia

Partially virilized female infants usually requre surgery to reduce the size of the clitoris, while retaining the nerve and blood supply to the glans, during the first year of life.

Rarer forms of CAH may present with inadequate virilization in male babies, or with hypertension—the chromosomes should always be checked in any baby with ambiguous genitalia as it is usually not possible by clinical examination to tell the genotypic sex of the baby. To make a definite diagnosis and to provide proper management, these babies must be referred to a centre of paediatric endocrinology.

Groin and scrotal swellings

These are quite common during the early days of life. They are usually due to one of two causes:

1 *Inguinal hernias* are quite common in the preterm baby. They seldom

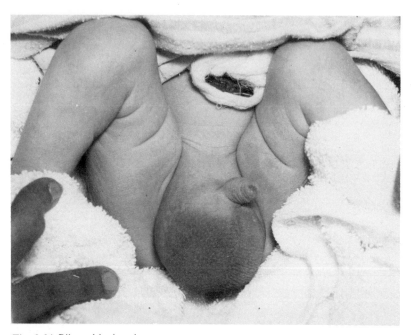

Fig. 9.24 Bilateral hydroceles

strangulate during the first few weeks of life, but almost never disappear spontaneously. They are best treated electively by herniotomy before the baby is discharged home.

2 *Hydrocele* (Fig. 9.24) (which unlike the inguinal hernia cannot be reduced and which transilluminates), in contrast, almost never needs treatment and resolves spontaneously over the succeeding months.

Testicular tumours and torsion of the testis are very rare. For information about undescended testes, see p. 71.

Urethral valves

These valves occur nearly always in male infants. They obstruct the outflow of urine from the bladder causing bladder, and sometimes renal, enlargement at birth (Fig. 9.25). For this reason it is always important to palpate these organs at the routine postnatal examination. The baby has a poor stream (dribbling) or may develop urinary tract infections. The diagnosis may be confirmed by excretion urography or cystography. Rather as in cystic fibrosis, the earlier the presentation the worse the prognosis, but the obstruction should be relieved surgically as soon as the diagnosis is made so as to minimize renal damage from infections and back pressure.

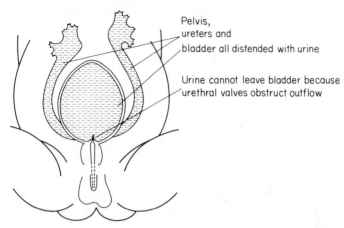

Pelvis, ureters and bladder all distended with urine

Urine cannot leave bladder because urethral valves obstruct outflow

Fig. 9.25 Urethral valves, an important cause of hydronephrosis in boys. Note the distended bladder, ureters and kidney pelves. From S. Wallis & D. Harvey (1979) *Nursing Times*, by permission of the authors and editor

Phimosis

Phimosis seems to be an imaginary congenital abnormality. There are no surgical, as opposed to social and religious, indications for circumcision in the newborn period. Unless parents hold strong religious convictions, it is worthwhile taking time to try and dissuade them from inflicting an unnecessary operation on their son. The operation carries a definite, although small, morbidity and mortality from anaesthesia, haemorrhage or infection.

Circumcision is often carried out without anaesthetic in the first two weeks of life using the plastic bell technique (Fig. 9.26) which reduces risks of haemorrhage. The baby, however, experiences some pain during the procedure. After the neonatal period the operation is best delayed at least until two years of age when the risks from general anaesthesia are extremely small.

Chromosomal Abnormalities

Down's syndrome (mongolism)

Down's syndrome is caused by having an extra chromosome 21 in the G Group (see Fig. 2.7). Its occurrence is nearly 2 per 1000 live births and it is the commonest cause of severe subnormality (IQ 50 or less) in the UK, accounting for about one-third of such children.

The incidence of the disease seems to be related in some way to ageing

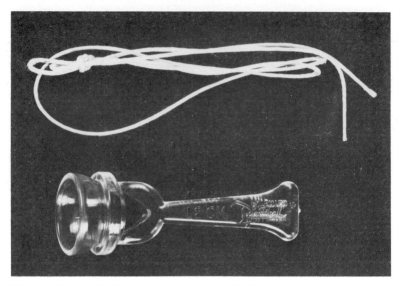

Fig. 9.26 The Plastibell for neonatal circumcision (*Hollister*)

of the maternal oocyte. Thus a woman below the age of 25 has less than a 1 in 2000 chance of giving birth to a baby with Down's syndrome whereas a woman over 45 has about a 1 in 50 chance (Fig. 9.27). It was thought that the age of the father was not relevant, but in one-third of cases the chromosome comes from him and increasing age possibly has a small effect on the incidence.

The physical features of babies with Down's syndrome are very characteristic so that even the mother may sometimes make the diagnosis at the delivery. The name mongolism was given to these babies because of the superficial resemblance that they have to oriental people, with almond-shaped eyes that slant upwards and outwards and inner epicanthic folds (Fig. 9.28). The term seems offensive and should not be used. Down's syndrome babies from oriental races look very similar to those in the West. Some oriental paediatricians have even called them 'international children' because they are the same in all parts of the world.

Other features of babies with Down's syndrome include: marked floppiness, which is in many ways the most characteristic feature; a skull flattened from front to back (brachycephaly) with a particularly flat occiput and a thin neck; a small mouth with a tongue that commonly protrudes (the tongue is of normal size unlike the large tongue of the cretin and protrudes because the mouth is small); the eyes commonly show speckling of the iris (Brushfield spots); broad hands with short fingers and a particularly short incurving little finger (clinodactyly); classically the palm shows a single (simian) crease and abnormalities of

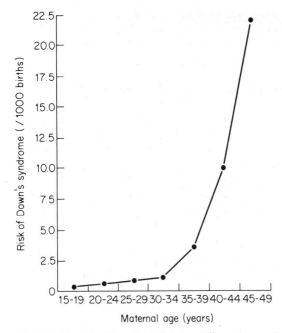

Fig. 9.27 The risk of Down's syndrome at different maternal ages

the dermal ridge patterns; and a wide fissure between the first and second toes (Fig. 9.29). Associated features include congenital heart disease, particularly ostium primum atrial septal defect and ventricular septal defect, and also gastrointestinal anomalies such as oesophageal atresia, duodenal atresia or imperforate anus.

Most babies with Down's syndrome have a triradius in the middle of the palm instead of the base of the hand. An auriscope is the best instrument for inspecting the hand.

It may be difficult to make an accurate clinical diagnosis in the first week. If there is any doubt, a chromosomal analysis must be performed. Although children with Down's syndrome are usually severely mentally handicapped, they can be happy and affectionate children. They do, however, place a considerable burden on their parents, particularly once they progress from the baby stage. There is no doubt, however, that from the child's point of view he is best brought up in the environment of his own family. For this reason it is probably best that such babies are given to the mother to cuddle straight after birth. The timing of telling the mother of the diagnosis and its implications cannot be rigidly laid down. In general, it is best to tell the parents early, but in very doubtful cases the results of chromosome studies should be awaited. It is a mistake to

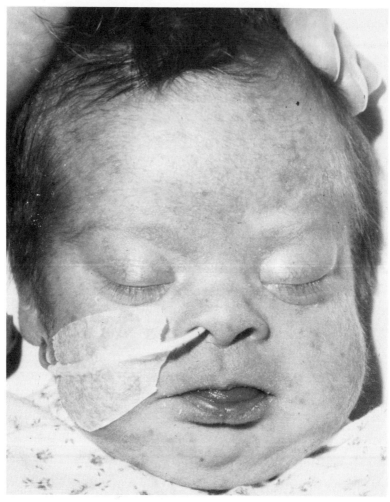

Fig. 9.28 The facies in Down's syndrome

remove the baby from the mother telling her that he is abnormal as he will then usually be rejected (see also Chapter 18).

Other trisomies

Trisomy 18 (Edwards' syndrome)

In this syndrome the extra chromosome is of number 18 from the E

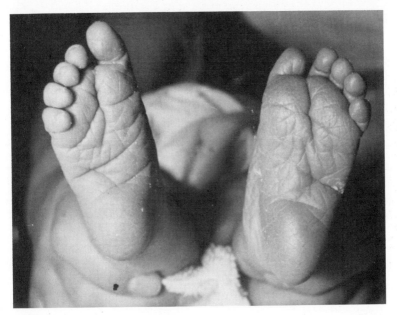

Fig. 9.29 The feet in Down's syndrome

Group (Fig. 9.30). It is much less common than Down's syndrome and the condition is often lethal during the early weeks of life. Characteristic features include a long narrow skull; low and malformed ears; prominent heels giving rise to the 'rocker-bottom' feet; and a short chest with broad spaced nipples (Fig. 9.31). Congenital heart disease is almost universal and is usually the immediate cause of death.

Trisomy 13

In Patau's syndrome the extra chromosome is in the D group, usually chromosome number 13. Again the head is abnormal, with low-set malformed ears, and there are cardiac anomalies. A characteristic feature is the cleft lip and/or palate. There may also be extra digits. Severe mental retardation is again universal.

Cri-du-chat syndrome

This is due to a partial deletion of the short arm of the fifth chromosome from the B group. The name derives from the kitten-like cry which these babies have during the newborn period. They lose this feature as they get older. These babies usually have small heads (microcephaly) and congenital heart defects. A related condition due to partial deletion of the

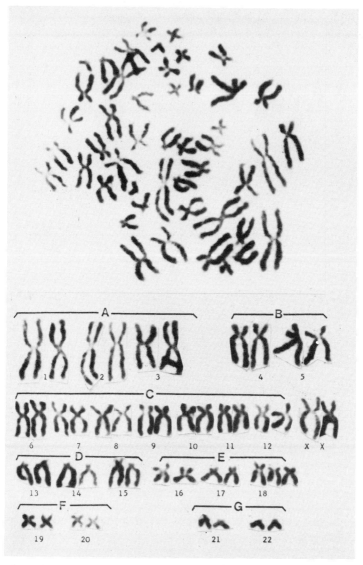

Fig. 9.30 The karyotype in Edwards' syndrome (trisomy 18)

short arm of the other B Group chromosome, number 4, is known as
Wolf's syndrome. These two syndromes have many features in common
but in Wolf's syndrome convulsions are a particular feature and may be
very resistant to treatment with anticonvulsants.

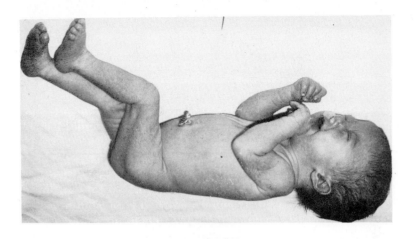

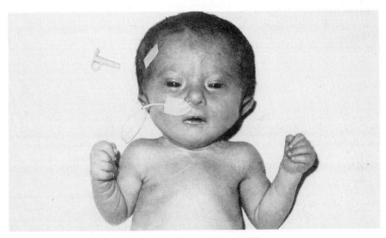

Fig. 9.31 A baby with Edwards' syndrome (trisomy 18)

In all these chromosomal anomalies, the birth weight of the infant is below that expected for his gestational age. In addition all such babies are severely mentally retarded.

Sex chromosome abnormalities

The sex chromosome anomaly which may be diagnosed in the newborn period is Turner's syndrome: in this condition, which is confined to females, there is only one female sex chromosome. This usually results in 'streak' ovaries and infertility. Diagnostic features in the newborn period include congenital lymphoedema of the extremities and a low birth weight for the baby's gestational age.

Further Reading

See Further Reading to Chapter 8

—10
Congenital Heart Disease

Babies with heart disease are often difficult clinical problems during the first week of life. A deeply blue baby may have cyanotic congenital heart disease, but this is often difficult to distinguish from a lung problem such as meconium aspiration with persistence of the fetal type of circulation. Some remarkable changes occur normally at birth and it is important to understand the circulatory changes if one is to attempt a diagnostic approach to congenital heart disease.

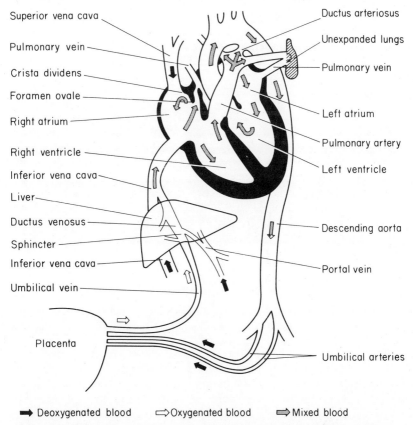

Fig. 10.1 The fetal circulation. Arrows indicate the direction of the blood flow. Adapted from J. Langman (1969) *Medical Embryology*, 2nd ed. Baltimore: Williams & Wilkins

Changes in the Circulation at Birth

A large part of cardiac output in utero (Fig. 10.1) is directed towards the placenta to allow gas exchange. The two umbilical arteries come from the internal iliac arteries, pass around the pelvis and up the abdominal wall to the umbilicus where they spiral through the umbilical cord to the placenta. Carbon dioxide is excreted across the placenta into the mother where her ventilation holds the $P\text{CO}_2$ at the same level in both the fetus' blood and her own blood; the value is around 5.5 kPa (40 mmHg). Oxygen passes across the placenta from the mother into the fetus. The mother's blood supply to the uterus flows into a lake of blood in the deciduum of the uterus with villi from the placenta in this lake. The oxygen passes across the placental membranes into capillaries and thence into the umbilical vein. This vein is, therefore, one of the few in the body which contain oxygenated blood. The vein spirals with the arteries in the umbilical cord and from the umbilicus passes upwards and backwards to join the portal vein underneath the liver. In adult life, the portal vein flows to the liver, but this organ can be bypassed in fetal life by a vein known as the ductus venosus, which connects the portal vein to the inferior vena cava. Therefore, most oxygenated blood passes direct from the placenta into the inferior vena cava and thence into the right atrium of the heart.

In the right side of the heart there is a fascinating mechanism for separating this stream of blood from the blood coming down the superior vena cava. A crescent-shaped hood directs the flow from the inferior vena cava through the foramen ovale into the left atrium. The foramen ovale is an opening in the wall between the two atria and has a valve which can be closed only from the left side of the heart. This mechanism allows oxygenated blood to pass directly into the left heart and thence into the left ventricle and out into the body.

Blood from the superior vena cava passes into the right atrium and then into the right ventricle and out into the pulmonary artery. In postnatal life it would then flow to the capillaries in the lung to take up oxygen and excrete carbon dioxide. However, this mechanism is not available in the fetus and the amount of blood flowing to the lungs is very small, mainly because there is constriction of the pulmonary arteries. A channel called the ductus arteriosus connects the pulmonary artery with the aorta. Therefore, in the fetus the lungs are bypassed because blood flows through this ductus into the aorta and to the lower part of the body where much of it flows to the placenta through the umbilical arteries.

Oxygenated blood flowing into the heart through the inferior vena cava is thus partially mixed with deoxygenated blood which reduces the $P\text{O}_2$. Blood in the aorta is also a mixture of oxygenated blood flowing out of the left ventricle and deoxygenated blood flowing through the ductus

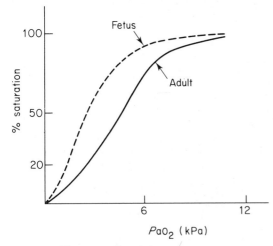

Fig. 10.2 The oxygen dissociation curve

arteriosus. The Po_2 in the fetus is much lower than that in later life, about 3 kPa (20–25 mmHg). The fetus can live with this low Po_2 because the oxygen dissociation curve of fetal haemoglobin is to the left of adult haemoglobin (Fig. 10.2). The position of the curve allows more oxygen to be carried by the blood at low tensions than in an adult who has haemoglobin A in his red cells. The dissociation curve is shifted by a number of factors, including acidaemia which moves the curve to the right. During labour, the blood gases and pH are relatively stable although there is a tendency for the pH to fall gradually from 7.4 to about 7.3; this is partly due to an accumulation of lactic acid due to the interruption of blood supply to the placenta during uterine contractions. At birth, there is often marked acidaemia, which is partly respiratory, because CO_2 cannot escape from the baby when the umbilical cord is compressed, and partly metabolic as a result of accumulation of lactic acid from hypoxia. The Po_2 values in cord blood are variable and may reflect a recent occlusion of the umbilical cord in a normal baby.

The first breath has always caused astonishment in those present at a birth, or dismay if it does not occur. A number of stimuli produce the first breath. In utero, a baby produces movements of the thorax during rapid-eye-movement sleep; these movements can be seen by ultrasound between one-third and one-half of the time. At birth, there is a sudden change to regular steady respiration that does not fail in a normal baby. Mild cooling, hypercarbia, hypoxia and physical stimuli probably combine together to start regular breathing (see Chapter 3).

As the lungs expand, there appears to be a mechanical effect on the pulmonary arterioles which dilate. This means that there is a flood of

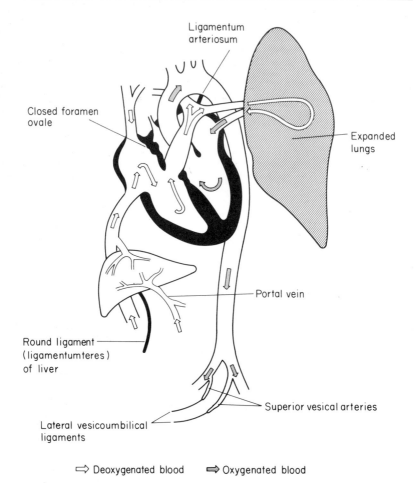

Fig. 10.3 The circulation after birth. Adapted from J. Langman (1969) *Medical Embryology*, 2nd ed. Baltimore: Williams & Wilkins

blood through the lungs; the pressure in the left atrium rises so that the valve of the foramen ovale closes. The wall of the ductus arteriosus is sensitive to the tension of oxygen in the blood; as this rises shortly after birth, the ductus closes. Interruption of the blood supply in the umbilical cord leads to closure of the ductus venosus. Eventually, the umbilical vein inside the body and the umbilical arteries become mere cords. These changes are shown in Fig. 10.3.

Shortly after birth the blood P_{CO_2} and pH return to normal adult values. There is a normal right-to-left shunt, mainly in the lung, during the first few days of life; the P_{O_2} does not therefore reach adult values

(13 kPa or 100 mmHg) until the end of the first week.

All the anatomical changes do not occur immediately. For instance a preterm baby may have a patent ductus arteriosus for many weeks after birth.

Signs and Symptoms in the Newborn Period

There are several possible presenting features, one or more of which is usually present:
1 tachypnoea
2 dyspnoea
3 cyanosis
4 tachycardia
5 murmurs
6 deterioration in feeding or taking longer over feeds
7 grunting.

Infants with any of these features should have a full cardiovascular examination. Cardiac failure is not always easily diagnosed in a small baby. The following are the most important clinical signs: a pale, anxious baby; tachycardia (more than 160/min), marked tachypnoea, usually over 60/min; crepitations; an enlarged liver (this is usually best felt in the middle of the epigastrium not in the right midclavicular line as in adults); peripheral oedema, seen in the eyelids, the hands or feet. The earliest sign of cardiac failure is often persisting unexplained tachypnoea.

The causes and management of cardiac failure are described below.

Several types of congenital heart disease may be extremely difficult to diagnose in the neonatal period. For instance, a ventricular septal defect may show no abnormal physical signs and the murmur often appears only after several weeks. Coarctation of the aorta classically produces femoral pulses which are absent or very difficult to feel, but during the period when the ductus arteriosus is still open there are strong pulsations which disappear only after several days. Some babies with cyanotic congenital heart disease such as Fallot's tetralogy are not cyanosed early in life.

In examining a baby for heart disease it is important to look for all the features of cardiac failure and to examine the peripheral pulses, particularly the femoral pulses, very carefully and repeatedly.

Investigations

Some investigations may help:

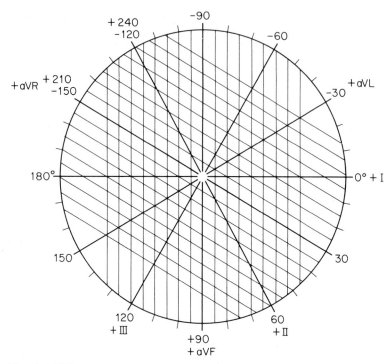

Fig. 10.4 ECG axes

Chest radiograph

It is difficult to take a chest radiograph in a standard way in the newborn period, so it is common to see radiographs that have not been centred properly or taken at the right distance. However, the films are often useful when they show a large heart. The breadth of the cardiac shadow in relation to the breadth of the thorax is rather greater than in an adult and is often a little over 50%. Although the heart may be large in a baby who has had asphyxia during birth, the films may be very useful if they show a very large heart which gives a clue to the diagnosis. One can also assess the number of blood vessels in the lung fields (oligaemia or hyperaemia). Some conditions have a characteristic shape to the cardiac shadow.

Electrocardiogram (ECG)

The electrocardiogram is difficult to assess in neonatal life because it changes so rapidly with age and many of the features are very different from those seen in adults or older children. It is reasonable to do standard leads (I, II, III, AVR, AVL and AVF) and a selection of chest leads; those often chosen are V4R, V1, V3 and V6. Without very small electrodes one cannot obtain intermediate chest leads.

Axis on standard leads. There is a marked right axis in normal babies. The axis is obtained in the same way as in older children; Fig. 10.4 demonstrates the axes in relation to the standard leads showing that lead I is 0°, lead III is + 120° and so on. A quick way of finding the approximate QRS axis is to look at the standard and V leads to find which one has R and S deflections which are almost equal. The QRS axis will then be 90° clockwise to that lead.

The mean QRS axis is about + 135° at birth and decreases to a mean of + 110° during the second, third and fourth weeks of the neonatal period (Fig. 10.5).

Left axis deviation is very abnormal at birth and is often the result of a conduction defect in the left ventricule; it is found in atrioventricular defects and tricuspid atresia.

T wave. The T wave is normally upright in the right precordial leads (V4R and V1) for at least 72 hours. A useful rule is that an upright T wave after that time is abnormal.

Right ventricular hypertrophy. The single most useful ECG sign is the upright T wave seen in right ventricular hypertrophy associated with an R/S ratio of greater than 1 in lead V1. Nevertheless it is sometimes difficult to be certain of right ventricular hypertrophy in the newborn period, and some other ECG features are summarized in Table 10.1.

Left ventricular hypertrophy occurs in conditions such as aortic stenosis. Criteria for its recognition are shown in Table 10.1.

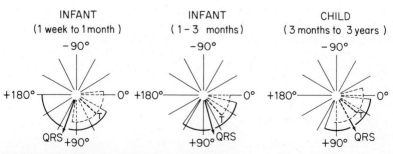

Fig. 10.5 Normal ECG axes in infants and young children.

Table 10.1 Criteria for evaluation of electrocardiograms in infants and children.

Right ventricular hypertrophy
1 R in V1 0–24 hours, 20 mm; 1–7 days, 29 mm; 8 days to 3 months, 20 mm; 3 months to 16 years 19 mm or more
2 S in V6 0–7 days, 14 mm; 8–30 days, 10 mm   } or more
  S in V6 1–3 months, 7 mm; 3 months to 16 years, 5 mm
3 R/S ratio in V1
  0–3 months, 6.5; 3–6 months, 4.0   } or more
  6 months to 2 years, 2.4; 3–5 years, 1.6; 6–15 years, 0.9

Left ventricular hypertrophy
1 S in V1, more than 20 mm at all ages
2 R in V6, 20 mm or more
3 Secondary T inversion in V5 or V6
4 Q 4 mm or more in V5, V6 or V7

Combined ventricular hypertrophy
Direct evidence of RVH + LVH
or RVH + Q of 2 mm or more in V5 or V6
or inverted T in V6 (after positive in right chest leads) + RVH

Right atrial hypertrophy
1 Peaked P waves, 3 mm or more in any one lead
2 Qr pattern in RV3 or V1

Left atrial hypertrophy
1 Bifid P in any lead
2 P duration of more than 0.09 seconds
3 Late inversion of P in V1 or more than 1.5 mm

Echocardiography

Echocardiography is now widely used. Advantages of the technique are that it can be done at the mother's bedside in the postnatal ward or in the special care nursery, so that the infant does not become cold or hypoxaemic moving to another department, and that the technique is non-invasive. It is important that it should be performed by somebody experienced in the technique so as to identify echoes from the various chambers and valves in the heart. It is now relatively easy to decide if the heart is structurally normal and, for example, to identify septal defects and pericardial effusion by the use of echoes. A normal 4-chamber echo is shown in Fig. 10.6. In many centres the majority of newborn babies now go to cardiac surgery without catheterization on the basis of the echo findings. However local expertise, experience and surgical practice will determine policy in individual centres.

Blood gases

An arterial sample (if possible from the right radial artery) from a baby breathing air and a further sample while breathing 100% oxygen for 10

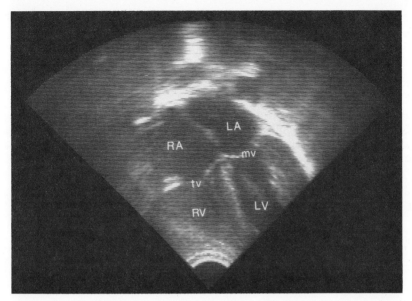

Fig. 10.6 A four-chamber echo of a normal heart (LA = left atrium, LV = left ventrical, RA = right atrium, RV = right ventricle, TV = tricuspid valve, MV = mitral valve)

minutes can provide very good evidence of a presence of a right-to-left shunt. In general, the arterial P_{O_2} rarely rises above 25 kPa in cyanotic heart disease but may easily rise above that in lung disorders. Unfortunately, the test may not be so valuable in the first few days when a baby is very ill with lung disease, but it is more useful from the age of about four days. The test may be dangerous as the ductus may close. It should only be done with careful monotoring and with prostaglandin immediately available.

Cardiac catheterization and angiocardiography

Many complicated types of congenital heart disease will need careful investigation before surgery is performed. These investigations must be performed in specialist units.

Types of Congenital Heart Disease

A useful distinction in considering congenital heart disease is between pink babies (acyanotic) and blue babies (cyanotic). In every case of central cyanosis there must be a right-to-left shunt, where some blood passes from the right to the left side of the heart without perfusing air-filled alveoli. In these situations, crying usually deepens the cyanosis. In acyanotic congenital heart disease there may be a left-to-right shunt, where blood passes back from the left to the right side of the heart and, therefore, passes through the heart twice during a single circulation; alternatively there may be a valvular abnormality. It is important to realize that any heart lesion may cause heart failure and this may lead to cyanosis even in acyanotic heart disease. Newborn babies with cyanotic heart disease are particularly prone to and vulnerable from hypothermia. Their environmental temperature should be kept at the upper end of the neutral range (see Chapter 5).

Common congenital heart defects are:
1 *Left-to-right shunt*
   Ventricular septal defect
   Patent ductus arteriosus
   Atrial septal defect
2 *Right-to-left shunt*
   Transposition of the great arteries
   Tetralogy of Fallot
   Pulmonary atresia
3 *Obstructive*
   Aortic stenosis
   Pulmonary stenosis
   Coarctation of the aorta
   Hypoplastic left heart

During the newborn period, babies who develop signs of congenital heart disease often have severe lesions with very complicated anatomical defects. For instance, coarctation of the aorta, although it theoretically has no shunt, is often associated with a ventricular septal defect. On the other hand, a ventricular septal defect may have no shunt at first as the right ventricular pressure is initially as high as that in the left ventricle (see below).

Left-to-Right Shunt

Ventricular septal defect (VSD)

This is the commonest congenital heart lesion. There is a window in the membranous or muscular septum between the two ventricles. It may often accompany other forms of congenital heart disease. Since the pulmonary artery resistance, and therefore right ventricular pressure, is much higher in the newborn than later in the first year of life, there may be very little shunt through the defect at first. The baby's heart sounds are usually quite normal in the newborn period and no murmur is heard.

As the pressure on the right side of the heart drops over the first few weeks, the characteristic pansystolic murmur is heard all over the praecordium. Large defects present, therefore, with heart failure around the second month of life. The chest radiograph is normal with small defects; with large ones there may be cardiac and left atrial enlargement with pulmonary plethora. There may be evidence of right or biventricular hypertrophy on ECG. 80% of VSDs close completely and spontaneously before eight years of age.

Ductus arteriosus

It is difficult to be certain whether persistent ductus arteriosus is a congenital heart lesion in the newborn period since all babies have a ductus at birth and preterm babies may have an open ductus for many weeks before it closes spontaneously. Characteristic signs are a continuous systolic and diastolic murmur below the left clavicle with left ventricular hypertrophy, a loud pulmonary second sound and a collapsing (bounding) pulse (check the systolic and diastolic blood pressures: the pulse pressure will be abnormally wide). The classical physical signs are often not present and only a systolic murmur may be heard. The chest radiograph and ECG are usually normal. In babies with rubella syndrome it is common for ductus arteriosus to persist and for there to be an additional septal defect. Delayed closure of the ductus arteriosus is very common in the preterm low birth weight baby. In the majority of cases, no treatment is required as the ductus closes spontaneously. In infants with respiratory distress syndrome, where oxygenation is variable and the Pao$_2$ is low, there is a tendency for the ductus to remain open. This may result in a right-to-left shunt if pulmonary resistance is high (especially if the baby is acidaemic), but more frequently a left-to-right shunt occurs and results in an increased cardiac output which can lead to chronic cardiac failure. Cyanosis may appear when the baby cries as the pressure in the right heart then exceeds that in the left.

Pharmacological agents have been investigated for their ability to close the ductus. Prostaglandins maintain the patency of the ductus (see under transposition below), and the prostaglandin synthetase inhibitor indomethacin has been used very successfully to obliterate the ductus in symptomatic babies with RDS (see also Chapter 6). Treatment with indomethacin is effective only in the preterm infant and never in the full-term infant with persistent ductus arteriosus. Complications have included oliguria and displacement of bilirubin from albumin. The place for indomethacin or surgical intervention in sick babies is not yet established, therefore, and meticulous supportive treatment is very important. Indomethacin should be given orally, 0.1 mg/kg once; the same dose is repeated after eight hours and a third dose of 0.2 mg/kg given 24 hours after the first dose. If there is no effect, more should *not* be given.

Atrial septal defect (ASD)

The common and less serious type of ASD in which there is a defect in the upper part of the septum (ostium secundum) presents only rarely in the newborn period. Babies with the more serious ostium primum defect in the lower portion of the septum often have associated abnormalities of the mitral valve or, more seriously, a common atrioventricular canal (endocardial cushion defects). Such babies may present in the early weeks of life with a harsh systolic murmur audible widely over the precordium, often associated with a thrill and a loud and widely split second sound. Babies with a common atrioventricular canal may also show early cyanosis and tachypnoea with rapid onset of cardiac failure (thus mimicking transposition of the great arteries) (see below).

Chest radiography shows general cardiomegaly and, in particular, left artrial enlargement, associated with increased pulmonary vascular markings (plethora). The ECG shows a characteristic pattern of left axis deviation with right ventricular hypertrophy and first degree heart block (prolonged P–R interval). Left atrial enlargement produces tall P waves.

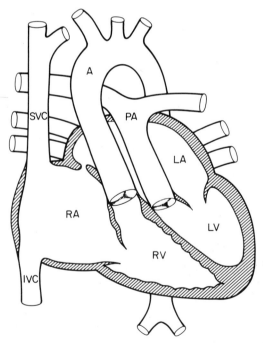

Fig. 10.7 Simple transposition of the great arteries. (LV = left ventricle; LA = left atrium; RA = right atrium; IVC = inferior vena cava; SVC = superior vena cava; A = aorta; PA = pulmonary artery)

There is a particular association between endocardial cushion defects and trisomy 21 (Down's syndrome, see Chapter 9).

Right-to-Left Shunts

Transposition of the great arteries

Transposition is a common cause of right-to-left shunt in the newborn period. It can cause profound cyanosis and is important because urgent treatment is needed to save the baby's life. The major arteries are reversed so that the pulmonary artery leaves the left ventricle and the aorta leaves the right ventricle. There are therefore two separate circulations, since blood returns to the lungs from the left side of the heart and blood returns to the body from the right side of the heart (Fig. 10.7). During fetal life there is, of course, mixing through the ductus arteriosus and the foramen ovale. There is very commonly an associated septal defect, for example at the ventricular level (Fig. 10.8) so that mixing can

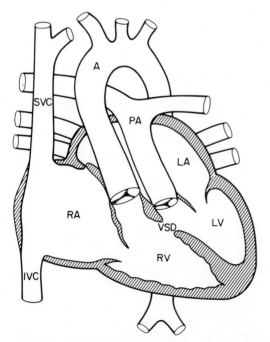

Fig. 10.8 Transposition of the great arteries, with associated ventricular septal defect (VSD). (For key see Fig. 10.7)

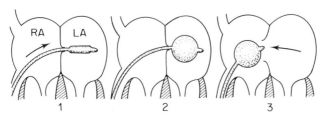

Fig. 10.9 Rashkind's atrial septostomy. 1, A catheter is passed into the right atrium and pushed through the foramen ovale into the left atrium. 2, A balloon at the tip of the catheter is inflated. 3, The catheter is withdrawn sharply so that the inflated balloon tears the atrial septum, allowing oxygenated blood to reach the systemic circulation. From S. Wallis & D. Harvey (1979) *Nursing Times*, by permission of the authors and editor

still occur after birth. However, many babies do not have any septal defect and mixing occurs only through the ductus arteriosus. When this closes, several days after birth, the baby may suddenly become deeply cyanosed and die. Cyanosis, irreversible by 100% oxygen, is characteristic. Tachypnoea develops within a few days, followed by increasing heart failure, cyanosis, acidaemia and death if untreated. Apart from the cyanosis, there are often no physical signs initially, although an ejection systolic murmur may be present. The ECG is usually normal at first but may later show left ventricular hypertrophy. The chest radiograph is said classically to show an 'egg on the side' appearance of the heart but is more often normal. When this diagnosis is suspected it is important to confirm the diagnosis by echocardiography, but cardiac catheterization is also necessary urgently because a balloon septostomy (Fig. 10.9) can be performed to provide mixing of the two circulations. A catheter with an inflatable balloon on the end is passed into the left atrium through the foramen ovale. The balloon is inflated and pulled back sharply to tear a hole in the atrial septum. A complete operation can be done towards the end of the first year but the balloon septostomy will enable the baby to survive until then.

Oxygen causes the ductus arteriosus to close. It is now usual to give a prostaglandin infusion to maintain an open ductus until the baby can be transferred to a neonatal cardiac unit. At present we recommend an intravenous infusion of prostaglandin E_1 (PGE$_1$), 0.1 µg/kg/min.

Pulmonary atresia and other forms of obstruction of the right ventricle together with septal defects

Babies with classical Fallot's tetralogy often present as an apparently uncomplicated ventricular septal defect and then later show cyanosis as the infundibular muscle proximal to the pulmonary valve becomes hypertrophied and obstructs the outflow to the right ventricle. The other features are an overriding aorta and right ventricular hypertrophy (Fig.

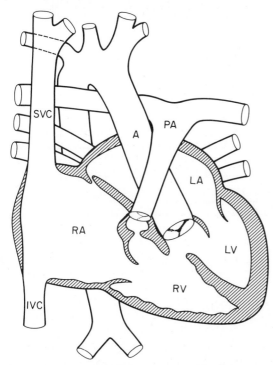

Fig. 10.10 Tetralogy of Fallot (For key see Fig. 10.7)

10.10). The more severe types of right ventricular outflow obstruction may produce symptoms of cyanosis in the newborn period. Sometimes the pulmonary artery and valve are completely obliterated, so that the lungs are perfused only through the ductus arteriosus (Fig. 10.11) and the baby becomes deeply cyanosed when this closes. If a baby becomes cyanosed, is given oxygen and then becomes even more deeply cyanosed, it is important to reduce the amount of inspired oxygen because this may save the baby's life. There is only a single second sound and a murmur may or may not be present. The baby is often very deeply cyanosed. The ECG shows marked right axis deviation and right ventricular and sometimes atrial hypertrophy. The chest radiograph shows a normally sized heart with a pulmonary artery 'bay' due to the small size of the main pulmonary artery; the apex of the heart is often said to be lifted up from the diaphragm. The lung fields are under-perfused (oligaemic) and therefore appear very translucent. A right-sided aortic arch is present in about 20% of cases.

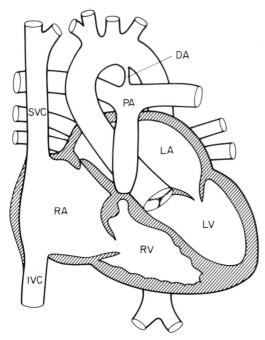

Fig. 10.11 Pulmonary atresia and ductus arteriosus. (For key see Fig. 10.7)

Total anomalous pulmonary venous drainage (TAPVD)

In this condition the pulmonary veins empty into the right side of the heart and then there is an additional right-to-left shunt at atrial or ventricular level so that the mixed oxygenated and deoxygenated blood is perfused both to the lungs and to the body. There are various subgroups of the condition but the most confusing and rarest is the type where the pulmonary veins empty into the inferior vena cava below the diaphragm, usually called the subdiaphragmatic type. There may be obstruction to the flow of these veins into the inferior vena cava. The ECG shows an axis to the right of normal and right ventricular hypertrophy.

The condition is easily confused with hyaline membrane disease, as the babies are deeply cyanosed, with a small heart on the radiograph and over-filled plethoric lung fields which may have the ground-glass appearance of hyaline membrane disease. Giving 100% oxygen is a very important aid in the differential diagnosis, as it hardly increases the arterial P_{O_2} in TAPVD. Unfortunately, the worst forms of RDS have such a large right-to-left shunt that 100% oxygen may not alter the P_{O_2}. Although this is a rare condition, it is a classic trap for anyone looking after ill newborn babies. The mortality is still between 15 and 50%. The

Table 10.2 Important causes of persistent cyanosis in the newborn period.

Pulmonary	Hyaline membrane disease
	Pneumonia
	Pneumothorax
	Diaphragmatic hernia
	Tracheo-oesophageal fistula
	Lobar emphysema
	Wilson–Mikity syndrome
Cardiovascular	Severe cyanosis (usually the presenting feature)
	Transposition of the great arteries
	Pulmonary atresia or severe pulmonary stenosis
	Tetralogy of Fallot
	Total anomalous pulmonary venous drainage (with obstruction of venous return)
	Tricuspid atresia
	Ebstein's anomaly of the tricuspid valve
	Mild cyanosis initially
	Hypoplastic left heart syndrome including aortic or mitral atresia, preductal coarctation of the aorta
	Truncus arteriosus
Cerebral	Cerebral oedema
	Intracerebral haemorrhage
Miscellaneous	Congenital methaemoglobinaemia
	Bilateral choanal atresia
	Vasomotor instability (peripheral cyanosis only)
	Sepsis, especially septicaemia (peripheral cyanosis only)
	Traumatic cyanosis

differential diagnosis of persistent cyanosis in the newborn is summarized in Table 10.2.

Obstructive Lesions

Coarctation of the aorta

Here there is an obstruction of the proximal aorta. There may be only a small narrowing after the ductus, usually called the adult type of coarctation, or there may be a much longer narrowing of the aorta, often proximal to the ductus, often called the infantile type of coarctation of the aorta. The left ventricle is often much smaller than normal and so the most severe forms of the condition may be called the hypoplastic left heart syndrome. A ventricular or atrial septal defect may be present as well. It is important to feel the femoral pulses in every baby, particularly when one is doing an examination for congenital heart disease. However, the femoral pulses may be easily palpable in a baby with coarctation of the aorta if the aorta is well perfused through a ductus arteriosus from the pulmonary artery. When the ductus arteriosus closes, the femoral pulses may disappear quite suddenly. If the narrowed segment of the aorta is quite small, it is often possible to resect it and replace it with a graft. Unfortunately many babies have a very long segment of narrowed aorta with a very small left ventricle so their prognosis is, at present, hopeless.

Hypoplastic left heart

In the hypoplastic left heart syndrome (Fig. 10.12) the baby is ductus dependent. When the duct closes there will be rapid deterioration over a few hours with a shock-like picture.

Valvular lesions

Many valvular lesions may be diagnosed in the neonatal period because they produce a murmur. Simple aortic or pulmonary stenosis produces an ejection systolic murmur. Luckily, these rarely produce cardiac

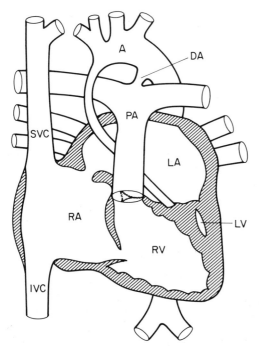

Fig. 10.12 Hypoplastic left heart syndrome with ductus arteriosus. (For key see Fig. 10.7)

Table 10.3 Causes of heart failure in the newborn.

Volume or pressure overload of the myocardium
Large left-to-right shunts
Left or right ventricular outflow obstruction
Total anomalous pulmonary venous drainage (with or without pulmonary venous
    obstruction)
Coarctation of the aorta and hypoplastic left heart syndrome
Anaemia
Severe hypertension (rare)

Primary depression or failure of myocardial contractility
Hypoxaemia and acidaemia
Electrolyte abnormalities, e.g. hypocalcaemia or hypokalaemia
Hypoglycaemia
Inflammatory myocardial disease (myocarditis)
Endocardial fibroelastosis
Coronary occlusive disease
Glycogen storage disease

Dysrhythmias with heart rate >220/min or <40/min

failure in the newborn but it is important to follow up any baby who has had a loud murmur. A very soft ejection systolic murmur is heard in 95% of newborn babies.

Cardiac Failure

Causes of heart failure in the newborn are shown in Table 10.3. Babies with evidence of cardiac failure should be managed as follows:
1 Restrict fluid intake to 120–150 ml/kg/day.
2 Give frusemide 1–2 mg/kg once or twice daily.
3 Digitalize (Table 10.4).
4 Nurse in a neutral thermal environment (at the lower end for babies with acyanotic heart defects and large left-to-right shunts) and tipped head up.
5 Give appropriate concentrations of added oxygen if necessary.
6 Consider sedation and ventilation.
   It is important to assess the effects of digoxin on the individual baby and to adjust the dose according to clinical response. In those on long-term therapy, remember to increase dosage according to weight.
   Check electrolytes and urea initially and regularly and give potassium supplements if needed. If digoxin toxicity is suspected, check digoxin levels.

Table 10.4 Digitalization in the event of cardiac failure.

Digitalization dose	Oral initially 20 μg/kg (0.02 mg/kg); then 10 μg/kg (0.01 mg/kg for 2 doses) Intramuscularly initially 15 μg/kg (0.015 mg/kg); then 8 μg/kg (0.008 mg/kg for 2 doses)
Maintenance dose	Oral 10 μg/kg/24 hours (0.01 mg/kg/24 hours) Intramuscularly 8 μg/kg/24 hours (0.008 mg/kg/24 hours) Give half maintenance dose every 12 hours Reduce dose slightly for infants <2 kg

Arrhythmias

Arrhythmias may cause heart failure in newborn babies.

Paroxysmal atrial tachycardia (PAT)

Many normal newborn babies achieve heart rates of 160–180/min or more when crying, but a persistent tachycardia of more than 180/min in a quiet or sleeping baby is an important clue to the diagnosis of PAT which may be confirmed by ECG. Often the rate may reach 300/min and congestive cardiac failure develops. Occasionally fetal tachycardia may cause intrauterine cardiac failure and the infant may then be born with peripheral oedema and hepatomegaly (hydrops fetalis, see p. 59 and p. 252). In attacks of PAT lasting more than a few hours, the baby becomes very ill with pallor, cyanosis, restlessness and irritability.

An attack may be aborted by vagal stimulation for example by massage over one carotid sinus in the neck, but the infant usually requires to be digitalized (see Table 10.4 for dose regimen) as recurrence is otherwise common. Therapy should be continued for about one year. In rare cases, or if there is severe circulatory failure, cardioversion (DC shock) may be necessary to abolish attacks. There is seldom any underlying structural heart disease in PAT.

Congenital complete atrioventricular block (congenital heart block)

Fetal bradycardia is usually a sign of hypoxia but occasionally the baby is found to have a persisting slow heart rate (often less than 60/min) after birth. This is due to a congenital defect in the main conducting system of the heart (bundle of His). The ventricles do not keep pace with the contraction rate of the atria and there is complete dissociation of the P waves and QRS complexes on the ECG.

About 30% of such babies have other associated structural heart defects, especially single ventricle, transposition of the great arteries or patent ductus arteriosus, so the prognosis depends on the severity of the associated lesion.

In the 70% without other abnormalities, the prognosis is good without treatment, although some patients need permanent pacemakers to prevent episodes of dizziness or syncope in later life.

There appears to be an important association with systemic lupus erythematosus in the mothers of many babies with congenital heart block.

Further Reading

Jordan, S.C. & Scott, O. (1981) *Heart Disease in Paediatrics*, 2nd ed. London: Butterworths.

Park, M.K. & Guntheroth, W.G. (1981) *How to Read Pediatric ECGs*. Chicago: Year Book Medical.

——11————————————

Birth Trauma

Severe birth trauma is now a rare complication in normal obstetric practice. However, minor trauma associated, for example, with rotational forceps deliveries, shoulder dystocia or breech delivery is still a problem. Preterm babies are at particular risk. Because of their small size they pass rapidly through the pelvis with little time for the skull to mould; the brain is only semi-solid and easily contused, with tearing of its septa such as the falx cerebri or tentorium cerebelli and resultant haemorrhage. The preterm blood vessels are also friable and easily torn. The advantages of caesarean section for many preterm deliveries have already been mentioned.

Bleeding may also result from hypoxia during delivery. Both trauma and hypoxia frequently coexist in a difficult labour. Venous distension or high blood pressure due to anoxia may be sufficient in itself to cause haemorrhage. There are often petechial haemorrhages throughout the brain or intraventricular haemorrhage.

Traumatic Cyanosis

Cyanosis is seen following difficult delivery, especially if the cord is tightly round the baby's neck. The appearance is frightening. The baby's face is bright blue or reddish-blue with petechial haemorrhages and ecchymoses. At first glance, the baby is thought to have cyanotic congenital heart disease, but closer inspection reveals no cyanosis below the neck and a pink tongue. Examination is otherwise normal. If you press on the face, the cyanosis does not fade. Parents need strong reassurance about the appearance of the baby and must be told that the bruising may take up to a few weeks to disappear completely. A watch should be kept for the development of jaundice as blood is reabsorbed.

Sometimes these babies have respiratory obstruction due to swelling so they need to be watched carefully in the first 24 hours. If the lips are very swollen the baby may need tube-feeding during this time.

Fat Necrosis

These areas of hard thickening occur under parts of the baby's skin that

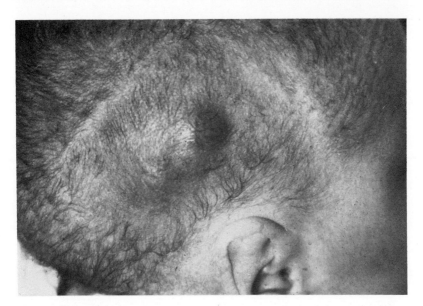

Fig. 11.1 Fat necrosis

have had pressure applied during delivery. They may occur over the mandible, in front of the ears, on the elbows or in the parietal regions (Fig. 11.1). Thus fat necrosis often follows forceps delivery, but may follow a normal delivery. Sometimes widespread fat necrosis is seen all down the extensor surfaces after asphyxia during delivery. Usually no treatment is necessary and explanation is all that is required. If large areas are involved they may become secondarily infected, requiring antibiotics. Occasionally, the parietal fat necrosis causes a discharging ulcer.

Cephalhaematoma

Bleeding between a skull bone and its outer covering (periosteum) is a common result of normal or complicated delivery and is due to mild shearing trauma (Fig. 11.2, see also Fig. 4.3). Most commonly one (or sometimes both) parietal bones are affected, rarely the frontal or occipital. The swelling is sharply limited by the suture lines which the blood is unable to cross. The swelling becomes visible as the moulding subsides and is a great source of worry to the mother. No attempt should be made to aspirate the haematoma because of the risk of introducing infection; it may take several weeks or even months to disappear and will meanwhile calcify

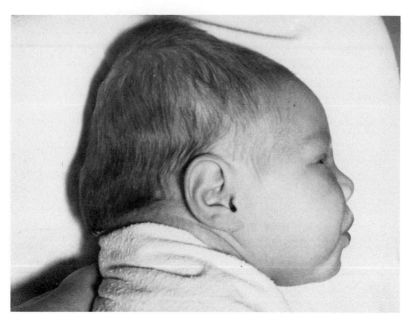

Fig. 11.2 Occipital and parietal cephalhaematoma

and go hard from the edge inwards, thus feeling like a depressed skull fracture after one to two weeks; the baby's head will later be a completely normal shape, but the baby may become jaundiced as blood is reabsorbed.

Subaponeurotic Haemorrhage

Unlike cephalhaematoma, which is common, subperiosteal and benign, subaponeurotic haemorrhage is rare and dangerous and extends widely into the areolar tissues of the scalp under the epicranial aponeurosis (the scalp). Babies particularly at risk include those born by ventouse extraction and African babies born by any means. It is possibly a manifestation of haemorrhagic disease of the newborn (see Chapter 13) but it does occur very early in life. Affected babies develop a boggy swelling of the scalp during the first two days of life with rapid onset of pallor, shock and subsequently, jaundice. The baby may lose a large part of his blood volume in this way. Treatment is by emergency blood transfusion (fresh frozen plasma may need to be given in the first instance) and intramuscular injection of 1 mg of vitamin K_1 to prevent further bleeding (vitamin

K dependent clotting factors II, VII, IX, X are low). The condition may be largely prevented by giving vitamin K_1 at birth to all babies following forceps or ventouse deliveries and all non-Caucasian babies. Many paediatricians feel that it is simpler and safer to treat *all* infants routinely with vitamin K_1 at birth. An oral dose of 1 mg is also effective.

Subdural Haemorrhage

Subdural haemorrhage is due to trauma and must be distinguished from intraventricular haemorrhage found in preterm babies who have been hypoxic. Subdural haemorrhage arises from a tear in the falx or tentorium, leading to rupture of and haemorrhage from the great cerebral vein (of Galen) or one of the other cerebral veins. The infant is often lethargic with apnoeic attacks, occasionally irritable and convulsing. The anterior fontanelle is often boggy or tense. Management is conservative with gentle handling, warmth, tube feeding and sedation if appropriate. The diagnosis may be confirmed by subdural tapping but often the haemorrhage is in the posterior fossa and may be missed. The value of therapeutic subdural taps is doubtful except in rare cases. The prognosis in those babies who survive the neonatal period is good, although some may be left with mental handicap or develop convulsions.

Nerve Injuries and Fractures

Depressed *skull fractures* are uncommon and are usually managed conservatively. Rarely, especially in breech delivery, there is associated intracranial bleeding with usually fatal results. Spinal cord injury is also uncommon.

Facial palsy (Fig. 11.3) is nearly always unilateral and may follow either forceps or, perhaps surprisingly, normal deliveries. When the baby cries the asymmetry is obvious, with the unaffected side drawn over. Often the lower lip alone is paralysed on one side. Sometimes, in addition, the baby may be unable to close the affected eye. In nearly all cases recovery is complete.

Brachial plexus nerve injuries are often associated with a fracture of the clavicle, but may occur independently. An upper plexus lesion (Erb's palsy) follows severe traction on the shoulders during breech delivery or may occur in large babies with shoulder dystocia; it results in an arm that hangs limply in pronation (waiter's tip position) and does not take part in the Moro reflex. Treatment is often unnecessary. It is probably not a good idea to pin the arm with the hand in supination alongside the

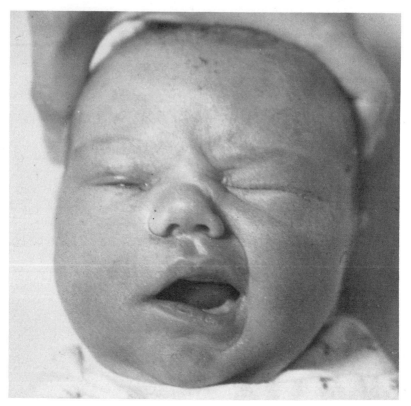

Fig. 11.3 Right facial palsy

infant's head because it is easy for someone to pick the baby up, forgetting the arm is pinned, and cause severe damage. Recovery usually takes place within a few weeks. Occasionally the phrenic nerve is damaged, producing unilateral diaphragmatic paralysis with dyspnoea and cyanosis.

Uncommonly, a lower brachial plexus lesion occurs (Klumpke's paralysis) with paralysis of the small hand muscles. It may be difficult to detect: there is loss of sensation on the inner forearm and medial three and a half fingers. Eventually there may be muscle wasting in the hand. It may be associated with damage to the cervical sympathetic nerves and Horner's syndrome (ipsilateral ptosis, enophthalmos and meiosis). The hand and forearm should be splinted in a cock-up position.

Radial nerve palsy may occur due to pressure on the nerve as it winds round the outer aspect of the elbow. An area of fat necrosis may overlie the nerve where it was compressed. A wrist drop may result and treatment is again by cock-up splint.

In the event of *fractures of the humerus or clavicle*, the baby does not move the affected arm and has an absent Moro reflex on that side. Crepitus may be felt over the bone. However, in many cases the result of the fracture is noticed only as a bump due to exuberant callus formation after a couple of weeks. Brachial plexus lesions may be associated. Usually no treatment is necessary, but splinting the arm with a tongue depressor sometimes relieves pain.

Fracture of the femur occurs rarely. Treatment is by gallows skin traction: suspending the baby's legs with strapping around the legs and ankles so that the buttocks are held just above the bed.

Sternomastoid Tumour

Occasionally a painless firm lump is noticed in the sternomastoid muscle on one or other side within a week or two of birth. No treatment is necessary. Torticollis is said to occur subsequently, but this is rare. For this reason physiotherapy (passive exercise) is sometimes given. The aetiology of the condition is unclear. However, it seems not to be due to traumatic haemorrhage as was once supposed.

—12—

Jaundice

In the 1970 British Births survey, about one in five newborn babies developed jaundice. At present about 15% have a peak plasma bilirubin over 200 μmol/l. To know why newborn babies become jaundiced and the particular importance of jaundice in the newborn, one must understand how bilirubin is formed and excreted from the body.

Bilirubin Metabolism

Haemoglobin is a constituent of red blood cells. Its most vital function is

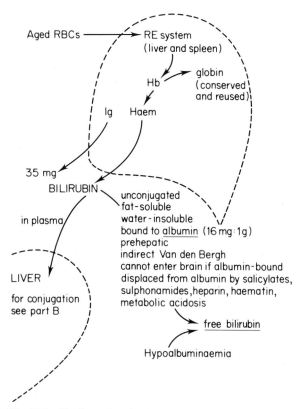

Fig. 12.1a The formation of bilirubin

the transport of oxygen to the tissues. Red cells have a life-span of 80–100 days in the neonate, compared to 120 days in the adult. At the end of their life the enzyme systems start to run down, and these aged cells are removed from the circulation by the reticuloendothelial (RE) system (specifically the liver and spleen). The contained haemoglobin is broken down into its two parts: globin, a protein which is conserved and utilized by the body; and haem, which cannot be reused and is degraded by a number of steps until it is excreted (Fig. 12.1). Bilirubin is a product of this degradation and its accumulation in the blood causes yellow staining of the skin and other tissues, thereby producing jaundice.

The first step in the conversion of haemoglobin (Fig. 12.1A) also takes place in the reticuloendothelial system and forms bilirubin (35 mg from each gram of Hb) which is fat-soluble and water-insoluble; it therefore

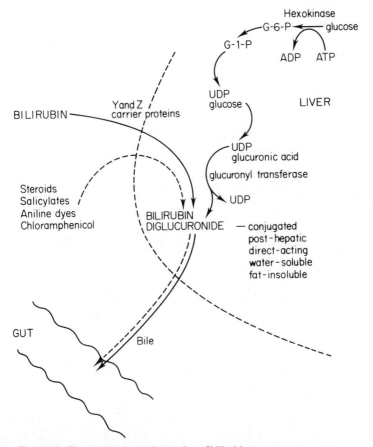

Fig. 12.1b The conjugation and excretion of bilirubin

cannot be excreted in bile or urine, but has a high affinity for fatty tissue and the brain. It does not travel free in plasma but is bound to the small protein albumin (16 mg bilirubin to 1 g albumin). It is also known as pre-hepatic, unconjugated or indirect-reacting bilirubin as it has not yet been conjugated in the liver and does not react directly with van den Bergh's reagent (a useful laboratory test) but has first to be split from its albumin. It travels bound to albumin in the plasma to the liver. Albumin-bound bilirubin cannot leave the blood and enter the brain. If there is too much unconjugated bilirubin in the plasma to be bound by albumin (i.e. the albumin-binding capacity of the plasma is exceeded), it may spill over into the brain and other tissues. In full-term infants this does not usually occur at serum bilirubin levels under 340 μmol/l unless there is present a substance which displaces bilirubin from albumin (e.g. drugs such as salicylates, sulphonamides, heparin, haematin formed during haemolysis, or the baby has a metabolic acidosis or hypoalbumin-aemia). Large amounts of bilirubin must be dealt with by the neonate's liver because during the early days of life there is a high rate of red cell destruction. This is related firstly to the shorter life of neonatal red cells and secondly to the high fetal and neonatal haemoglobin levels (18–19 g/dl) enabling the fetus to maintain an oxyhaemoglobin of 11 g/dl (see Chapter 5, the early anaemia of the preterm baby). Clearly, therefore, there will be a high bilirubin load to excrete. Late clamping of the cord leading to placental transfusion may exacerbate the problem.

The albumin-bound bilirubin enters the liver cells (Fig. 12.1B) with the aid of two carrier proteins, Y and Z. Once in the cell, the molecule is converted by a series of enzyme reactions which require glucose and oxygen to form the bilirubin diglucuronide. This last step, conjugation, is catalysed by the enzyme glucuronyl transferase. Bilirubin diglucur-onide is thus known as conjungated, post-hepatic or direct-acting bili-rubin (as it reacts directly with the van den Bergh reagent). Other substances are excreted by the same pathway as bilirubin (Fig. 12.1B) and should not be given to the newborn baby, e.g. steroids, salicylates, aniline dyes in nappies and chloramphenicol (chloramphenicol may need to be used if the baby has meningitis). Thus hypoxia or hypoglycaemia in the perinatal period may compromise bilirubin conjugation. Bilirubin diglucuronide is water-soluble and fat-insoluble. It cannot therefore enter the brain and cause damage. It is excreted via the bile into the gut and, being water-soluble, can also be excreted in the urine.

The capacity of a normal newborn baby to excrete a given bilirubin load is only about one-fiftieth of that of an adult. In the fetus the bilirubin is excreted across the placenta in unconjugated form and conjugated bilirubin does not cross. At birth, therefore, a change to a new mechan-ism is necessary. This helps to explain why so many normal babies become jaundiced. The preterm baby is even more likely to become jaundiced (see Chapter 5). Reasons include a relative glucuronyl transferase deficiency in the neonate's 'immature' liver, deficiencies in the Y and Z carrier proteins, and the strain of a high bilirubin load to excrete. It is probably incorrect to look upon immaturity as the cause of jaundice however. It is more logical to think of the preterm baby as not expecting to have to change his mechanism of bilirubin excretion so soon.

All babies, therefore, have hyperbilirubinaemia by adult standards, and in many normal babies frank jaundice appears (for this to occur plasma bilirubin levels must exceed 80 μmol/l in Caucasian infants). Jaundice usually reaches a maximum at three to six days.

Jaundice requires further investigation and possibly treatment when:
1 jaundice appears during the first 24 hours of life
2 jaundice persists after two weeks of age
3 the bilirubin level is above 250 μmol/l
4 there is a conjugated hyperbilirubinaemia (above 30 μmol/l)
5 jaundice is present in an ill baby.

In all these situations, medical advice should be sought without delay and the baby examined and investigated.

Table 12.1 Some important causes of jaundice.

Pre-hepatic	Hepatic	Post-hepatic
Unconjugated bilirubin	**Unconjugated bilirubin**	**Mixed conjugated and unconjugated bilirubin**
Haemolytic disorders	Breast milk jaundice	*Extrahepatic obstruction*
Rhesus isoimmunization	Congenital hypothyroidism	Congenital biliary atresia
ABO incompatibility	Hereditary glucuronyl	Choledochal cyst
Red cell enzyme defects	transferase deficiency	Bile plug syndrome
(e.g. glucose-6-phosphate		
dehydrogenase deficiency	**Mixed conjugated and**	
and pyruvate kinase	**unconjugated bilirubin**	**Unconjugated bilirubin**
deficiency)	*Inborn errors of metabolism*	*Increased enterohepatic*
Hereditary spherocytosis	Cystic fibrosis	*circulation*
	Galactosaemia	Paralytic ileus
Infections	Tyrosinaemia	High intestinal obstruction
Septicaemia	Alpha-l-antitrypsin	(e.g. pyloric stenosis,
Urinary tract infections	deficiency	duodenal atresia)
Meningitis	Fructosaemia	
Bruising, haematomas	*Hepatitis*	
Cephalhaematoma	Rubella	
Bruising during breech	Cytomegalovirus	
delivery	Toxoplasmosis	
	Herpes simplex	
Polycythaemia	Syphilis	
Twin transfusion syndrome	Hepatitis B	
Maternofetal transfusion	Listeriosis	
Delayed clamping of cord	Coxsackie virus	
Infants of diabetic mothers		

Table 12.2 Drugs and metabolic factors that increase the danger of neonatal jaundice.

Drugs that compete for albumin-binding sites
Sulphonamides
Salicylates
Heparin
Intravenous diazepam (the sodium benzoate carrier rather than the drug itself)

Reduced bilirubin binding capacity results from
Drugs, as above
Haematin (derived from haemolysis)
Acidosis
Hypoxia
Hypoglycaemia
Low albumin levels (preterm babies)

Drugs interfering with glucuronyl transferase
Novobiocin

Causes of Jaundice

The possible causes of neonatal jaundice classified according to aetiology are listed in Tables 12.1 and 12.2. Some of these conditions are discussed in detail below.

Apart from the physiological jaundice of many newborn babies (described above), the most important common causes of jaundice are:
1 *Red cell incompatibility*, usually due to either rhesus haemolytic disease or ABO incompatibility, where jaundice usually appears within the first 24 hours.
2 *Infections*, usually urinary tract or septicaemia, which seldom cause jaundice in the first 72 hours.
3 *Breast milk*. At one time this was thought to be the result of a steroid in breast milk. It seems more likely that the milk contains an enzyme, which split conjugated bilirubin in the gut. Therefore, unconjugated bilirubin is absorbed leading to jaundice. Jaundice due to breast milk is never a reason for stopping breast feeding (see below).

There are a number of rarer causes of jaundice which it may be important to exclude. Some, such as hypothyroidism, galactosaemia, bile duct atresia or viral hepatitis, cause prolonged jaundice (see below).

Investigation of Jaundice

Bilirubin estimation

All babies who appear more than mildly jaundiced should have a plasma bilirubin estimation: this means a full-term baby whose bilirubin looks more than 170 μmol/l by clinical estimation or any jaundiced preterm baby. Any baby who appears jaundiced during the first 24 hours of life must have an urgent bilirubin estimation.

Estimation of conjugated bilirubin

This must be done at least once during the course of jaundice in any baby who needs bilirubin estimations. If the conjugated bilirubin is more than 30 μmol/l a search should be made for the cause. The most important causes are rhesus incompatibility, congenital bile duct obstruction, $α_1$-antitrypsin deficiency, cystic fibrosis, intrauterine viral infection or an inborn metabolic error such as galactosaemia.

Mother's blood group and tests for antibodies or haemolysins

The mother's notes must always be reviewed to ensure that a rhesus problem has not been overlooked. The tests are done as a routine during the antenatal period, but may have been missed if the mother booked very late.

Baby's blood group and Coombs' test in albumin and saline

These tests should be done by the laboratory on any baby who is jaundiced.

Baby's haemoglobin

This should also be checked on any jaundiced baby—if jaundice is due to haemolysis the baby may become anaemic.

Additional tests

Additional tests may be needed if there are clinical indications or if the bilirubin level is more than about 250 μmol/l and otherwise unexplained.

Check the notes to see if there is a possible cause for jaundice such as *cephalhaematoma, bruising* or a *preterm* or *difficult delivery*. Make certain the laboratory have looked for spherocytes and done a *reticulocyte count*. Ask about a family history of spherocytosis. A reticulocyte count of more than 10% in the absence of blood group incompatibility should be repeated at one week and, if still more than 10%, should be investigated to be certain that there is no inherited haemolytic anaemia, for example pyruvate kinase deficiency.

Glucose-6-phosphate dehydrogenase (G-6-PD) assay should be requested for any baby with a bilirubin over 200 μmol/l whose parents originated from southern Europe, Asia or Africa. The assay should be done on any child whose mother is believed to be a carrier for G-6-PD deficiency or on any girl whose father has the condition.

Reducing substances in the urine should be tested to exclude galactos-aemia. If a reducing substance is present, arrange sugar chromatography.

Urine culture can be taken by suprapubic aspiration or from a clean catch specimen. *Blood culture* or *lumbar puncture* might be necessary in some cases where infection is suspected. *Swabs* from obviously infected areas are valuable, as is an ear swab after prolonged rupture of membranes. Routine swabbing is not helpful as it can provide evidence only of colonization rather than infection.

IgM and cytomegalovirus (CMV), toxoplasma and rubella antibody titres should be estimated. A raised IgM (especially in cord blood) is valuable evidence of intrauterine infection. Jaundice, especially in a small-for-dates infant with other stigmata, may be due to CMV, toxoplasmosis or congenital rubella.

T_4 *and TSH* estimations will exclude hypothyroidism (see below).

Albumin binding of bilirubin (ABB) may be measured. Unconjugated bilirubin is carried in the blood bound to albumin. When all the binding sites are saturated, the amount of free bilirubin increases and it is thought that kernicterus then occurs. If we could estimate the bilirubin level at which a baby's albumin were saturated, it would be possible to plan individual treatment for jaundice instead of relying on bilirubin levels. Unfortunately the present methods are complex and require several millilitres of blood; therefore the estimation cannot be done routinely. ABB measurements are available in certain specialist units; in some situations, e.g. cord blood from a rhesus baby or at the beginning of an exchange transfusion, they are particularly useful.

Persistent jaundice

Bilirubin levels above 150 μmol/l at two weeks of age should be investigated. It is important to determine whether the bilirubin is conjugated or unconjugated, as ordinary physiological jaundice may otherwise merge unnoticed into obstructive jaundice. The investigation of prolonged jaundice must include looking for evidence of intrauterine infection and of galactosaemia and haemolysis. Primary hypothyroidism will now be detected as it is routinely screened for in the United Kingdom. Check that the Guthrie test has been done and the TSH level is not raised (see Chapter 4). A not-infrequent cause of prolonged jaundice seems to be breast feeding. It is likely that some mothers excrete an enzyme in their milk which unconjugates bilirubin in the gut. It is, of course, important to exclude the other serious causes listed above before making this diagnosis. Breast milk jaundice is generally harmless and is emphatically *not* a reason for stopping breast feeding.

Management of Jaundice

General measures

There is good evidence that early feeding after birth will reduce the prevalence of jaundice. The feed chart should be checked; if there is any indication that the baby has not had enough feeds—marked loss of weight, high packed cell volume, signs of dehydration or poor milk intake—adequate feeds should be given. The baby can be put to the breast frequently or given three-hourly bottle feeds. There is no evidence that supplementing breast feeding with water or dextrose solutions will prevent jaundice appearing or make it disappear quicker. It could decrease the success of breast feeding by undermining the mother's confidence and reducing the amount of suckling. Jaundice appearing in the first 24 hours is due to blood group incompatibility until proved otherwise and requires urgent investigation. An infection should be treated vigorously with antibiotics.

Plotting the level of jaundice

All babies with rhesus disease, jaundice in the first 24 hours or a plasma bilirubin over 300 μmol/l should have a bilirubin chart (Fig. 12.2). A horizontal line should be drawn on the chart at the plasma bilirubin which would be an indication for exchange transfusion (ET) in that baby, because of a danger of kernicterus (see below). Depending on the rate of rise, which is linear, you can decide when to do another bilirubin estimation or whether to do an ET. Remember that it generally takes about three hours to organize an exchange.

Techniques for lowering plasma bilirubin levels

In cases where bilirubin levels are rising rapidly or are already dangerously high, exchange transfusion is the treatment of choice (see below). In less urgent situations other techniques for lowering serum bilirubin have been employed.

Phenobarbitone

Phenobarbitone is metabolized by the liver. Its metabolism causes induction of many liver enzymes, including glucuronyl transferase essential for the conjugation of bilirubin. There is good evidence that phenobarbitone given to mothers from the 32nd week of pregnancy will result in infants who are less jaundiced. However, the development of severe neonatal jaundice is often not predictable, so that this is of little practical value. Treating the newborn baby with phenobarbitone from

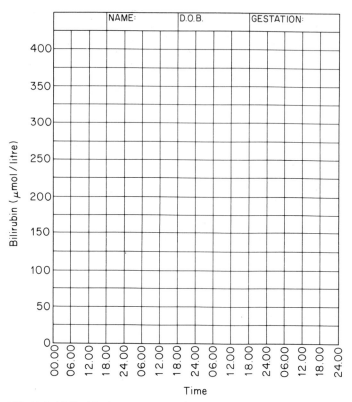

Fig. 12.2 A bilirubin chart

birth will reduce the bilirubin level at four days or later, but we do not recommend it as it makes the baby very sleepy and more effective techniques are now available.

Phototherapy

The chance observation in the pathology laboratory at Rochford Hospital, Essex, that jaundiced serum left in sunlight over the lunch hour was considerably paler led to the placing of babies in sunlight to reduce their jaundice; this was successful. It was found subsequently that the bilirubin molecule maximally absorbs light of wavelength 450 nm (the visible blue part of the spectrum) and in so doing is broken down to a number of non-toxic photodegradation products which the baby can easily excrete. It is possible that the light also has an effect on the excretion of bilirubin by the liver. In practice, blue light is not often used since it makes all babies look cyanosed and this prevents the recognition of cyanosis in a sick baby. Fluorescent lights have a high output at the visible blue part of the spectrum while giving the infant a relatively normal skin appearance. They are readily available commercially.

There is good evidence that phototherapy is effective in reducing jaundice (or slowing the rate of worsening in severely affected babies) by breaking down bilirubin in the skin and skin capillaries. There are side-effects, but these are not usually very serious: skin rashes and loose green stools (due to the excretion of biliverdin and other photodegradation products) are common. Because of the additional water lost in this way and through the skin, an extra fluid intake of 30 ml/kg/day should be given. Extra calories are needed to counteract intestinal hurry. Weight, urine output and osmolality or specific gravity should be checked and the fluid intake further increased if necessary. Conventionally, infants' eyes are protected during treatment although there is no good evidence that damage would otherwise occur—retinal damage has been reported in animals. It is important to explain phototherapy to mothers and warn them that their baby's eyes will be covered, otherwise needless anxiety will be caused. Phototherapy must not be used as an excuse for separating mother and baby; the phototherapy machine should be used alongside the mother's bed. She should feed and cuddle the baby in the normal way. It has recently been found that it is as effective to give phototherapy intermittently (say one hour in three) and this reduces the incidence and severity of side-effects. The baby's temperature should be recorded every 3–4 hours (small babies could become hypothermic without a heat shield; big babies could overheat unless the incubator thermostat is turned down to minimum or off altogether). The baby should be nursed naked and turned at intervals to allow maximal skin exposure to the light.

Any baby whose jaundice is not being adequately controlled by phototherapy will need an exchange transfusion. However, the use of phototherapy has reduced the frequency with which exchange transfusion need be performed. Our criteria for the use of phototherapy would be a bilirubin of 340 μmol/l in a term baby, with correspondingly lower thresholds in preterm, small-for-dates or sick infants, e.g. 150–180 μmol/l at 28 weeks and 200–240 μmol/l at 34 weeks gestation. It is sensible to treat rhesus babies with phototherapy from birth and it could also be used early for a preterm baby with bruising or any baby in an incubator.

Intravenous albumin

It may sometimes be useful to give a baby an intravenous albumin transfusion, especially if there is a delay in obtaining blood for exchange transfusion. It reduces the likelihood of kernicterus by increasing the bilirubin-binding capacity of the blood. It is confusing because its use *increases* the plasma bilirubin level as conventionally measured, although the baby is safer.

Exchange transfusion (ET)

Indications. Estimate the danger level for kernicterus in the baby. The following are reasonable guidelines:

Gestation	Bilirubin (μmol/l)
39 weeks or more	380
35–38 weeks	350
31–34 weeks	280
30 weeks or less	240

The danger level may be lower if the baby is ill, is very acidaemic or has had a drug which competes with bilirubin for the albumin binding sites (see Table 12.2). Some other units use lower values because this will prevent kernicterus found at autopsy but there is no good evidence that lower values must be taken in order to prevent clinical kernicterus; indeed some would think these criteria overcautious. The indications in haemolytic disease are shown in Table 12.3.

Technique. Exchange transfusion is usually done in the special care baby

Table 12.3 The management at birth of haemolytic disease (HDN).

Hb (g/dl)	Coombs'	Diagnosis	Procedure
Above 15	Negative	Unaffected	None
Below 15	Negative	Fetal haemorrhage	May need simple transfusion
14–16	+	Mild HDN	May need phototherapy. May need simple transfusion later
12–14	++	Moderate HDN	Phototherapy. Exchange transfusion if jaundice appears in first 24 hours and if bilirubin rises more than 80 μmol/l in 12 hours
7–11	++	Severe HDN	Early exchange transfusion. Phototherapy
Under 7	+/−	Hydrops	Immediate venesection to reduce venous pressure followed by extended controlled replacement with packed blood; treatment of cardiac failure and respiratory support

unit. Exceptions include the infected baby or the hydropic infant requiring urgent transfusion in the labour ward. In most cases the need for exchange can be anticipated in good time to order fresh blood (see below), obtain a warm incubator or an overhead heater and set up the necessary equipment for monitoring ECG, temperature and blood pressure. Sterile techniques must be used. The baby must be kept warm and relatively immobile; it is convenient to restrain the hands and feet. Before starting, the baby's stomach should be emptied and a nasogastric tube left in place.

The umbilical cord is cut transversely about 1 cm from the skin. It is then usually an easy matter to insert into the single vein a 5 French or 8 French gauge catheter. The catheter is advanced until blood comes back (about 10 cm) (but see Fig. 12.3). It is convenient to use the cannulae in commercial exchange transfusion packs which also contain sterile disposable giving sets, tubing, waste bag, four-way tap and Luer-lock syringes.

Blood is always first removed from the baby before the same volume is transfused. In this way the baby's blood volume is always normal or 10–20 ml below normal (which is safer than being too high). In most babies 10 ml aliquots are used. In babies weighing 3 kg or more 20 ml aliquots may be used but 5 ml aliquots should be used for very small or sick babies. Donor blood should be Rh-negative and preferably of the same ABO group as the baby's (O rhesus-negative in extreme emergencies). It is best that it is fresh (less than two days old) because the intrinsic rate of haemolysis is then less, and also the plasma potassium concentration is normal. It should be compatible with the mother's serum. The

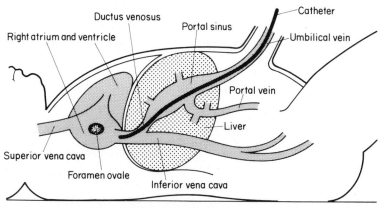

Fig. 12.3 The umbilical vein and its connections in the neonate. The position of the umbilical venous catheter is shown. Note how easy it would be to push it accidentally into the right atrium. From S. Wallis & D. Harvey (1979) *Nursing Times*, by permission of the authors and editor

total volume of blood exchanged is 180 ml/kg body weight. Partially packed blood (semi-concentrated red cells) should be used. The procedure is summarized in Fig. 12.4 and Tables 12.4 and 12.5.

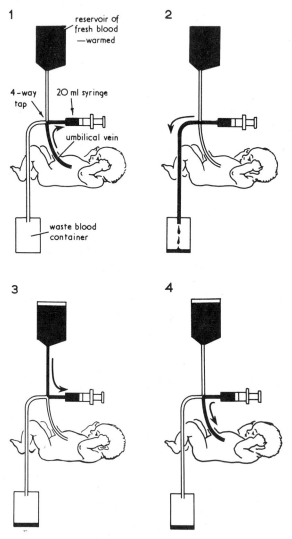

Fig. 12.4 Exchange transfusion. 1, Blood is drawn out into a syringe via an umbilical vein catheter. 2, This blood is discarded into a waste container. 3, Fresh blood warmed to body temperature is drawn into the syringe. The blood is cross-matched for compatibility with blood from the baby's mother. 4, This blood is injected slowly. The process is repeated until twice the baby's blood volume has been exchanged. From S. Wallis & D. Harvey (1979) *Nursing Times*, by permission of the authors and editor

Table 12.4 Exchange transfusion: materials and technique.

Materials needed

'Pharmaseal' exchange transfusion tray

Cut-down pack

Gown and gloves

Ampoule of normal saline

Fine silk sutures on a cutting needle

Chlorhexidine in spirit

Antibiotic spray

Large scalpel blade and handle

Blood warmer and blood warming coil

Blood bottles

Sequestrene × 2

Heparin 2 ml × 2

Blood culture bottles × 2

Technique

1 Place baby on Resuscitaire under heat-shield; connect skin temperature probe and turn to servo control; connect ECG monitor; gently restrain the limbs
2 Put on a gown, prepare tray, prime a suitable venous catheter with saline
3 Run the blood through the giving set. This is connected to the warming coil which in turn is attached to a four-way tap
4 Clean the umbilicus and cord clamp with chlorhexidine in spirit
5 Insert purse-string suture around base of cord (avoiding blood vessels and not piercing skin)
6 Cut cleanly through cord 1 cm above skin with a single slice of the scalpel blade. Pinch base to prevent blood loss
7 Identify vein and dilate gently
8 Insert the venous catheter. Stop as soon as there is a free flow of blood back from the vein
9 Tie the catheter to the purse-string suture to prevent it falling out

Table 12.5 Exchange transfusion – method.

1 Slowly withdraw 20 ml blood from the baby (less in a preterm baby). The nurse records 20 ml 'blood out' on sheet; send examples for pre-exchange haemoglobin, plasma urea and electrolytes, calcium, bilirubin, sugar and blood culture
2 Draw up 10 ml (see text) of fresh blood and inject slowly into the baby, watching ECG monitor and baby's condition. The nurse records '10 ml in' on sheet
3 Continue to exchange 10 ml blood at a time: the four-way tap is designed so that if properly connected you continue to turn it clockwise (from baby to waste to fresh blood and back to baby). Keep the baby in at least 10 ml deficit throughout. Each cycle should take about three minutes, depending on the baby's condition
4 At the end of the exchange send samples of the last 'blood out' for post-exchange haemoglobin, plasma urea and electrolytes, calcium, bilirubin, blood culture and sugar. Then slowly restore the deficit until the total 'blood in' equals the total 'blood out'
5 Check the post-exchange bilirubin *before* removing the catheter: it may be necessary to continue the exchange transfusion
6 Check the blood gases and correct a severe metabolic acidaemia if necessary with intravenous sodium bicarbonate
7 Remove the catheter. Send the tip for culture. Pinch the base of the cord until there is no further bleeding. Put a *small* sterile gauze dressing on the umbilicus in such a way that any bleeding will be apparent. It is best to avoid stitching the stump unless *really* necessary

The purpose of the exchange is:
1 to correct anaemia
2 to remove damaged and antibody-coated red cells
3 to remove unfixed antibody and
4 to remove bilirubin from plasma and tissues

Dangers include:
1 Haemorrhage from disconnected tubing.
2 Thrombosis or embolism due to air or clots.
3 Infection leading to septicaemia.
4 Hypocalcaemia. This is because citrate is used to preserve blood. It binds calcium, thus lowering the amount of ionized calcium in the blood. In spite of this, calcium measured in the usual way will be normal. Some doctors inject 1 ml of 10% calcium gluconate intravenously after every 100 ml of blood exchanged.
5 Hyperkalaemia is not a problem with fresh blood, but potassium leaks out of *old* red cells into the plasma.
6 Hypothermia. Infused blood should be warmed by passage through a heating coil in a water bath or preferably a proper blood warmer at body temperature. It is important to do the procedure under a heater.
7 Cardiac arrhythmias associated with electrolyte disturbances or rapid injection or withdrawal of blood.
8 Hypoglycaemia.
9 Trauma or perforation of the umbilical vein at insertion of catheter.
10 Late portal hypertension due to venous thrombosis.

To help prevent some of these problems, blood is taken from the first withdrawn syringeful and checked for Hb, PCV, urea and electrolytes, calcium, sugar and bilirubin. Bilirubin estimation is repeated at the halfway stage and the full investigations repeated at the end.

A complete cycle takes place as follows: 5, 10 or 20 ml of blood is slowly and gradually withdrawn from the baby; the syringe and four-way tap to which it is attached is turned through 90° clockwise so that the portal to the waste bag is open and the blood is rapidly ejected; the syringe is then turned clockwise through a further 90° and the same volume of donor blood is rapidly drawn up. The syringe is then turned clockwise through 180° and the donor blood slowly injected into the baby. The cycle is then repeated (see Table 12.5). The slower the exchange the more efficient the mixing of bloods and the more effective the procedure. For this reason, and to avoid cardiovascular disturbance, blood must be withdrawn from and injected into the baby slowly. It is useful to pause after injection and before withdrawal to allow further equilibration to take place. In practice, each cycle should take about three minutes.

Obviously, the earlier part of the exchange is more effective than later, by which time a high proportion of donor blood is being re-exchanged. There should therefore be no hesitation in stopping an exchange either temporarily or permanently if there is deterioration in the baby's condition.

Indications for stopping are:
1 heart rate less than 100 or more than 180/min
2 cyanosis
3 arrhythmias
4 obvious discomfort.

At least one assistant is required: a nurse who will monitor the baby's temperature, pulse rate and general condition during each cycle, and keep a 'score' of volumes withdrawn and infused. After each withdrawal or infusion the operator calls, for example, '10 out' or '10 in'. The nurse totals these volumes as the exchange proceeds and is able to correct the doctor if there is confusion as to whether blood is due to be withdrawn or infused next. Such mix-ups are made less likely by the syringe always having to be turned clockwise, but it is easy to lose concentration during such a repetitive procedure. A bilirubin estimation should always be done two to four hours after an ET to be certain that the bilirubin has not risen above the exchange indication level again, as in severely affected babies more than one exchange is sometimes necessary. As with the first exchange this is decided on the rate of rise of bilirubin and total bilirubin level. However, there is always a sudden rapid rise after ET and so the rate of rise from the post-exchange specimen to one a few hours later is not a good indication of the subsequent rate of rise. We have seen babies who needed eight exchange transfusions in all. Subsequently, exchanged babies may become anaemic as transfusion may cause red cell production to be depressed for some weeks. Following exchange transfusion the baby should be monitored carefully for at least four hours in case of arrhythmias or hypoglycaemia. Babies who have had an exchange transfusion must have their haemoglobin levels checked weekly in the outpatient department and a simple top-up transfusion may be necessary.

The emergency treatment of hydrops fetalis by exchange transfusion is described in Chapter 3.

Conditions causing Jaundice

Some conditions causing jaundice will now be discussed in greater detail.

Haemolytic disease

Excess haemolysis in the neonatal period may result from incompatibility between fetal and maternal blood groups. The incidence of the different types of disease varies in different parts of the world. In Britain, Rhesus incompatibility is common but becoming less so now that it can be prevented and ABO incompatibility is common, but often mild. G-6-PD deficiency (an inherited red cell enzyme abnormality) is common in many parts of the world, for example east Asia and Greece.

Rhesus incompatibility

Approximately 85% of Caucasians carry Rh antigen on their red cells and are therefore Rh+. The remainder have no Rh antigen and are therefore Rh−. If a Rh− mother gives birth to a Rh+ baby (the antigen coming from the Rh+ father), and if their ABO groups are similar, Rh+ fetal cells entering the mother's circulation during late pregnancy or parturition may sensitize her. She responds by forming Rh antibodies. When she is next pregnant with an Rh+ baby these antibodies, which are IgG immunoglobulins, are able to cross the placenta. They do so and destroy the fetal red cells. Initial sensitization usually occurs in this way but may occur during a miscarriage or if a Rh− woman is inadvertently transfused with Rh− incompatible (Rh+) blood.

In fact there are three pairs of Rh genes, C, D and E. D is the most important and Rh+ means D+. A father may be Rh− or Rh+. If Rh+, he may be heterozygous (Dd) or homozygous (DD). If homozygous, all his children will be D+; if heterozygous, only half of them will be D+ and therefore at risk. Among Caucasians, one marriage in seven is between a Rh− woman and a Rh+ man, but only six babies in every 1000 born are affected by Rh disease. This is probably because many spouses are of unlike groups in the ABO system. This means that fetal red cells entering the maternal circulation are destroyed by naturally occurring haemolysins in the mother's blood, because of their ABO incompatibility with the mother, before they can cause sensitization. The disease is rare in east Asia because almost all the population are D+.

Problems can occasionally occur in D− women who have the C or E Rhesus antigen. On routine testing they are Rh− but sensitization may occur and may be all the more serious because diagnosis is delayed. C− incompatibility can be severe; E incompatibility is usually mild.

Fetuses are affected to different degrees depending on the strength of the maternal antibody response. Accordingly, there are different modes of presentation. In the most severe cases there is marked haemolysis in utero with fetal anaemia, cardiac failure and oedema. The liver and spleen, which are sites of fetal erythropoiesis, are considerably enlarged. Such babies are often stillborn or occasionally born prematurely with the signs of hydrops fetalis: pallor, gross oedema and hepatosplenomegaly. (The term hydrops is derived from the Greek *hydor* meaning water, and was used by Celsus in AD 30). The prognosis is poor and immediate exchange transfusion (see above) provides the only chance of survival. The emergency treatment of hydrops fetalis in the labour ward is discussed in Chapter 3. Less severely affected babies look normal at birth, although liver and spleen may be palpable. However, within a few hours of birth they become clinically jaundiced with increasingly high levels of unconjugated bilirubin.

Management. This is also summarized in Table 12.6.

Prevention is important. Red cells from the original Rh+ fetus which sensitizes the Rh− mother usually cross the placenta during labour or at birth and Rh antibodies take several weeks to develop. Sensitization is more likely if there has been an antepartum haemorrhage or in cases of retained placenta requiring manual removal. Antibody formation can be prevented if an intramuscular injection of 100 µg of anti-D immunoglobulin is given soon after the birth or miscarriage of a Rh+ fetus in order to destroy the Rh+ red cells. Thus, anti-D antibody both causes the illness and provides a means of preventing it.

Before delivery all pregnant women must have their ABO and Rh blood groups determined early in pregnancy. If they are Rh−, their blood should be checked regularly throughout pregnancy for Rh antibodies. A rising antibody titre suggests that the fetus is Rh+ and is being increasingly affected.

If the Coombs' antibody titre rises above 1 : 8 the severity of the disease may also be monitored using a technique developed by Liley. Amniotic fluid is obtained at amniocentesis by the 28th week of pregnancy and is examined spectrophotometrically. The bilirubin molecule absorbs light maximally if the light has a wavelength of 450 nm (this absorption is the optical density of bilirubin). If the optical density of normal bilirubin-free liquor is plotted on a logarithmic scale against wavelength, a straight line is obtained (Fig. 12.5). However, in the presence of bilirubin there is a 'hump' in the graph at 450 nm. The size

Table 12.6 Management of Rh disease.

1 Do Rh and ABO grouping at booking
2 If Rh-negative, measure Rh antibody titre and repeat throughout pregnancy
3 Check father's genotype if antibodies are present to see if he is homozygous or heterozygous
4 Amniocentesis by 20 weeks gestation if Coombs' antibody titre greater than 1:16. Spectrophotometry; repeat as indicated
5 Intrauterine transfusion, preterm elective delivery, exchange transfusion as indicated
6 *At birth.* Give 100 µg anti-D immunoglobulin intramuscularly to immunized Rh-negative mother within 48 hours of birth, miscarriage or abortion of a Rh-positive infant. Do Kleihauer test and give larger dose if there is a lot of fetal blood in the mother's circulation

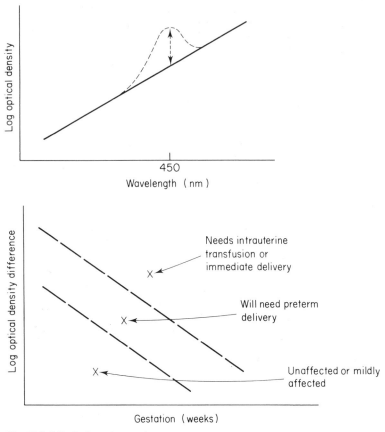

Fig. 12.5 Liley's charts (see text)

(vertical height) of the hump is proportional to the amount of bilirubin in the liquor and this indicates the severity of the disease. By plotting this difference in optical density logarithmically against the gestational age of the fetus, Liley was able to determine how the pregnancy should be managed. He divided the graph into three zones. In the lower zone are mildly affected babies who may be allowed to go to term. In the middle are babies with moderately severe disease. The amniocentesis may be repeated at intervals to provide further guidance.

The moderately affected babies should be delivered at an optimal time which is a compromise between the complications and risks of preterm delivery, on the one hand, and those of haemolytic disease on the other. The usual time for delivery is between 34 and 37 weeks.

Severely affected babies may be delivered electively very early (28–33 weeks gestation) but the combination of haemolytic disease with extreme prematurity has a high morbidity and mortality. An alternative is to transfuse these babies in utero with Rh− blood compatible with that of the mother. This is possible because red cells are rapidly absorbed from the fetal peritoneal cavity. A cannula, aimed under radiographic control or ultrasonic screening, may be directed through the fetal abdominal wall and blood is then injected. The transfusion temporarily corrects fetal anaemia by providing Rh− red cells which are not haemolysed. It may have to be repeated several times before delivery. No controlled trial of its effectiveness has been carried out, however, and there is still some doubt as to its value in reducing mortality. This is because the technique carries a risk for the fetus, particularly fetal bleeding which may result in intrauterine death. However, babies born alive are much less likely to be anaemic and have a better prognosis.

At birth, clamp the cord at once and cut it 5 cm (2 in) from the umbilicus. Collect cord blood and arrange tests for blood group, direct Coombs' antiglobulin test (to detect the presence of antibody on the baby's red cells), bilirubin concentration, haemoglobin and packed cell volume. On the basis of these results a decision is made about further management (see Table 12.3). Mildly affected babies are placed under phototherapy (see above) and their bilirubin level checked four-hourly. Severely affected babies require early exchange transfusion. This is indicated if there is a strongly positive Coombs' test with either haemoglobin less than 12 g/dl or haemoglobin greater than 12 g/dl but cord bilirubin greater than 85 μmol/l.

It should be realized that a false-negative Coombs' test is found in some severely affected babies who have received several intrauterine transfusions. These babies' red cells have been largely replaced by transfused Rh− donor blood, hence the negative test result.

Phototherapy in a Rh-affected baby should be started at birth. There is good evidence that it will reduce the number of exchange transfusions. The rate of rise of bilirubin is observed carefully. As a rough guide, a rate of rise greater than 6 μmol/l/h means that exchange transfusion will be necessary. Plotting the bilirubin levels on a chart against time from birth provides a visual guide to the rate of rise. It is useful to choose a level which you think would be dangerous for the baby and to draw a line across the chart. You can then predict when the baby's bilirubin would cross the line and you take action in good time. Exchange transfusion is discussed above.

ABO incompatibility

ABO incompatibility is common but usually mild. It frequently presents with jaundice within 24 hours of birth. Any baby jaundiced at this time must have his blood group and Coombs' test checked. Classically the syndrome occurs in Group O mothers with Group A or B infants. Unlike in Rh disease, the Coombs' test is usually negative (although it may be positive in albumin), the anaemia is less severe and the antibodies that cause haemolysis occur naturally without previous sensitization. These antibodies are IgG immunoglobulins and are known as alpha- and beta-haemolysins. They are able to cross the placenta from mother to baby and destroy his group A or B cells respectively. They may be detected in maternal serum to confirm the diagnosis. Treatment is dependent on the rate of rise and absolute level of the serum indirect bilirubin and is either by phototherapy or by exchange transfusion as described above. Some mothers have haemolysins which are IgM immunoglobulins. These cannot cross the placenta and therefore do not cause haemolysis in the baby.

Glucose-6-phosphate dehydrogenase (G-6-PD) deficiency

G-6-PD is an important enzyme in red cells as well as in leucocytes and other cells. A deficiency of the enzyme makes the red cells liable to haemolyse in certain situations. It happens after taking some drugs (e.g. sulphonamides, primaquine, nitrofurantoin) or during an infection. Many African, West Indian and American Negroes have such an enzyme defect; it is also common among inhabitants of Mediterranean countries who in addition may haemolyse if they eat broad beans, a condition known as favism. The condition is inherited as a sex-linked recessive, like haemophilia. Thus males are usually affected while females are carriers. However, newborn babies who are G-6-PD-deficient may have spontaneous haemolysis (in the absence of any exogenous precipitating factor). In addition, newborn baby girls may be affected, although not usually as severely as boys.

G-6-PD deficiency is the commonest indication for exchange transfusion in the Far East. In Britain, it must be considered in the differential diagnosis of neonatal jaundice when treating babies of Oriental, Negro or Mediterranean stock. G-6-PD may be checked easily in most laboratories.

Treatment is as for other causes of haemolysis and exchange transfusion is often necessary.

Many drugs that cause haemolysis in susceptible patients are excreted in breast milk and a mother who is breast-feeding must take care to avoid them. Mothers should be warned not to store nappies or baby clothes with naphthalene mothballs as this substance will cause haemolysis following absorption through the skin. When the baby goes home, his mother should be given a list of drugs that he should avoid in the future and a copy should be sent to the family doctor with the discharge summary (Table 12.7). It is important to remember that babies with high reticulocyte counts may have falsely high G-6-PD levels as reticulocytes

Table 12.7 Drugs which may cause haemolysis in G6PD-deficient subjects.

Aminoquinolines (antimalarials) Primaquine Pamaquin Chloroquine Pentaquine	*Analgesics* Acetylsalicylic acid (aspirin) Phenacetin (Acetophenetidin) Acetanilid Paracetamol
Sulphones Dapsone Sulphoxone Thiazosulphone Diaminidiphenyl sulphone (DDS)	*Miscellaneous* Vitamin K (water-soluble analogues) Naphthalene (moth balls) Probenecid Dimercaprol (BAL) Methylene blue Acetylphenylhydrazine
Sulphonamides Sulphanilamide Sulphacetamide Sulphafurazole Sulphisozaxole Sulphamethoxypyridazine Salicylazosulphapyridine	Phenylhydrazine *p*-Aminosalicylic acid (PAS) Nalidixic acid Neoarsphenamine Quinine Quinidine Chloramphenicol Isoniazid
Nitrofurans Nitrofurantoin Furaxolodine Nitrofurazone	Trinitrotoluene Broad beans (*Fava*)

have more G-6-PD than mature red cells. Even normal babies may have reticulocyte counts of up to 7% on the first postnatal day, while babies who are haemolysing may have considerably more. In such babies with G-6-PD deficiency, blood taken during the early days of life may not exclude the diagnosis; blood taken later will show low G-6-PD levels.

Others

Congenital spherocytosis, a hereditary disease in which red cells are small and spherical rather than disc-shaped, may sometimes present in the newborn period. There is usually a family history of jaundice or gallstones. The neonatal jaundice which may result is generally mild but may need exchange transfusion.

Beta-thalassaemia hardly ever presents in the newborn as it is due to defective beta-chain haemoglobin production, and fetal haemoglobin (which makes up nearly all the baby's haemoglobin at birth) contains two alpha and two gamma (but no beta) chains. It is only when sufficient adult haemoglobin (alpha$_2$–beta$_2$) is produced during the second half of the first year of life that the condition may present.

In contrast, the less common *alpha-thalassaemia*, in which alpha chains are synthesized abnormally, produces abnormalities both in fetal life and later. If a fetus inherits the alpha-thalassaemia gene from both parents and is thus homozygous severe hydrops develops in utero. Its haemoglobin is made up entirely of gamma chains and is known as haemoglobin Bart's. Such babies often die in utero; a few reach term and may survive for a short time.

Obstructive jaundice

Obstructive jaundice is much less common than non-obstructive jaundice in the neonatal period. The differentiation between the two usual causes, hepatitis and biliary atresia, is frequently impossible without the use of special tests at specialist units, including the use of ultrasound and liver biopsy. Obstructive jaundice is characterized by a high level of conjugated bilirubin, pale stools and dark urine due to the presence of bile.

Biliary atresia

Biliary atresia may be either extrahepatic or intrahepatic (possibly secondary to hepatitis in some cases). Infants present with increasingly severe jaundice, which may, however, vary in intensity. The liver is enlarged and firm. Tests show that the bilirubin is conjugated and that the urine contains bilirubin but no urobilinogen. Distinction from hepatitis is often difficult. The prognosis is poor as only a small number prove to be operable. In the few infants in whom corrective surgery is possible it is important that the diagnosis is made before liver damage has taken place (by about two months of age).

Hepatitis

Hepatitis may be due to one of several organisms in the newborn, e.g. the viruses of hepatitis A and B, cytomegalovirus, herpes simplex, rubella or toxoplasmosis. Many of these are transplacentally acquired. In some cases the jaundice is part of a wider syndrome of disease more or less specific to the infecting organism. In the majority of cases, however, no cause is found. About 70% recover spontaneously. Results indicating severe hepatitis include markedly abnormal liver function tests. High IgM levels in cord blood or blood taken shortly after birth are good non-specific evidence of intrauterine infection. (IgM levels greater than 20 mg/100 ml are abnormal.) Compliment-fixation tests showing a rise in antibody titre to a specific organism may also be significant. In some cases, where there are low levels of α_1-antitrypsin in the blood, the hepatitis may progress irreversibly to cirrhosis and hepatic failure (see below).

α_1-Antitrypsin deficiency

Deficiency of α_1-antitrypsin is responsible for a significant proportion of cholestatic jaundice in infants, perhaps 5–30%. It is an autosomal recessively inherited condition although not all affected individuals will show clinical manifestations. Many different genetic variants exist. α_1-Antitrypsin is a glycoprotein synthesized in the liver which normally inhibits many enzymes which break down protein. It is thought that its lack allows a damaging process (however initiated) in the liver to continue unchecked.

Some infants deteriorate rapidly with ascites and hepatic failure within months. In others the course is more chronic with persisting conjugated hyperbilirubinaemia and, usually, cirrhosis by adolescence. Diagnosis is by finding low α_1-antitrypsin levels in serum and tissue fluids. Electron microscopy shows amorphous cytoplasmic granules in the liver cells.

The variety of clinical associations with the homozygous state makes genetic counselling difficult but the severity of the disease tends to be consistent in an individual family. It is now possible, using fetal blood sampling techniques, to identify the protease inhibitor phenotype sufficiently early in pregnancy to offer termination to parents who have already had a severely affected infant.

Hypothyroidism

This condition is discussed in Chapter 4.

Galactosaemia

Prolonged neonatal jaundice with predominantly conjugated hyperbilirubinaemia may be a presenting feature of galactosaemia. There may also be hepatomegaly and cataracts with poor feeding or vomiting and failure to thrive. The condition is due to the absence of the enzyme galactose-l-phosphate uridyl transferase which converts galactose to glucose. This causes toxic galactose to accumulate in the blood and damage the liver (sometimes causing haemorrhages as well as jaundice) and central nervous system leading to blindness and mental retardation. The galactose is excreted in the urine where it is detected by a positive Clinitest (Clinistix, which detect glucose, will be negative) and by sugar chromatography. There will also be proteinuria and abnormal aminoaciduria. The diagnosis is confirmed by finding a deficiency of the enzyme in the red cells. Treatment is by excluding the lactose in milk from the diet (lactose is made up of galactose and glucose) by feeding with a proprietary low-lactose milk. Growth and development then take place normally. Vitamin supplements are necessary and the mother must subsequently be given a diet sheet telling her which foods must not be given to her baby. Galactosaemia is inherited as an autosomal recessive condition and the recurrence rate in subsequent pregnancies is one in four. The diagnosis can now be made antenatally by culturing amniotic cells (see Chapter 2). When there is a family history, cord blood should always be tested.

Fructosaemia

This rare inborn error of metabolism appears when fructose or sucrose, from which it is derived, are included in the baby's diet. It can present with neonatal jaundice and bleeding. Today it is likely to present later because sucrose is less used in artificial milk formulae. The urine contains reducing substances and hypoglucosaemia is common.

Kernicterus

It has been said that high unconjugated levels of bilirubin which exceed the albumin-binding capacity of the baby's plasma are dangerous, as bilirubin is able to enter the brain and cause damage. This condition is known as kernicterus. There is no unequivocally safe level of serum bilirubin. Levels of 380 μmol/l are usually safe in term babies; levels of 180 μmol/l could damage an ill baby of 28 weeks gestation. One of the problems is that kernicterus is sometimes seen at post-mortem when only very mild jaundice was present in life (serum bilirubin as low as 100 μmol/l). It is known that this post-mortem kernicterus can be prevented by treating jaundice at very low levels of bilirubin, but we do not know how important this is. It is important to check bilirubin levels and relate them to the gestational and chronological ages of the baby and to his general condition. Plotting levels graphically is useful. Logically, the albumin-binding capacity of a baby's blood would be the most helpful measurement, but it is difficult to do in practice (see above).

Free unconjugated bilirubin enters the brain and causes damage by interfering with specific neuronal enzyme activities, particularly in the basal ganglia, corpus striatum and thalamus. Liver conjugation of bilirubin with glucuronic acid renders it fat-insoluble, unable to enter the brain and therefore non-toxic.

Clinically, affected babies are lethargic and poor feeders. They may subsequently become floppy or hypertonic, with head retraction and convulsions. The Moro reflex is abnormally stereotyped with only extension and no adduction. If the infant survives, he is often mentally handicapped, is prone to convulsions and, by two years of age, shows the signs of athetoid cerebral palsy with high-tone deafness.

The appearance of neurological signs in a deeply jaundiced baby is an indication for immediate exchange transfusion, with Group O rhesus-negative blood if necessary. Kernicterus should be exceedingly rare in properly organized neonatal units.

Further Reading

Clarke, C.A. (1975) *Rhesus Haemolytic Disease*. Lancaster: MTP Press.

Liley, A.W. (1961) Liquor amnii analysis in management of pregnancy complicated by rhesus sensitisation. *American Journal of Obstetrics and Gynecology*, *82*, 1359.

Mowat, A.P. (1979) *Liver Disorders in Childhood*. London: Butterworths.

Mowat, A.P. (1981) Current developments in chronic liver disease. In *Recent Advances in Paediatrics*, ed. D. Hull, pp 137–156. Edinburgh: Churchill Livingstone.

Mowat, A.P. (1985) Congenital abnormalities of bilirubin metabolism. *Hospital Update*, *11*, 921–930.

Odell, G.B. (1980) *Neonatal Hyperbilirubinaemia*. New York: Grune and Stratton.

—13

Bleeding Disorders

Bleeding in the newborn infant may be due to local causes including trauma, asphyxia or infection or may result from failure of haemostatic mechanisms. Local haemorrhages may be due to local causes or they may occur secondarily to general haemostatic failure. As in the adult, the newborn infant has two mechanisms in the blood for preventing bleeding: platelets and coagulation factors. In the healthy full-term newborn infant the platelet count is usually in the adult normal range. However, around one third of babies on an intensive care unit will have platelet counts below 100 000. Counts of 80 000 or less are found in some babies but this will not cause haemorrhage. The range is very wide in healthy newborn babies. Some factors (V, VIII and fibrinogen) are in the low normal adult range. Factors synthesized in the baby's liver, which depend on adequate levels of vitamin K, are low at birth by adult standards and their levels become even lower during the first few days of life. This is because vitamin K is made by bacteria in the gut. At birth the gut is sterile and only gradually becomes colonized with bacteria during feeding. The process takes longer in breast-fed than bottle-fed babies. The normal postnatal drop in these factors (II, VII, IX and X) can be prevented by giving vitamin K_1 to newborn babies. Preterm babies have low levels of nearly all clotting factors and their platelet count reaches adult levels only by about 30 weeks gestation. In addition, their blood vessels are fragile and easily damaged so they bleed and bruise easily.

Causes of Neonatal Bleeding

The conditions which cause bleeding in the newborn infant may be classified as follows:

Generalized bleeding tendency

Deficiency of coagulation factors may result from:
1 Exaggeration of the temporary drop in vitamin K dependent factors which occurs after birth. This is *haemorrhagic disease of the newborn* and responds to the administration of vitamin K. It is most common in breast-fed babies or those not given vitamin K as a routine. It is now less common in the neonatal period but may be seen later following gastro-

intestinal upset with or without antibiotic treatment.

2 Failure of liver synthesis. Bleeding due to this condition does not improve with vitamin K but is usually temporary.

3 Congenital disorders of coagulation factor synthesis, e.g. haemophilia (Factor VIII) or Christmas disease (Factor IX). These conditions are permanent.

Deficiency of platelets may be due to:

1 Impaired production, often associated with skeletal abnormalities. Fanconi's anaemia may present as isolated thrombocytopenic purpura at this age.

2 Excessive destruction. This may be secondary to maternal drugs, such as the thiazide diuretics, to maternal idiopathic thrombocytopenic purpura, when maternal antibodies cross the placenta, to maternal systemic lupus erythematosus or to intrauterine infection (e.g. toxoplasmosis or rubella). Platelet antigen incompatibility is being increasingly recognized; 98% of the population are antigen (PLA_1) positive, 2% negative. An iso-immune response may occur in the PLA_1 positive offspring of PLA_1 negative mothers—an analogous situation to rhesus disease.

Isolated thrombocytopenic purpura may be seen with serious infection e.g. intrapartum acquisition of β-haemolytic streptococci (confirmed by high vaginal swab from the mother).

Combined deficiencies, with low levels of both platelets and coagulation factors, are found when both are used up in the process of disseminated intravascular coagulation (DIC). This almost always occurs in infants who are already extremely unwell with hypoxia, hypothermia or severe rhesus disease. Clots may form within the circulation in very ill babies and the platelets and clotting factors cannot then be replaced quickly enough to prevent profuse bleeding into the tissues.

Local causes

Local causes of bleeding include:

1 loose clamp or ligature on umbilical cord, or premature attempts to dislodge the cord remnant

2 birth trauma causing, for example, cephalhaematoma or subcapsular liver haematoma

3 subaponeurotic haemorrhage (see Chapter 11)

4 gastrointestinal bleeding due to volvulus, fissure or polyp

5 intraventricular haemorrhage in hypoxaemia

6 intrapulmonary haemorrhage in hypothermia.

The commonest cause of bleeding in an otherwise well infant is haemorrhagic disease of the newborn. In the sick infant it is probably DIC.

The causes of local haemorrhage classified by site are summarized in Table 13.1.

There are three common clinical situations in which there is neonatal bleeding unassociated with haemostatic failure in the baby. *Vaginal bleeding* in newborn girls is common and is due to the baby's withdrawal from the maternal circulating oestrogens. The mechanism is therefore analogous to the normal period in the post-pubertal girl or withdrawal bleeding when coming off the contraceptive pill. Parents should be warned to expect this and reassured that it is harmless if it does occur.

Table 13.1 Causes of local bleeding according to site.

Site of bleeding	Possible clinical associations	Possible haemostatic deficiencies
Umbilicus	Trauma, infection, loose clamp or ligature	Haemorrhagic disease of the newborn; Factor VII or XIII; fibrinogen
Skin petechiae	Asphyxia (cord around neck, facial petechiae)	Thrombocytopenia
Bruising	Trauma	Any coagulation deficiency
Gastrointestinal tract	Swallowed maternal blood, anorectal trauma	Haemorrhagic disease
Pulmonary	Kernicterus, small-for-dates, hyaline membrane disease	Disseminated intravascular coagulation
Intra-abdominal	Breech delivery causing ruptured liver or spleen	
Genito-urinary	Urinary tract infection, renal vein thrombosis	Haemorrhagic disease
Scalp	Vacuum extraction, subaponeurotic haemorrhage in African babies	Haemorrhagic disease Factor VIII deficiency
Intracranial subdural	Trauma	
Intracranial subarachnoid	Infection	DIC, any haemostatic defect
Intracranial intraventricular	Prematurity, hyaline membrane disease and possibly alkali therapy	
Circumcision wound	Bad surgical technique. Less common with Plastibell circumcision unless the string is not pulled tight	Any haemostatic defect; for example haemophilia may present in this way

Table 13.2 Apt's test.

1 Dissolve two drops of adult blood in half a test tube of water
2 Dissolve sufficient of the specimen to be tested in the same volume of water so that the colour obtained matches
3 Dissolve two drops of baby's blood in the same volume of water
4 Increase the volume of each solution by about one fifth by adding 1% NaOH
5 Wait for one or two minutes
6 Within this time the tube containing adult blood changes from pink to yellow-brown as the alkali denatures the adult haemoglobin. The fetal blood remains pink
7 Compare the colour of the specimen tube and identify the specimen as of fetal or maternal origin

Haemorrhage from the umbilical cord may be due to infection or to the cord ligature being too loose or too tight or having slipped. Most usually, however, it is due to fiddling with the partially separated cord, before it is ready to separate. This practice should be discouraged. Finally, *haematemesis or melaena* in the neonate is most commonly due to swallowed maternal blood. This may have been swallowed either during delivery or from cracked nipples during breast feeding. The blood can sometimes be shown to be of maternal origin if the haemoglobin is denatured by alkali (Apt's test, Table 13.2). Do *not* assume that swallowed blood is the cause; examine the baby carefully and if indicated do a plain abdominal X-ray to exclude a volvulus.

Blood Loss before Birth

Causes of fetal haemorrhage include caesarean section with an anterior placenta praevia, abruption with tearing of blood vessels on the fetal side of the placenta, transplacental fetomaternal transfusion and trauma at artificial rupture of membranes. It is thought that fetomaternal transfusion occurs in up to 50% of pregnancies. In 10% the loss to the fetus is between 0.5 ml and 40 ml, but it may be as high as 100 ml or more in 1%. Fetal haemorrhage should be suspected if there is loss of bright red blood from the mother's vagina before delivery. The diagnosis may be confirmed by tests (see Apt's test above) which differentiate fetal and maternal red cells by making use of the fact that fetal haemoglobin is resistant to alkali. The same technique can be used in Kleihauer's test to search for fetal cells in the mother's blood. Treatment is urgent if the baby is pale or shocked at delivery; it involves early delivery and clamping of the cord, followed by blood transfusion, with Group O rhesus negative blood if necessary. Fifty per cent of placental blood crosses into the baby in the first 15 seconds following delivery.

History and Examination

In all cases, a careful history must be taken from the mother of her general health, anticoagulant therapy given, or other drugs taken during pregnancy such as aspirin or phenytoin, which may lower the levels of vitamin K dependent clotting factors. The birth history should be checked for evidence of trauma. The mother should be asked specifically about contact with rubella or other infections; whether there is a family history of bleeding tendency; about the infant's health until now; whether the baby is breast fed; and if vitamin K was given.

The baby should be examined carefully. First his general circulatory state must be assessed; his colour should be observed; and his pulse and respiration rates and blood pressure measured. The liver and spleen should be palpated to detect any enlargement, and any congenital malformations should be noted. Bruising and petechial haemorrhages should be looked for. If localized bleeding has occurred from the umbilicus, the cord clamp should be checked, as sometimes this becomes loose as the cord shrinks after birth.

If there is bleeding beneath the scalp the head develops a generalized boggy swelling. Measurement of the head circumference is useful because the difference between the head circumference at birth and later will give an indication of the amount of blood lost into the scalp. Check that the baby has not had heparin in, for example, a blood transfusion.

Investigations

1 *Group and cross match* blood in case transfusion is required.

2 *Haemoglobin (Hb) and packed cell volume* are measured to help assess severity of blood loss.

3 A *platelet count* is taken. A count below $80–100 \times 10^9$/litre is abnormal in the newborn. If the count is below 30×10^9/litre there is a serious risk of bleeding.

4 *Clotting studies*. Thrombotest measures factors II (prothrombin), VII, IX, and X, the vitamin K dependent clotting factors. Prothrombin time tests for deficiencies of factors II, V, VII and X. Partial thromboplastin time tests for deficiencies of factors VIII (low in haemophilia), IX (Christmas factor), XI and XII. It will be prolonged if the prothrombin time or the thrombotest is prolonged. If it is prolonged specific assays of individual factors may be necessary. Fibrinogen degradation products are elevated when fibrin clots formed in the circulation are broken down. They are usually raised when there is disseminated intravascular coagulation.

5 *Apt's test* distinguishes swallowed maternal blood from fetal blood when it appears unchangd in vomit or stools. (Maternal blood is sometimes swallowed at birth or occasionally when the mother's breast milk is blood-stained.) The test is based on the fact that adult haemoglobin is more readily denatured by alkali than fetal haemoglobin and turns a brown colour (Table 13.2).

Management

Local bleeding

Any obvious local cause of bleeding from, for example, the umbilicus should be stopped with firm pressure and then a cord clamp or a purse-string suture applied.

Transfusion

A baby who is pale and breathless, whether newborn or with a history of blood loss, needs urgent transfusion. Blood should be taken for investigation but the results should not be waited for. An intravenous transfusion of Group O rhesus-negative blood is set up immediately (plasma can be used if blood is not readily available). Shock is corrected by giving 10 ml/kg by rapid injection over the first 10 minutes; the infusion is then slowed down.

If the volume of blood loss is not known, give about 30 ml/kg initially; haemoglobin and packed cell volume measurements are then repeated. If there has been bleeding into the scalp, a rough guide is that 35 ml of blood should be given for each centimetre by which the head circumference exceeds that measured at birth. Alternatively, calculations can be on a ml/kg basis.

A pale baby who is not breathless or shocked should be observed carefully with half-hourly pulse, respiration, and blood pressure measurements. If bleeding is continuing internally he may suddenly deteriorate and need a transfusion.

Most babies with a haemoglobin of less than 10 g/dl at birth will need a transfusion.

It is helpful and useful to know the blood group of staff members so that appropriate fresh blood can be quickly obtained in an emergency. The donors should, of course, be screened with a serological test for syphilis, HBsAg and HIV (AIDS virus). Some doctors have been concerned about the possibility of transmitting cytomegalovirus (CMV) by transfusion and it is wise to give CMV-negative blood. It is possible to test for CMV antibodies, but 60% of the population are positive and this reduces the number of donors. Unless donors are screened repeatedly a recent infection would not be detected.

Vitamin K

In all cases vitamin K_1 (Konakion) 1 mg intravenously or intramuscularly is given after blood has been taken for investigation. If there is severe bruising, an intravenous injection is better, because intramuscular injection may produce a large haematoma.

If the platelet count is less than 100 × 10^9/litre

Check whether the mother has been unwell or her platelet count is low. A mother who has systemic lupus erythematosus or thrombocytopenic purpura may produce a transient secondary thrombocytopenia (deficiency of platelets) in her baby. Healthy mothers may also pass antiplatelet antibodies across the placenta, resulting in transient thrombocytopenia in their babies. These babies are usually well apart from petechial haemorrhages in the skin or mucosae. If the platelet count remains low the bone marrow should be examined.

Examine the infant carefully. Congenital malformations are sometimes associated with bone marrow dyscrasias, for example Fanconi's anaemia, where there is pancytopenia associated with upper limb malformation, and the radial aplasia thrombocytopenia syndrome. These diagnoses are confirmed by bone marrow examination. Enlargement of the liver and spleen with thrombocytopenia occurs with intrauterine infection. The baby should be screened for rubella, cytomegalovirus, toxoplasmosis and syphilis. Thrombocytopenia is usually transient in these conditions.

Sick preterm infants are most likely to develop *disseminated intravascular coagulation (DIC)*, particularly those with septicaemia or hypoxia and acidosis secondary to respiratory distress syndrome or rhesus disease. In this condition the platelet count is low, the prothrombin and partial thromboplastin times are prolonged and fibrinogen degradation products elevated. It is most important to treat the precipitating illness vigorously with antibiotics, artificial ventilation and oxygen or exchange transfusion as indicated. The coagulation disorder is treated with transfusions of fresh plasma containing clotting factors and platelets. Fresh blood can be used if the haemoglobin level has dropped. If fibrinogen levels have dropped (below 1 g), cryoprecipitate is useful.

In practice a mixture of infusions is often useful in DIC, e.g. platelets (1 unit) with fresh frozen plasma (10 ml/kg), cryoprecipitate (10 ml/kg) and sometimes blood. The volumes infused must be watched carefully. Coagulation studies must be repeated 1–2 hours after all products have been infused.

If the platelet count is normal but clotting times abnormal

A prolonged prothrombin time or thrombotest less than 10% of normal is probably due to haemorrhagic disease of the newborn, a temporary deficiency of vitamin K dependent clotting factors. Vitamin K_1 (Konakion) 1 mg intramuscularly or intravenously should be given. The diagnosis is confirmed if the prothrombin time or thrombotest returns to normal within 12 hours. A prothrombin time or thrombotest remaining abnormal after an injection of vitamin K_1 confirms a deficiency of clotting factors. If the infant is well it is probably due to an inherited deficiency of a clotting factor. The family history should be checked. The partial thromboplastin time will be prolonged. By repeating this test after adding small amounts of different clotting factors, one can determine which clotting factor is deficient. If the infant is sick he may have a reduction of clotting factors due to severe liver disease, e.g. secondary to fructosaemia or galactosaemia. The urine can be checked for reducing substances using a Clinitest tablet.

The mother should always be asked if she has taken anticoagulants or any other drugs which could interfere with the production of clotting factors in the baby. During the last few weeks of pregnancy most mothers taking anticoagulants are changed from taking coumarin type drugs, for example warfarin, to heparin which does not affect the fetus. Mothers on anticonvulsants should be given vitamin K at the onset of labour.

The baby may have had too much heparin during a blood transfusion or from heparinized saline in an umbilical arterial catheter. This can be reversed using protamine (dose 1 mg for each 100 units of heparin, maximum 50 mg).

Further Reading

Hathaway, W.E. & Bonnar, J. (1978) *Perinatal Coagulation*. New York: Grune & Stratton.

Miller, D.R., Baehner, R.L. & McMillan, C.W. (ed) (1984) *Blood Diseases of Infancy and Childhood*, 5th ed. St Louis: C.V. Mosby.

Oski, F.A. & Naiman, J.L. (1982) *Hematologic Problems in the Newborn*, 3rd ed. Philadelphia: W.B. Saunders.

Rivers, R. (1980) Bleeding disorders in the newborn infant. *Journal of Maternal and Child Health*, 5, 334.

Zibursky, A. (ed) (1984) Perinatal Hematology. *Clinics in Perinatology*, *11*, 249–513. Philadelphia: W.B. Saunders.

—14————————————

Neurological Disorders

Neurological disorders remain an important problem in the preterm baby. As many as 40% will have evidence of intraventricular haemorrhage (IVH). Eighty per cent of sick newborns have a subependymal bleed. Nonetheless, around 95% of preterm babies will attend normal schools. The price for very many more normal survivors is a few more surviving with handicap.

Neurological disorders may be conveniently categorized as shown in Table 14.1. They may be considered as primary malformations (e.g. aqueduct stenosis) or as secondary deformations (destruction of structures already formed). Some conditions are described in other chapters.

Hydranencephaly

In this condition the cerebral hemispheres are largely absent and the skull vault contains a watery fluid. The diagnosis should be considered in a baby with a large or abnormally shaped head or who is exhibiting abnormal behaviour. It may be recognized by transilluminating the head in a darkened room when it will glow brightly. The diagnosis is confirmed by ultrasound. The condition is thought to be due sometimes to severe hydrocephalus and sometimes to infarction or malformation.

The prognosis is usually hopeless, but the extent to which these babies are able to perform basic functions, such as suckling, is surprising and instructive. A few of the post-hydrocephalus group do relatively well. The decision whether to shunt such babies is sometimes a difficult one.

Midline Abnormalities over the Spine

A naevus or hairy patch over the spine may cover an underlying spinal cord abnormality (e.g. meningocele; see Chapter 9) or an abnormality of the vertebrae (spina bifida occulta). Assess the neurological findings in the lower limbs and bladder and anal sphincter function. Occasionally, a plain radiograph will reveal diastematomyelia in which a bony spur bisects the spinal cord.

It is common to find shallow coccygeal pits, which are harmless. Sacral or higher pits should be investigated. Rarely a deep pin-sized hole is

Table 14.1 Neurological abnormalities.

Structural CNS abnormalities
Hydrocephalus (see Chapter 9)
Microcephaly (see Chapter 9)
Hydranencephaly
Anencephaly (see Chapter 9)
Myelomeningocele (see Chapter 9)
Other midline abnormalities
   Dermal sinus
   Hairy patch
   Naevus
Degenerative diseases

Abnormal neurological behaviour unassociated with overt structural abnormalities
Cerebral irritation
Cerebral depression ± respiratory failure
Fits
Floppy baby
Kernicterus (see Chapter 12)
Meningitis (see Chapter 16)
Subarachnoid haemorrhage
Babies born to drug-addicted mothers

Traumatic lesions
Peripheral nerve palsies (see Chapter 11)
Brachial plexus palsy (see Chapter 11)

found which communicates with the theca and is therefore a portal of entry for bacteria which will cause meningitis. These lesions should be sought at the routine postnatal examination and the baby referred urgently to a neurosurgeon.

A pit can be examined with an auriscope which will often enable the floor to be seen and a sinus to be excluded.

Progressive Degenerative Diseases

Most of these conditions do not present in the newborn period, but Werdnig–Hoffmann progressive spinal paralysis (see below) may appear at or within a few weeks of birth.

Cerebral Irritation

It is often difficult to know the significance of findings such as hypertonia, exaggerated reflexes and tendon jerks, tremor and a high-pitched cry. They may be associated with perinatal hypoxaemia, with or without intraventricular heamorrhage or kernicterus. They often seem to have a good prognosis and some of them may be due to headache. Serious signs include poor sucking, convulsions and apnoeic attacks. New neurological examinations are being developed as a guide to prognosis. Particular attention is being paid to the baby's ability to look at objects. It is helpful to distinguish between the irritable, bad tempered, inconsolable baby who does not cuddle or like being handled (because of headache or other pain), who may have a cerebral cry and has a good prognosis, from the jittery baby who may exhibit jaw, ankle, finger or hamstring clonus. These latter babies may have metabolic upset (hypocalcaemia, hypomagnesaemia, hypernatraemia with thirst), may have drug withdrawal (mother on heroin) or may have a thyrotoxic mother.

Cyanotic attacks with apnoea carry a bad prognosis as does the need for tube feeding for more than about four days.

Cerebral Depression

Diminished spontaneous movements, hypotonia and depressed reflexes, if prolonged, may carry a serious prognosis. Brief periods may follow a very difficult or traumatic delivery. Hypotonia may occur in kernicterus.

Fits

Fits are common in newborn babies and are a great source of anxiety both to parents and to the nurses and doctors. There are many causes, some peculiar to the newborn, but very often a clinical diagnosis can be made, base-line investigations ordered and appropriate treatment started before the results are available. It is a mistake to expect newborn babies to have grand mal fits of the kind that occur in adults, with an aura, tonic and clonic phases associated with incontinence or tongue-biting. It may be difficult to recognize fits, particularly in the preterm infant, in whom cycling movements, paroxysmal sucking, apnoeic attacks, jitteriness or athetoid movements may be considered normal. In addition, some sick or preterm babies may show abnormal behaviour which is a manifestation of prolonged convulsions. Asphyxia is still a very common cause of fits and can itself lead to biochemical abnormality, for instance hypoglycaemia or hypocalcaemia.

In general there are three types of convulsion in the newborn baby:

Tonic or major fits occur at any gestational age, including the preterm baby usually in the first 24 hours of life. They often represent severe brain damage and may be found following severe asphyxia, intraventricular haemorrhage, kernicterus and some metabolic disorders. The baby lies rigidly and hypertonic. There is usually no clonus but sometimes it may be present and sustained. The prognosis is bad.

Many *clonic fits* start focally with the baby fully conscious, but they may gradually become generalized and the baby may lose consciousness or become cyanosed. Such fits are rare in the preterm baby. The focal fits may represent a localized response to asphyxia or birth trauma, while generalized clonic convulsions are often seen in generalized biochemical disorders, for example hypoglycaemia or hypocalcaemia. These fits often start between 24 hours and 48 hours of life and have a less bad prognosis.

The fit most easily missed is known as the *fragmentary* or *primitive fit*. These manifest themselves by such things as cycling leg movements, recurrent apnoeic attacks and nystagmus or as primitive reflexes.

The distinction between jitteriness and true convulsions is sometimes thought to be blurred. In practice, they can usually be differentiated; in jitteriness there is tremor with rapid alternating movements of equal rate in each direction whereas fits are rapid contractions of specific muscle groups associated with slow relaxation of others so that they show a fast and slow phase. Jitteriness can be stopped by bending the limb; it starts

Table 14.2 Important causes of convulsions in the newborn.

Metabolic	Birth asphyxia
	Hypocalcaemia
	Hypomagnesaemia
	Hyperbilirubinaemia
	Hyperammonaemia
	Hypernatraemia
	Hyponatraemia and water intoxication
	Pyridoxine dependency
	Organic acidurias
	Galactosaemia
	Aminoacidopathies
	Alkalaemia
Intracranial haemorrhage	Asphyxia with intraventricular haemorrhage
	Trauma with subdural or subarachnoid haemorrhage
	Haemorrhagic disease
	Non-accidental injury
	Platelet deficiency
Infection	Intrauterine: cytomegalovirus, toxoplasmosis, rubella
	Meningitis/encephalitis
	Septicaemia
	Gastroenteritis
Genetic	Cerebral malformations and dysplasias
Drug withdrawal	

again if the limb is stretched. This will help to differentiate such things as slow hamstring clonus from a fit. It must be remembered, however, that some causes are common to both.

The major causes of neonatal convulsions are listed in Table 14.2.

In many cases the diagnosis may be suspected from a brief history and examination. For example, in the small-for-dates baby, suspect hypoglycaemia; in the very jaundiced baby, suspect kernicterus; if there has been heavy maternal sedation, suspect drug withdrawal. Fits associated with hypoglycaemia often occur in babies who are small-for-dates or babies of diabetic mothers (large-for-dates). Such babies should have routine monitoring of blood glucose by strips and should be fed early to prevent such a situation developing (see Chapters 5 and 15). Hypoglycaemia is not a diagnosis in itself. If there is no obvious cause, a blood sample during hypoglycaemia to measure insulin, lactate, ketone bodies, branched chain amino acids, growth hormone and cortisol is crucially important for diagnosis and in planning long-term treatment.

Hypocalcaemia used to be common around the end of the first week of life in artificially fed babies given baby milks with high phosphate loads. Currently available baby milks are more physiological and this problem is now seldom seen. Now, fits at the end of the first week are not always accompanied by hypocalcaemia and when they are found there is often no demonstrable cause. Hypocalcaemia is seen during the first few days of life in preterm babies, but is hardly ever associated with convulsions. Low plasma calcium values in Asian babies often indicate a significant degree of osteomalacia from vitamin D deficiency in their mothers; ask the obstetricians to check the mother's calcium, phosphate and alkaline phosphatase. Hypocalcaemic fits are sometimes seen in the severely stressed baby, for instance those with septicaemia.

The relationship between calcium and magnesium levels is very variable. Magnesium is necessary for parathyroid hormone to be released from the parathyroid gland. Some babies with low plasma calcium levels also have low magnesium levels.

Either a high or a low plasma sodium (more than 150 mmol/l or less than 120 mmol/l) may be associated with fits. Sodium has sometimes been given to the baby orally or intravenously by mistake. A low plasma sodium occurs during the first day when the mother has been given intravenous dextrose with oxytocin, and also occurs in tiny babies under 1 kg who pass too much sodium in the urine.

A history of trauma or intrapartum asphyxia is a frequent finding in babies who convulse within the first few days of life. There are usually other associated neurological abnormalities.

Management

Review the history

Check the notes for evidence of maternal diabetes, endocrine disorders, osteomalacia, infection, hypertension or pre-eclampsia, and whether there was prolonged rupture of membranes, difficult labour, instrumental delivery or fetal hypoxia. Note the Apgar scores and the milk the baby has received.

Examine the baby

Observe the infant's behaviour and note abnormal posture or movements, tone, pattern of respiration and nature and frequency of the cry. Look for external evidence of difficult birth, e.g. conjunctival haemorrhages, chignon (from ventouse), forceps blade marks, cephalhaematoma or traumatic cyanosis. Note any infected areas or signs of infection. Feel the fontanelle to ensure that it is not full or bulging and measure the head circumference and compare it with previous measurements.

Examine the baby's eyes with an ophthalmoscope to exclude cataracts, choroidoretinitis or haemorrhages. Transilluminate the skull.

Investigations

1 Check the blood glucose monitoring strips and measure the true blood glucose level if it is low.
2 Take blood for a full blood count, platelet count, packed cell volume and blood culture. Blood is also needed to screen for congenital infections such as cytomegalovirus, rubella and toxoplasma titres and to test the IgM level. Biochemical tests on blood include glucose, calcium, electrolytes and urea; magnesium, phosphorus and bilirubin may be measured in some cases. Blood gas studies should also be performed.
3 Urine must be taken for estimation of protein and reducing substances, amino acid chromatography, microscopy, culture and sensitivity and virus culture.
4 Swab obviously infected areas only and send for culture.
5 Examine the cerebrospinal fluid (CSF) by lumbar puncture to diagnose meningitis. Cisternal or ventricular taps are only very rarely necessary. Lumbar puncture to detect blood in the CSF is often of little practical help, because it is common to do a traumatic tap and blood in the ventricles may not have leaked into the subarachnoid space. Normal CSF in the newborn is often yellow and the range for protein, sugar or cells is wide (see Appendix). CSF protein concentrations in preterm babies may be even higher.
6 Real-time ultrasound, if available, may detect intracranial haemor-

rhages, particularly intraventricular bleeding. CAT scan, if available, is also useful. An electroencephalograph (EEG) may be useful for prognosis and to see if paroxysmal behaviour is due to cerebral arrhythmia. Twenty-four-hour EEG monitoring is sometimes used in preterm babies but EEGs are difficult to interpret in this age group. One should not expect a routine adult EEG department to be able to do so—spike and episodic activity is commonly seen in a normal baby's EEG.

Treatment

If a cause is found, treat it. If fits recur or continue, whether or not the underlying cause is found, give anticonvulsants. Ensure careful attention to nutrition, temperature control, respiratory status and metabolic balance.

Hypocalcaemia or hypomagnesaemia. In an emergency give 10% calcium gluconate 0.2 ml/kg slowly intravenously. Watch for cardiac arrhythmias or bradycardia. In most cases oral correction is adequate and safer: 10% calcium gluconate 100 mg/kg (about 1 ml) before each feed. It is sometimes necessary to correct hypomagnesaemia before the hypocalcaemia becomes correctable; a suitable dose is 50% magnesium sulphate 0.2 mg/kg intramuscularly or intravenously in an emergency or magnesium sulphate or chloride by mouth.

Hypoglycaemia. If symptomatic, give intravenous dextrose 0.5 g/kg in 10% solution. This should be given into a large vein to reduce the risk of thrombosis. If asymptomatic hypoglycaemia is found, early feeding may raise the blood glucose before the onset of symptoms, provided feeds are being absorbed. Blood sugars should be checked with blood glucose monitoring strips.

Meningitis. See Chapter 16.

Anticonvulsants. To abort prolonged or recurrent fits, paraldehyde 0.1 ml/kg by deep intramuscular injection can be given; diazepam (intramuscular or intravenous) is also useful, but the dose which controls the fits may produce severe respiration depression or apnoea. Paraldehyde can be given in the same dose rectally. The use of intravenous diazepam also carries the theoretical risk of increasing hyperbilirubinaemia by displacing bilirubin from its binding sites by the sodium benzoate component of injectable diazepam. It is commonly said that paraldehyde must be drawn up in glass syringes. This is not true provided that the drug is used immediately. It is only if the drug is drawn up in a plastic syringe and allowed to stand for some time that a reaction with the syringe may take place.

For long-term control the drug of choice in the newborn baby is probably phenobarbitone, 1–2 mg/kg six-hourly orally after one intramuscular loading dose of 10 mg/kg. A problem with the drug is that its half-life is extremely variable in the newborn baby, ranging between 72 and 400 hours, so that accumulation may occur. It is important, therefore, to measure blood levels and adjust the dose accordingly. Chloral (10 mg/kg, six-hourly orally) is probably best used for jitteriness rather than true convulsions. Sodium valproate (starting dose 20 mg/kg/day orally in three divided doses; maximum 50 mg/kg/day) has turned out to be a much less useful drug in the control of neonatal convulsions than had been hoped. It is best not to use phenytoin as it may interfere with brain growth during this critical period of particularly rapid growth. Rectal diazepam can cause apnoea.

Cerebral oedema. It is wise to restrict fluids. Steroids and mannitol are now much less used.

Prognosis

Prognosis varies with the cause. Most convulsions in the newborn stop eventually with or without treatment, so this is no cause for optimism in itself.

Fits with hyperbilirubinaemia (kernicterus) may lead to deafness and choreoathetosis. Hypoglycaemia with fits, if long uncorrected, is associated with mental retardation and cerebral palsy but early diagnosis and treatment will prevent this and prolonged hypoglycaemia should not now occur. Hypocalcaemic fits carry a very good prognosis, except that the children often have hypoplasia of dental enamel.

Bad prognostic signs include tonic fits in the first 24 hours, prolonged or recurrent fits despite treatment, associated neurological abnormalities and marked diffuse EEG abnormalities. It is true to say that many babies do surprisingly well, but, if hypocalcaemia is excluded, up to 50% of other babies who had convulsions as newborn babies used to die or show a later handicap. Modern obstetric practices, with reduction in the incidence and severity of intrapartum asphyxia, together with intensive treatment post-partum, mean that 80% of babies with problems relating to birth injury or asphyxia are now normal subsequently.

The pertussis component of the triple vaccine should be omitted in all babies who have had neonatal fits. This is because the very small risk of developing encephalitis that the vaccine may carry is theoretically increased in these babies.

The Floppy Baby

Hypotonia is a common finding in ill babies, for instance those with severe respiratory distress, septicaemia or kernicterus, or for a short period after difficult or traumatic delivery. It is a normal finding in extremely preterm babies. In such circumstances the reason for the floppiness is usually obvious and asphyxia is still the commonest cause.

Rarely, floppiness is the presenting feature in an otherwise well baby. It is useful then to check whether there is weakness, shown by lack of movement as well as flaccidity. The most likely cause of a flaccid paralysis is *Werdnig–Hoffmann disease* (spinal muscular atrophy or progressive spinal paralysis); in modern obstetric practice spinal cord injury or transection is very rare.

Werdnig–Hoffmann disease is inherited in an autosomal recessive manner and is due to loss of motor neurons in the spinal cord. The onset is often before birth and the mother may report only a few fetal movements. The infant gradually loses the ability to suck and develops breathing difficulties as the muscles of respiration become affected. Signs in the newborn include absent deep reflexes with muscle and tongue fasciculation. The disease is progressive, leading to death within a few years. No specific treatment is possible, apart from physiotherapy, although considerable support must be given to the family. Muscle biopsy characteristically shows the atrophy of denervation. Genetic counselling is essential.

The most important differential diagnosis is *benign congenital hypotonia*. The cause of this condition is unknown but, as the name implies, it gradually improves during the first years of life. Unlike in Werdnig–Hoffmann disease, the deep reflexes are present and there is no fasciculation. Muscle biopsy is normal.

Rare causes of floppiness in the newborn include *congenital myopathies* (chronic and non-progressive, diagnosable by muscle biopsy); *glycogen storage diseases* affecting the CNS (e.g. Type II, Pompe's disease, recessively inherited); *organic acidaemias* (where signs of respiratory failure rapidly develop; recessively inherited, diagnosable from plasma and urine amino acid chomatography). Two commonly missed causes are *dystrophia myotonica* in the mother [diagnosed by electromyography (EMG) of the mother's thenar eminence], and *Prader–Willi* syndrome (where there are pronounced neonatal feeding difficulties, and later obesity, cryptorchidism, hypogonadism, mental retardation and, sometimes, diabetes mellitus).

Floppiness is a particular characteristic of children with *Down's syndrome* (see Chapter 9) but cases are usually recognized from their other features.

Some babies born to mothers with myasthenia gravis have temporary floppiness with sucking and respiratory difficulties. The diagnosis is confirmed by the intravenous injection of edrophonium chloride 1 mg (Tensilon 0.1 ml) which leads to rapid improvement. Maintenance therapy with neostigmine or prostigmine (1–5 mg orally with feeds) is then necessary and can be reduced gradually as improvement occurs (see also p. 128).

Intracranial Haemorrhage

There are many different possible sites of bleeding within or around the brain (see also Chapters 6 and 11).

Periventricular haemorrhage (PVH). This is now known to be common following hypoxaemia, but if severe is often fatal. Affected babies suddenly deteriorate and often become floppy with marked bradycardia, unresponsiveness and respiratory arrest. The condition occurs characteristically in babies under 32 weeks gestation. It seems that the haemorrhage starts from capillaries in the germinal layer in the lateral wall of the lateral ventricles. Such capillaries, already maximally dilated by hypoxia and hypercapnia, may easily rupture either because of a sudden rise in osmolality from a large or rapid injection of alkali or following hypertensive episodes caused by hypoxia, pneumothorax, or unnecessary handling of the infant. The post-mortem appearances are shown in Fig. 14.1.

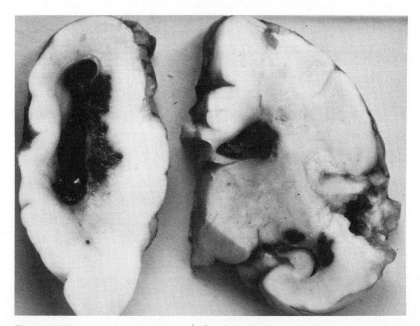

Fig. 14.1 The post-mortem appearances of periventricular haemorrhage

Thus PVH is particularly likely to follow a hypoxic insult to the immature brain. Sequential ultrasound examinations of a sick baby will identify bleeds in 40–50% with around 10% developing hydrocephalus. In these babies it is now important to monitor intracranial pressure—increased pressure will reduce cerebral perfusion.

Subarachnoid haemorrhage. This is usually secondary to severe hypoxaemia and IVH but it may occur in an otherwise normal baby. Sometimes it is the result of an arterial malformation. There is a particular risk of hydrocephalus in survivors.

Intracerebral haemorrhage. This is most commonly the result of an extension of severe germinal layer haemorrhage and intraventricular haemorrhage. It is also a feature of very severe generalized illness, such as Gram-negative septicaemia, cold injury, hypoxaemia, meningitis or severe rhesus incompatibility. There is often evidence of disseminated intravascular coagulation. Most babies will die and a high proportion of the survivors will be brain-damaged. Autopsies of babies who have suffered intrapartum hypoxia show tiny haemorrhages scattered through the brain.

Periventricular leucomalacia (PVL). This is now recognized to be an important form of ischaemic damage to the neonatal brain. It may follow severe birth asphyxia or prolonged apnoea in the term baby but is more usually seen in the preterm baby where it is a significant cause of subsequent neurological handicap.

It is thought to occur as a result of hypotensive episodes during apnoea or hypoxaemia. The periventricular region is particularly vulnerable to the resulting circulatory impairment because it is a boundary zone between different supplying blood vessels.

It is still difficult to recognize in life with the currently available imaging techniques but it is possible to see characteristically echo-dense areas on ultrasound which correspond to areas of fresh necrosis. Serial ultrasound scanning can define the progression of the lesions to echo-free cystic areas. As PVL involves destruction of tissue which would have become white matter it can prevent development of corticospinal motor pathways, resulting in spastic hemiplegia or quadriplegia.

Subdural haemorrhage. This results from trauma especially during difficult instrumental delivery (see Chapter 11).

Babies Born to Drug-Addicted Mothers

This is an increasingly recognized problem in many developed countries.

About 70% of babies born to mothers taking heroin or methadone will show signs of withdrawal. Some are only mildly affected, others severely affected; the babies born to methadone addicts show more frequent and severe signs than those of heroin-addicted mothers.

The likelihood of the baby being affected is related to maternal consumption and how long she has been an addict. However, babies born to heavily addicted mothers may be normal while those born to light users may show serious signs of withdrawal. The closer to delivery the last dose the more likely the baby is to be affected.

Although 70% will show signs of withdrawal only 40% will have signs severe enough to require treatment. Two-thirds of those showing signs will start to have them in the first 24 hours, 90% by 48 hours and most of the others within the next two days. Initial signs of withdrawal are rare after 10 days of age, but withdrawal signs of barbiturate abuse are often very late. Infants showing mild signs initially may suddenly show severe signs later, but life-threatening illness occurs within the first week. The mortality is about 3%.

| Name : |
| Score baby 6 hourly |
| Score according to the following scale : |
| 0 = Absent |
| 1 = Mild to moderate |
| 2 = Severe |

SIGN	TIME											
TREMOR												
IRRITABILITY												
HYPERTONICITY/ HYPERACTIVITY												
VOMITING												
HIGH PITCHED CRY												
SNEEZING												
RESPIRATORY DISTRESS												
FEVER												
DIARRHOEA												
SWEATING												
CONVULSIONS												
TOTAL												

Fig. 14.2 Clinical score for infants born to drug-addicted mothers. Consider treatment if the score increases above 4 or 5.

It is important to consider meningitis, hypocalcaemia, and hypoglycaemia in the differential diagnosis.

Signs of withdrawal include the following, in the order of frequency:

1 tremors
2 irritability
3 hypertonicity
4 vomiting
5 high-pitched cry
6 sneezing
7 respiratory distress
8 fever
9 diarrhoea
10 sweating
11 mucus secretion
12 convulsions
13 yawning

Treatment consists of giving a sedative drug. Many recommend chlorpromazine as the drug of choice, given as 2.2 mg/kg/24 hours in four divided doses either orally or by injection. Full dosage is given for two to four days then decreased at two-day intervals if baby's condition (according to clinical score) permits (Fig. 14.2). Some paediatricians use opiates in the first week as they effectively suppress the signs during the dangerous phase of the illness.

Further Reading

Brown, J.K. (1973) Convulsions in the newborn period. *Developmental Medicine and Child Neurology*, *15*, 823.

Brown, J.K. (1976) Infants damaged during birth: pathology. And: Infants damaged during birth: perinatal asphyxia. In *Recent Advances in Paediatrics*, 5, ed. D. Hull. Edinburgh and London: Churchill Livingstone.

Han, D. (1979) Neonatal neurology. In *Paediatric Neurology*, ed. F.C. Rose, Oxford: Blackwell Scientific.

Levene, M.I., Williams, J.L. & Fawer, C.-L. (1985) Ultrasound of the infant brain. In *Clinics in Developmental Medicine*, *92*. (Spastics International Medical Publications.) Oxford: Blackwell Scientific.

Volpe, J.J. (1977) Neonatal neurology. In *Clinics in Perinatology*, *3*, Philadelphia: W.B. Saunders.

Wigglesworth, J.S. (1984) Brain development and its modification by adverse influences. In *Clinics in Developmental Medicine*, *87*, 12–26 (Spastics International Medical Publications.) Oxford: Blackwell Scientific.

―15―

The Large-for-Dates Baby

Large-for-dates babies are, by definition, heavier than the 90th centile for gestational age. Some are normal babies at the heavy end of the spectrum with tall and large parents.

Diabetes Mellitus

The common pathological diagnosis among large-for-dates babies is that their mothers are diabetic or pre-diabetic. These babies have a characteristic appearance which may point to previously unsuspected impairment of glucose tolerance in an asymptomatic mother. About one in every thousand pregnant mothers has diabetes, while about one in a hundred are gestational diabetics.

A generation ago, the achievement of pregnancy in a diabetic was rare and the results in terms of perinatal mortality very poor, with a high stillbirth rate. The perinatal morbidity and mortality in such infants is still higher than in normal pregnancies but careful control of diabetes during pregnancies has reduced the mortality and morbidity dramatically. In many series perinatal mortality is now less than 5%.

Infants of diabetic mothers (IDM) have a strong resemblance to one another (Fig. 15.1). They are large and fat, tend to lie in the frog position typical of preterm babies and often develop hyaline membrane disease. They have a two to three times greater incidence of congenital malformations than babies of normal pregnancies. It is not clear why these babies have more abnormalities; it may be a result of the metabolic disorder or could be from treatment, perhaps from insulin. The frequency of congenital malformation in diabetic pregnancies does not seem to be falling however. Glucose seems to be teratogenic in animal experiments, and poor diabetic control is associated with an increased risk of spontaneous abortion.

The large size of the IDM is thought to be secondary to maternal (and hence fetal) hyperglycaemia. Insulin produces fat deposition and stimulates growth. Not all babies of diabetic mothers are large-for-dates; when there is placental insufficiency from complicated diabetes the baby may be small-for-dates. There is now good evidence that careful control of blood glucose concentrations in pregnancy (less than 7 mmol/l) results in babies of normal weight, who do not develop hypoglycaemia. If, as seems likely, poor maternal metabolic control in the first 6–8 weeks of pregnancy

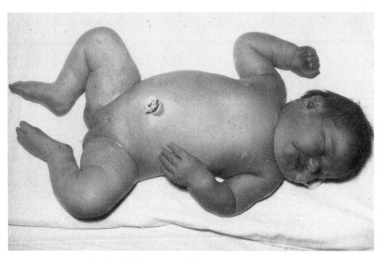

Fig. 15.1 A large-for-dates baby from a diabetic mother

predisposes to the development of congenital malformations, education and counselling of diabetics is necessary before conception, and indeed before a pregnancy is planned. In some areas pre-pregnancy clinics have been set up for this purpose. Some physicians admit diabetic women to hospital during the last two months of pregnancy, but equally good results have been obtained by careful control as out-patients. The optimal delivery date is unclear. Thirty-eight weeks gestation seems a reasonable compromise at present.

Sustained fetal hyperinsulinism means that such babies are at risk of hypoglycaemia after birth as their blood sugar falls rapidly. The period of greatest risk is between two and eight hours. It should be anticipated by routine two-hourly monitoring using blood glucose strips estimations and prevented by early feeding. (Detailed management is as for small-for-dates babies, see Chapter 5.) In some babies whose mothers have received oral hypoglycaemic agents such as chlorpropamide, there may be very prolonged and severe hypoglycaemia requiring intravenous therapy with glucose. In a baby who is well, it is important to resist the temptation to give intravenous glucose during the first 12 hours because this will only increase the plasma insulin and thus increase the tendency to hypoglycaemia.

Other problems to which these babies are susceptible include:
1 hypocalcaemia
2 hyperbilirubinaemia (due to prematurity, polycythaemia, increased red cell breakdown and traumatic delivery of a big baby)
3 Hyaline membrane disease or apnoeic attacks (much more rarely seen

than a few years ago as metabolic control during pregnancy has improved)
4 Congenital abnormalities (including congenital heart disease). Sacral agenesis is one congenital abnormality that occurs more commonly in babies of diabetic mothers (see above)
5 Renal vein thrombosis
6 Shoulder dystonia leading to Erb's palsy.
The aetiology of many of these conditions remains obscure. The paediatrician should always be informed when a diabetic is in labour and the baby is best supervised in an intermediate care nursery with the monitor for at least the first 24 hours.

The prognosis for babies of a diabetic mother is very good. The overall perinatal mortality varies in recent series between about 23 and 46 per 1000—if the problem of major congenital abnormalities were overcome it would be close to that in the non-diabetic population. Ultimately children of diabetic mothers are almost all of normal height, weight and intelligence in later childhood. They do, however, have an increased risk of developing diabetes mellitus themselves. If good, and improving, results are to continue close cooperation between diabetologist, obstetrician and neonatologist is crucial.

Other Causes

Rarer causes of a baby being large-for-dates are:
1 *Beckwith's syndrome.* These babies are heavy at birth because of a large liver and kidneys (organomegaly). The tongue is also enlarged and protrudes and there is a characteristic transverse crease in the ear lobe. There is often herniation of the gut into the base of the umbilical cord or even frank exomphalos or gastroschisis (see Chapter 9). The head circumference is usually on a very much lower centile than the length and weight. Hypoglycaemia is common; treatment is analogous to the management of hypoglycaemia in small-for-dates babies (see Chapter 5). There is an increased risk of having subsequent babies with the syndrome.
2 *Nesidioblastosis of the pancreas.* Persistent hypoglycaemia (beyond about 7 days) in a large-for-dates baby may be due to this diffuse abnormality of the pancreas which causes hyperinsulinism. Ketones will be absent from blood and urine. Very high glucose infusion rates may be necessary to prevent hypoglycaemia. Drugs such as diazoxide can be used to inhibit the excessive insulin release, but, in most cases, subtotal (about 95%) pancreatectomy is necessary. These babies are best managed in speciailist centres.
3 *Transposition of the great arteries* (see Chapter 10). It is not clear why these babies are large.

Further Reading

Babson, S.G., Pernell, M.L. & Benda, G.I. (1980) *Diagnosis and Management of the Fetus and Neonate at Risk*, 4th ed. St Louis: C.V. Mosby.

Cornblath, M. & Schwartz, R. (1976) *Carbohydrate Metabolism in the Neonate*, 2nd ed. Philadelphia: W.B. Saunders.

Cowett, R.M. & Schwartz, R. (1980) The infant of the diabetic mother. *Pediatric Clinics North America 29*, 1213–31. Philadelphia: W.B. Saunders.

Elliott, K.M. & O'Connor, M. (1979) *Pregnancy Metabolism, Diabetes and the Fetus*, Ciba Foundation Symposium 63. Amsterdam: Excerpta Medica.

Gillmer, M.D.G., Oakley, N.W. & Persson, B. (1984) Diabetes mellitus and the fetus. In *Fetal Physiology and Medicine*, eds Beard, R.W. & Nathanielz, P., pp 211–254. New York: Marcel Dekker.

Lang, M.A. (1985) The nursing management of neonates born of diabetic mothers. *Practical Diabetes, 2*, 16–17.

Pederson, J. (1967) *The Pregnant Diabetic and her Newborn: Problems and Management*. Baltimore: Williams and Wilkins.

Rahman, F.R. & Swift, P.G.F. (1985) Neonatal management of the infant of a diabetic mother. *Practical Diabetes, 2*, 11–15.

Steel, J.M. (1985) The pre-pregnancy clinic. *Practical Diabetes, 2*, 8–10.

Steel, J.M., Parboosingh, J., Cole, R.A., Duncan, L.P.J. (1980) Pre-pregnancy counselling: a logical prelude to the management of the pregnant woman. *Diabetes Care, 3*, 371–373.

Sutherland, H.W. & Stowers, J.M. (eds) (1984) *Carbohydrate Metabolism in Pregnancy and the Newborn*. Edinburgh: Churchill Livingstone.

Wright, A.M. (1984) Diabetes in pregnancy. In *Recent Advances in Diabetes*, ed. Nattrass, M. & Santiago, J. V., 239–254. Churchill Livingstone: Edinburgh.

—16

Infection

Newborn babies are particularly susceptible to infections; sometimes these are caused by microorganisms which do not cause trouble at any other time of life. This is because of the relative immaturity of the newborn baby's immune responses and because of his vulnerability to certain infections acquired in utero from the mother.

Infections may be acquired in utero, during delivery or postnatally. The conventional signs and symptoms of infection detectable in older children or adults are usually absent. Furthermore, infections which in older children are localized to an organ or system are frequently complicated by septicaemia or meningitis in the newborn and the rate of spread and deterioration may be extremely rapid.

Defences against Infection

There are a number of specific and non-specific defences which the newborn baby possesses to combat infection. Non-specific defences include the skin, which forms a barrier to invading organisms, phagocytosis by macrophages and the inflammatory response. The specific immune response consists of the production of antibodies in response to a specific antigenic stimulus. An antigen is a substance (e.g. an infecting microorganism) which stimulates the production of specific proteins (antibodies) by lymphocytes and plasma cells. The antibodies so formed help to protect the host from possible damage from that antigen. Antibody may be bound to cells (lymphocytes) or may be free in the plasma (humoral antibodies derived from plasma cells, the immunoglobulins). The immunoglobulins are divided into several subclasses according to their properties and several of these are relevant to the incidence and nature of neonatal infection (see below).

Cellular immunity is effective from birth, hence we can immunize infants with BCG at birth. This is not surprising as the newborn baby has a high peripheral lymphocyte count at birth and indeed for the next two or three years. Humoral immunity develops more slowly, however (Fig. 16.1).

The IgG subclass of immunoglobulins contains antibodies to most bacteria and viruses which the mother has already encountered. Of the various immunoglobulins only IgG can cross the placenta. This is because of its small molecular weight and therefore size and because of

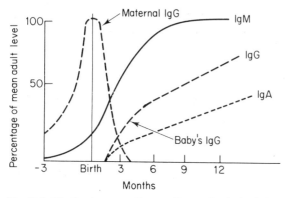

Fig. 16.1 The development of humoral immunity during infancy

specific binding sites which the molecule possesses. IgG crosses the placenta from the third month of pregnancy onwards, so that in full-term infants the IgG levels are similar to those in the mother. (This is not so in the preterm infant and is one reason why he is particularly vulnerable to infection.) These passively acquired antibodies are gradually destroyed over the first three months of extrauterine life. At the same time there is a gradual increase in the baby's own IgG synthesis; IgG levels do not reach those of the adult until about three years of age. There is, therefore, a physiological trough at about three months of age when maternally acquired IgG is disappearing and the baby's own IgG is being produced only gradually; therefore babies of this age are particularly at risk. IgG levels fall from about 1000 mg/100 ml at birth to about 400 mg/100 ml at three months.

Full-term newborn babies are thus passively protected against such common pathogens as streptococci, pneumococci, meningococci and *Haemophilus influenzae*. They are protected against tetanus and diphtheria toxins and viruses such as measles, rubella and mumps.

IgM is a larger molecule which does not cross the placenta. It is this immunoglobulin fraction which is responsible for combating Gram-negative bacterial infections, the most common of which is *E. coli*. IgM synthesis begins slowly in the fetus. It starts at about 20 weeks gestation and by term has reached only about 10% of adult levels (less than 20 mg/100 ml). If the fetus has been infected, a high level of IgM is found at birth; this is used as a non-specific marker of intrauterine infection. It is the low neonatal IgM levels which allow *E.coli* to be such a common and dangerous pathogen for these babies—at no other time of life does *E.coli* commonly cause meningitis—and at present Gram-negative bacteria are the commonest causes of infection.

IgA does not cross the placenta and is synthesized by babies only after birth. However, it is present in very high concentration in maternal colostrum and breast milk. It protects breast-fed infants (in conjunction with another substance present in breast milk called lactoferrin) from gastroenteritis caused by pathogenic *E.coli*. This is one of the reasons why breast feeding is so good for the baby: the incidence of gastroenteritis is very much lower in the wholly breast-fed infant than in bottle-fed babies (see Chapter 7). Lactoferrin is efficient at binding iron, as its name implies; *E.coli* need iron for growth and replacation, and, therefore, breast milk suppresses the growth of *E.coli* which is then more easily destroyed by the IgA.

Classification of Infections

It is convenient to classify infections in the newborn according to the time at which the infection was acquired.

Antenatally acquired

1 *Viruses* which cross the placenta: coxsackie, rubella, poliomyelitis, variola, vaccinia, cytomegalovirus.
2 *Spirochaetes*: syphilis.
3 *Protozoa*: toxoplasmosis.
4 *Bacteria*, e.g. tuberculosis, typhoid, listeriosis.

Acquired during delivery

1 *Ascending vaginal infections*. These occur with prolonged rupture of membranes. This may lead to amnionitis with placentitis and fetal septicaemia or to a congenital pneumonia following inhalation of organisms.
2 *Gonococcal ophthalmia*. This has become more common again recently. At one time prophylactic Credé (silver nitrate) drops were given to all newborn babies. This unfortunately caused chemical conjunctivitis in many babies and since treatment with systemic and intraocular penicillin proved to be very effective routine use of the drops was stopped. Some paediatricians now feel that Credé drops should be given to all babies whose mothers have not attended for antenatal care.
3 *Herpes*. This is usually of type 2 (genital). The mother has no natural immunity to transfer to the fetus because the herpes live in the vagina and are therefore extracorporeal in terms of the mother's own immune responses. Neonatal herpes is often a fulminating and fatal infection.
4 *Candidiasis* (thrush) acquired from the mother's vaginal infection.
5 *Listeriosis* (see below).
6 *Group B streptococci* (see below).
7 *Chlamydia* can cause severe ophthalmia and pneumonia. It is difficult to grow and special cultures must be taken.

Postnatally acquired

Examples in this group are *E.coli*, staphylococci, *Klebsiella* sp., *Enterobacter* sp., *Serratia* sp., Group B streptococci.

Prevention of Infection

Prevention of neonatal sepsis is very important:

1 Infected or potentially infected babies must be adequately supervised in a separate isolation unit or cubicle. (In some types of infection, e.g. urinary tract infection, isolation is not usually considered necessary; in contrast gastroenteritis, for instance, is very infectious indeed.)

2 Hand-washing before and after handling each baby is the single most important procedure. Basins in the isolation unit must be fitted with elbow taps to avoid contamination. There is no evidence that the wearing of gowns and gloves reduces the spread of infection but disposable gloves could be used during procedures where there is great danger of infecting the baby such as tracheal toilet. Masks are also unnecessary. Any doctor or nurse with a sore throat or other infectious illness or fever should not be on the unit. Sometimes a doctor who feels well may carry an organism such as the virus Echo 11 which can cause serious illness among newborn babies. Disposable paper towels should be used for hand drying.

3 Floors, incubators and lockers must be cleaned regularly. Dirty nappies and dirty linen should be disposed of separately into colour-coded covered bags. A regular supply of clean nappies is necessary. Disposable ones are usually best.

4 There must be facilities for aseptic preparation and storage of feeds. A modern milk kitchen or the use of prepacked feeds is suitable.

5 Crowding infants too closely together, either because of pressure of admissions or, for example, under a phototherapy unit, should be avoided.

6 Antibiotics should be used appropriately and sensibly with good laboratory back-up. Overuse of powerful antibiotics will only lead to the development of resistant organisms.

7 Babies admitted from home or other units should be regarded as potentially infected and not admitted to the main unit until proved otherwise.

8 Breast feeding should be encouraged.

9 Babies must be examined daily by the nursing staff for signs of minor infection, such as a red umbilicus, sticky eyes, septic spots or oral candidiasis.

10 There is no evidence that unrestricted visiting by healthy adults and their children increases the infection rate on the nursery. However, all those with an active infection should keep away.

Diagnosis

The diagnosis of neonatal infection is difficult. Fever is not essential for the diagnosis (infected babies are equally likely to be hypothermic) and signs are often non-specific, for example poor weight gain or weight loss, reluctance to feed, vomiting, jaundice, lethargy, irritability, tachypnoea, apnoea or collapse. Owing to the rapid spread from a localized infection to generalized septicaemia, delay in diagnosis may be extremely serious. Certainly morbidity and mortality are reduced by early diagnosis and treatment. It is worth remembering that any deterioration after the first two or three days in a hitherto healthy baby is most likely to be due to infection until proved otherwise. For all these reasons, the concept of the infection screen has grown up.

At the first suspicion of infection, the following investigations should be carried out:
1 Full white cell count and differential (usually haemoglobin is done at the same time). Neutropenia is as likely a finding in septicaemia as neutrophilia.
2 Platelet count. A low count may be the first sign of septicaemia.
3 Blood culture (from an antecubital vein using a 23 gauge butterfly, not from the umbilical or femoral veins).
4 Suprapubic sample of urine (if possible) for culture and sensitivities. Failing this a bag urine specimen.
5 Swabs from any obvious infected area. Other swabs may just show what organisms have colonized the baby and do not necessarily show infection.
6 In an *ill* baby, CSF should be obtained by lumbar puncture and tested for protein and sugar content, culture and sensitivities.
7 Blood-gas analysis and biochemical studies (glucose, calcium, urea and electrolytes, bilirubin) may also give valuable information.

The infection screen must not be thought of as a substitute for full clinical examination of the infant, since local signs may well be present, e.g. a red umbilicus, a painful, swollen limb in osteitis or a bulging fontanelle in meningitis.

Treatment of Infections

Treatment, like diagnosis, is a matter of urgency. In ill babies antibiotics should be started before the *results* of the investigations are known. Many units think that the drugs of choice are penicillin and gentamicin. Penicillin is particularly effective against streptococci while gentamicin is bactericidal to staphylococci and Gram-negative organisms.

Gentamicin should not be given intravenously because of the danger of toxic blood levels which might damage the infant's hearing. It is essential to check plasma gentamicin levels in infants being treated so as to ensure that adequate therapeutic amounts are being given and that toxic levels are not being reached. It is usual to take blood just before an injection and

Table 16.1 Daily antibiotic dosage for neonates.

Drug	Route	Preterm infants and term infants less than seven days (/kg/day)	Term infants more than seven days (/kg/day)
Penicillin	i.v., i.m.	100 000 units divided six-hourly (increase in meningitis, Group B β-haemolytic streptococcal infection)	150 000 units divided six-hourly
Ampicillin	i.v., i.m.	62.5 mg divided six-hourly	100 mg divided six-hourly
Flucloxacillin	i.v., i.m., oral	62.5 mg divided six-hourly	75 mg divided eight-hourly
Mecillinam	i.m.	40 mg divided six-hourly	40 mg divided six-hourly
Azlocillin Mezlocillin	i.v., i.m.	100 mg divided eight-hourly	150 mg divided eight-hourly
Carbenicillin	i.v.	½–1 hour infusion 300 mg divided eight-hourly	½–1 hour infusion 300–400 mg divided six or eight-hourly
Cefuroxime	i.m.	30 mg divided twelve-hourly	30 mg divided twelve-hourly
Cefotaxime	i.m.	100 mg divided twelve-hourly	150 mg divided eight-hourly
Gentamicin†	i.m.	6 mg divided twelve-hourly; 4.5 mg every 18 hours for <7 days or <1000 g	7.5 mg divided twelve-hourly
Amikacin†	i.v., i.m.	15 mg divided twelve-hourly	15–22.5 mg divided twelve-hourly
Chloramphenicol†	i.v.	Day 1, 50 mg divided twelve-hourly. Then 25 mg divided	Day 1, 75 mg divided twelve-hourly. Then 50 mg divided

Table 16.1 Daily antibiotic dosage for neonates (*contd*)

Drug	Route	Preterm infants and term infants less than seven days (/kg/day)	Term infants more than seven days (/kg/day)
		twelve-hourly (may be four-to-six-hourly)	twelve-hourly (may be four-to-six-hourly)
Fusidic acid	i.v.	20 mg continuous infusion	20 mg continuous infusion
Cotrimoxazole	oral*	1 ml paediatric suspension (sulphamethoxazole 40 mg/ml; trimethoprim 8 mg/ml)	
Metronidazole	rectal, i.v.	20 mg divided six-hourly	20 mg divided six-hourly
Flucytosine†	oral	120 mg divided six-hourly	120 mg divided six-hourly
Miconazole	i.v.	30 mg divided twelve-hourly	30 mg divided twelve-hourly
Piperacillin	i.m., i.v.	200 mg divided twelve-hourly	200 mg divided twelve-hourly
Ticarcillin	i.m., i.v.	225 mg divided eight-hourly	300 mg divided six-hourly
Latamoxef	i.m., i.v.	100 mg divided twelve-hourly	150 mg divided eight-hourly
Ceftazidime	i.m., i.v.	50 mg divided twelve-hourly	50 mg divided twelve-hourly
Tobramycin†	i.m., i.v.	4 mg divided twelve-hourly	6 mg divided eight-hourly
Netilmicin	i.m., i.v.	5 mg divided twelve-hourly	5 mg divided eight-hourly
Rifampicin	i.v.	10 mg divided six-hourly	10 mg divided twelve-hourly
Erythromycin	i.v. (slow)	40–60 mg divided six-hourly	40–60 mg divided six-hourly
Vancomycin†	i.v. as 60 minute infusion	30 mg divided twelve-hourly	30 mg divided twelve-hourly
Acyclovir	i.v. as 60 minute infusion	15–30 mg divided eight-hourly	15–30 mg divided eight-hourly

* Not to be given to jaundiced babies
† Levels need to be assayed

about one hour afterwards. Satisfactory levels should be 5–12 µg/ml (peak) and less than 3 µg/ml (trough). An important rule is that antibiotics should be stopped after 48 hours if there is no bacteriological or clinical evidence of infection.

At present, we use cefotaxime as 'blind' therapy and change to more specific therapy if pathogenic bacteria insensitive to this antibiotic are isolated. Ceftazidime or cefotaxime and gentamicin may be necessary in severe infections. The drugs can be withdrawn after 48 hours if the infant is well and cultures are negative. Each unit should decide on antibiotic policy after discussion with the microbiologists. The antibiotics chosen should be appropriate for the flora in the hospital. A guide to daily antibiotic dosages for the newborn is given in Table 16.1.

It is interesting to look back on how the incidence and type of neonatal infections has changed over the last 40 years. At that time epidemics of gastroenteritis due to Gram-negative organisms were common in newborn baby nurseries. This was largely due to the failure to realize the importance of sterile preparation of feeds and of precautions against spreading infection from one baby to another. In the 1950s and 1960s, the incidence of Gram-negative infections fell because these simple precautions were taken. This led to an increase in the number of staphylococcal infections, which, although they often produced only minor illnesses, occasionally led to epidemics of severe sepsis with a high mortality. These infections were often acquired from nursing and medical staff. In the last 20 years the incidence of staphylococcal infections has fallen, owing partly to antibiotic use, but also to regular hand washing with hexachlorophane soaps before and after handling babies and to the use in many units of hexachlorophane baths. Two problems arose, however, with the widespread use of hexachlorophane: if used in high concentration it is absorbed through the newborn preterm baby's skin to produce toxic effects to the nervous system; second, its use has encouraged the spread of Gram-negative infections so that it is these which are now most common. Chlorhexidine is a substance which kills Gram-negative organisms and many paediatric units are now using a combination of hexachlorophane and chlorhexidine solutions or dusting powders to suppress both Gram-negative and Gram-positive infections. If hexachlorophane baths are used it must be carefully washed off each day.

A number of specific conditions, and infections caused by specific organisms or groups of organisms, will now be described in greater detail.

Septicaemia

The invasion of the bloodstream by actively dividing organisms may follow localized infection by many organisms (see for example under group B β-haemolytic streptococcal and water-borne infections) but at present Gram-negative septicaemia due to infection by enteric Gram-negative rods including *E.coli* is the most common. There may be, but need not be, evidence of a preceding localized infection such as urinary tract infection, pneumonia or meningitis. The role of *Staph epidermidis* in septicaemia is now more important. The diagnosis depends on blood culture, but antibiotics should be started before the results are available if the infant is ill.

Meningitis

Since 1981, in the UK, Group B streptococci have replaced *E.coli* as the commonest cause of meningitis in the newborn baby. These two now account for more than 70% of cases. Other causative organisms include staphylococci, pneumococci, *Listeria monocytogenes* and *Candida albicans*. The onset is often insidious with poor feeding, drowsiness and vomiting as the only signs. Convulsions are a late sign, as are a bulging fontanelle or head retraction. Neck stiffness is rare. It is a grave mistake to wait for neurological signs before suspecting meningitis. Lumbar puncture should be a screening test whenever systemic infection is suspected, which is to say in most ill babies.

Remember that normal cerebrospinal fluid shows a great variation in the neonate. The fluid is often yellow and this may be due both to the relatively high protein content (up to 1000 mg/l is within the normal range and it may be two or three times this in normal preterm babies) and to the presence of bilirubin in the jaundiced baby. Yellow CSF is by no means diagnostic of kernicterus and is found at relatively low serum bilirubin levels. Up to 20 cells per μl (if all lymphocytes) may normally occur.

If meningitis is suspected, treatment should be started before culture results are available. A standard regime is intravenous penicillin (up to 150 000 units/kg four- to six-hourly) and intravenous chloramphenicol is best given 8–12 hourly, as 4–6 hourly results in low serum concentrations (50 mg/kg/day for 48 hours, then 25 mg/kg/day). Gentamicin, though commonly prescribed, does not seem particularly useful in this situation—it does not cross the blood–brain barrier and is poorly effective when given intrathecally or even into the ventricles.

Chloramphenicol blood levels must be monitored to avoid both inadequate dosage and the grey baby syndrome (circulatory collapse and death) where there is a very high blood concentration of chloramphenicol. When the organism and its sensitivities are known, the least appropriate of these drugs may be discontinued. The newer cephalosporins may turn out to be very useful for treating Gram-negative bacterial meningitis in the newborn.

Meningitis is an extremely serious condition in the newborn with a high mortality. Complications in survivors include subdural effusions, mental retardation, deafness and isolated cranial nerve palsies.

Pneumonia

Congenital pneumonia acquired by the inhalation of infected liquor presents with respiratory distress during the early hours of life. It is often associated with prolonged rupture of membranes.

Aspiration pneumonia was particularly common in preterm babies in whom sucking, swallowing and cough reflexes are poorly developed. It may follow sucking or careless tube feeding and lead to sudden onset of choking and cyanosis.

Pneumonia may be due to infection with other specific organisms, for example *Chlamydia* or staphylococci.

Uncommonly air-borne *bronchopneumonia* occurs in the neonate, acquired as in older children.

Treatment is by oxygen, antibiotics and other supportive treatment as indicated.

Gastroenteritis

Gastric infection is rare in the wholly breast-fed baby. Outbreaks are most often due to rotavirus and sometimes to pathogenic *E.coli*. It is likely that both infections may be asymptomatic in many babies. In some, however, there is rapid deterioration and dehydration. Treatment is by stopping oral feeding and giving intravenous fluid replacement. Antibiotics are not indicated; they do nothing to improve the clinical course and tend to encourage the growth of resistant strains. The only exception to this rule is in the baby in whom septicaemia has developed.

Necrotizing enterocolitis

The cause of this serious illness is still a mystery. There are probably several aetiological factors acting together. We can now identify certain babies as being particularly at risk. They include those who are preterm, weigh less than 2000 g, have suffered perinatal asphyxia or hypoglycaemia or have had hyaline membrane disease, septicaemia, hypothermia, congenital heart disease or exchange transfusions. The syndrome is less likely in babies taking milk from the breast but may occur in those babies fed expressed breast milk from a milk bank or those who are being complemented with artificial feed. Colostrum seems to have a particular protective value. Other important associations are a history of umbilical arterial or venous catheterization, and nasojejunal feeding.

It is probable that necrotizing enterocolitis develops in the following way: a primary insult, such as hypoxaemia, hypoglycaemia or hypothermia, leads to reduced blood flow to the gut. This, perhaps coupled with hypertonic or artificial feeds, produces mucosal oedema and ulceration. In the baby who is not being suckled, the absence of such factors as

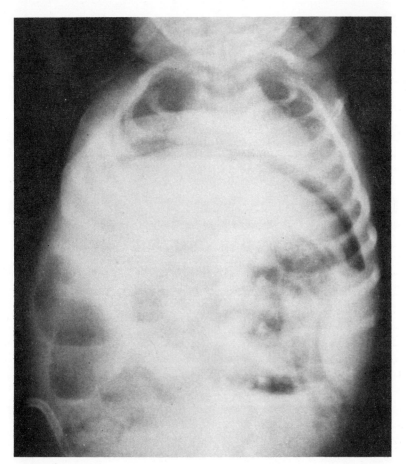

Fig. 16.2 Necrotizing enterocolitis

IgA and lymphocytes in colostrum, plus the colonization of the bowel with Gram-negative organisms such as *E.coli* and *Klebsiella*, leads to invasion of the bowel wall, portal system and bowel lymphatics by these organisms and others such as *Clostridium* and *Bacteroides*. Affected babies become systemically unwell both because of resultant endotoxin release leading to disseminated intravascular coagulation and collapse and through septicaemia with bowel necrosis and peritonitis.

In the early stages clinical signs are non-specific. Failure of temperature control is an important clue and this is followed by gradual abdominal distension and blood in the stools. Bile-stained vomiting develops, but constipation rather than diarrhoea is usual initially. Unless treatment is started promptly at this stage, there is rapid deterioration, collapse and death. Initially, radiographic changes are confined to dilatation of small loops of bowel with or without fluid levels. Later, probably following invasion of the bowel wall by gas-producing organisms, gas is seen within the bowel wall (pneumatosis intestinalis) or the portal tract (Fig 16.2). Once perforation occurs, free air is seen under the diaphragm in an erect abdominal radiograph.

The platelet count and plasma sodium concentration are usually low.

Management is initially conservative. Oral feeds should be discontinued and a wide-bore nasogastric tube passed passed into the stomach and left on continuous drainage with additional hourly gentle aspiration of stomach contents to decompress the bowel. Fluid should be given intravenously. Care must be taken to maintain a normal body temperature. Samples of blood and stool should be sent for culture and antibiotics should then be started. The most effective combination is usually intravenous penicillin and intramuscular gentamicin. Because of the frequent presence of *Bacteriodes* and other anaerobic organisms, most paediatricians add intravenous metronidazole. *Klibsiella* species are often found, so the use of an aminoglycoside antibiotic, such as gentamicin, is essential.

As there is considerable loss of fluid from the damaged bowel it is easy to underestimate the volume needed for adequate replacement. Transfusion with fresh blood (10–20 ml/kg body weight) over one or two hours may help re-establish normal blood pressure and ensure good perfusion of potentially necrotic bowel. Progress should be checked clinically by the baby's general condition and examination of the abdomen including measurements of girth, and radiologically by serial abdominal radiographs (lateral decubitus views with the baby lying on his left side are most useful). About three-quarters of affected babies will survive on this regimen provided diagnosis is prompt.

Surgery should be considered if the urine output drops, if abdominal distension increases, if there is free air in the peritoneal cavity on the radiograph or if there is a palpable abdominal mass. Whether the baby then survives depends largely on the length of necrotic bowel which has to be resected and hence on the amount of viable bowel that is left.

Late complications, of both medical and surgical treatment, include bowel strictures, presenting either as recurrent intestinal obstruction or as recurrent septicaemia, and diarrhoea. This may be due to a secondary lactose intolerance or may follow resection of the terminal ileum (where bile salts are primarily reabsorbed). It is usual to continue intravenous alimentation for one week after the last blood-stained stool. Small epidemics of the condition occur; when one case is diagnosed it is useful to test the stools of other babies in the ward. A positive test for blood is an indication for careful observation.

The overall survival rate is now about 60–70%.

Urinary tract infection

The only sign of a urinary tract infection in the neonate may be poor weight gain, jaundice or vomiting. This is the only time of life when such infections are commoner in boys than girls. Suprapubic aspiration is the best way to make the diagnosis as there is then no possibility of contamination of the specimen by organisms on the perineum. Septicaemia may supervene if the diagnosis is delayed. The diagnosis of a true urinary tract infection in either sex in infancy is adequate grounds for radiological examination of the urinary tract. Ultrasound has now largely replaced intravenous pyelography but micturating cystography should still be carried out. This is to detect the presence of any underlying anatomical abnormality which may be predisposing to infection, and the presence of reflux.

Hepatitis

Hepatitis may be caused by a number of organisms, for example viruses such as that of serum hepatitis, cytomegalovirus (CMV), rubella or herpes simplex, and protozoa such as toxoplasmosis, or it may be found as a complication of septicaemia with bacteria such as *E.coli*. CMV, rubella and serum hepatitis are acquired transplacentally, while herpes simplex is acquired during passage down the birth canal.

Characteristically, the baby is jaundiced with pale and heavily bile-stained (dark) urine. The liver is often palpably enlarged. The differential diagnosis from other causes of obstructive jaundice may be extremely difficult (see Chapter 12).

Ophthalmia

The most common organisms are staphylococcus, *E.coli*, *Mycoplasma hominis*, *Chlamydia* (the TRIC agent) and, increasingly once more, beta-lactamase-producing (i.e. penicillin resistant) strains of the gonococcus. Purulent ophthalmia, which is a notifiable disease, should not be confused with the common sticky eye, although the latter may progress to ophthalmia. The fluid that bathes the surface of the eye normally drains down into the nose via the tear duct which leads from the inner canthus of the eye. The tear duct is an extremely fine passage in the newborn baby and is easily blocked by sticky secretions. This results in the sticky eye, which needs mopping with normal saline while the tear duct is gently massaged towards the nose. If this is not done, the stasis may lead to infection with one of the organisms mentioned above. Such infections are best treated, after a swab has been taken, with chloramphenicol or neomycin eyedrops. If chlamydial cultures are not taken prior to treatment then neomycin should be used, as chloramphenicol will not cure chlamydial infection but will make it impossible to isolate the organism.

In a severe purulent ophthalmia, especially in babies whose mothers have not attended for antenatal care, gonococcal or chlamydial infection should be suspected. This is potentially dangerous and needs extremely vigorous treatment. Penicillin drops should be instilled into the eyes as soon as a swab and smear have been sent for confirmation and then every five minutes for the first two hours, then quarter-hourly for 12 hours, half-hourly for 12 hours and so on. It is important during this time to treat with systemic penicillin in addition.

In all cases of ophthalmia it is worth remembering that the baby should be treated on his side with the worse affected eye downwards so that infection is not spread needlessly from the infected to the good eye. When treating it is sensible to treat both eyes simultaneously.

Tetanus

Neonatal tetanus is discussed in Chapter 19.

Breast abscess

Breast abscess is now uncommon in nursing mothers but sometimes occurs in newborn babies. It must not be confused with the common, harmless breast enlargement in the newborn (sometimes confusingly called mastitis). If a widespread abscess forms over the anterior chest wall (Fig. 16.3) surgical drainage may be necessary.

Omphalitis

As the cord separates there is often a little redness of the edge of the skin. Any more widespread erythema is a sign of infection, particularly if there is also a discharge of pus, and should be treated with antibiotics. The cord is colonized with bacteria shortly after birth, but the numbers of organisms can be reduced by applying an antiseptic. If these are used the cord separates later. Severe infection of the umbilicus (see Fig. 16.4) may spread through the umbilical vein to the liver.

Group B β-haemolytic streptococcal infection

Infection by this group of organisms has become more widely recognized in recent years. The organisms are commonly found in the maternal birth canal and can be very difficult to eradicate from the vagina by antibiotic treatment. Ascending infection may result in early onset streptococcal disease in the neonate, since the organism can pass across the membranes

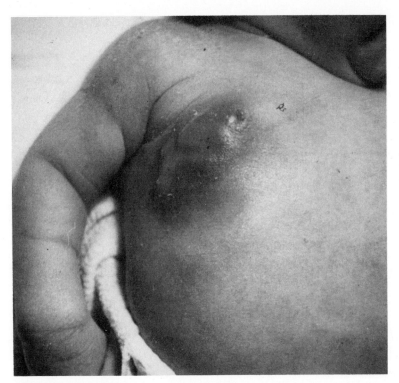

Fig. 16.3 Breast abscess

into amniotic fluid. They may be inhaled during passage of the fetus down the birth canal leading to sudden collapse during the first 48 hours of life with additional signs of respiratory distress (see Chapter 6). Alternatively they may cause meningitis during the early weeks of life.

Mortality is still high. As the organisms are relatively penicillin-resistant, treatment must be with high-dose penicillin (100 000–150 000 units/kg six-hourly intravenously or intramuscularly) and gentamicin. Some units have even given one injection of long-acting penicillin to every newborn baby in an attempt to prevent the condition. We do not give penicillin prophylaxis or treat healthy babies colonized with Group B streptococci.

The infection should be suspected in any baby who becomes severely ill within the first 48 hours of life, paticularly those with respiratory distress. However, other organisms such as *Klebsiella* may produce similar catastrophic illnesses.

Gram-negative infections

These organisms remain common and important pathogens in the newborn. The reasons for this are discussed in the early part of the chapter (p. 288). As well as the commonly recognized infections due to *E.coli* there are many reports of infections in newborn babies caused by *organisms transmitted in water*. This is probably due to the use of incubators with built-in water tanks, resuscitation tables with water manometers, indwelling catheters for prolonged intravenous alimentation, water-filled heating coils for warming blood and contaminated sinks. It is a good idea to change the water in humidifiers daily to prevent colonization by such organisms.

The most important organism causing such infections is *Pseudomonas aeruginosa* which is particularly likely to affect ill or preterm babies who are being ventilated. Skin lesions looking like red rings are signs of septicaemia, and diarrhoea is sometimes an early sign, but sudden or insidious deterioration in a small or sick baby may be the first warning. Gentamicin is effective against most strains of the organism, but ceftazidime or other drugs may be necessary for resistant types. Autoclaving effectively sterilizes equipment which would otherwise harbour organisms. We now see unusual infections in babies on intravenous alimentation; *Serratia marcescens* and *Enterobacter* sp. are becoming a particular problem and are difficult to treat.

Staphylococcal infection

Today staphylococcal infections are usually less virulent than in the past. This is partly because of the appropriate use of antiseptics and antibiotics, but the staphylococci colonizing newborn babies are probably less virulent than they were.

Staphylococcus aureus has long been recognized as an important pathogen in the newborn. *S.epidermidis* is now thought to be important as well. Types of infection particularly associated with staphylococci include:

1 *Omphalitis*. See above (p. 300). A high incidence of colonization with staphylococci correlates with the incidence of clinical infection. Serious inflammation of the umbilicus with pockets of pus or peeling of the skin is now uncommon. (Fig. 16.4).

2 *Pustules*. Pustules are probably the commonest sign of staphylococcal infection in the newborn. They often occur around the neck or in the axillae. Unlike the pustules in toxic erythema, staphylococcal pustules are rare before the third day of life and contain neutrophils, not eosinophils, if a smear is taken from a lesion.

3 *Bullous impetigo (pemphigus neonatorum)*. Large vesicles, without erythema, containing clear yellow fluid.

4 *Scalded skin syndrome* (Ritter's disease, toxic epidermal necrolysis).

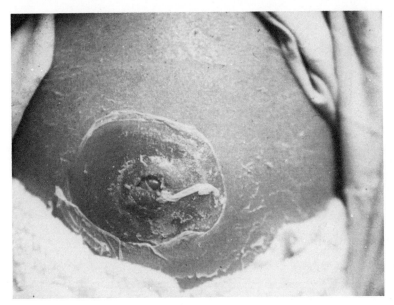

Fig. 16.4 Severe periumbilical infection

This is a much more extensive infection of the skin leading to widespread desquamation with raw areas. It is probably due to an exfoliative toxin produced by certain types of staphylococci (e.g. phage types 71 or 55/71) (Fig. 16.5).

5 *Otitis media.* This condition is probably underdiagnosed in the newborn. It should be considered in any ill baby, or one with an unexplained fever.

6 *Pneumonia.* Staphylococcal pneumonia is now rare in the newborn. It may lead to abscesses or emphysematous bullae. It is common in severe cystic fibrosis.

7 *Septicaemia.* This is now more commonly seen following an invasive procedure, for example the insertion of an umbilical arterial catheter through a contaminated umbilicus. However, any minor infection such as a pustule or paronychia is a potential source of septicaemia and should be taken seriously. A septicaemia may lead to *osteomyelitis* or *infective arthritis* with potentially severe damage to bones and joints.

8 *Meningitis.* Recurrent staphylococcal meningitis should suggest the presence of a midline congenital sinus connecting skin and CSF. It may be necessary to shave the head to seek carefully any sign of a track which could communicate with the subarachnoid space.

Any baby with a proven staphylococcal infection should be isolated from other babies in the hospital. The prevalence of colonization can be

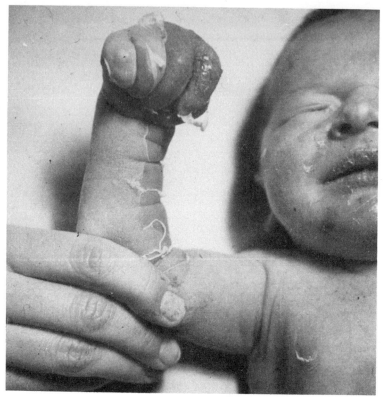

Fig. 16.5   The scalded skin syndrome (toxic epidermal necrolysis)

reduced by the use of chlorhexidine spirit and hexachlorophane powder on the umbilicus. Hand washing using a chlorhexidine/hexachlorophane liquid is important.

Local treatement may be adequate, for example the treatment of pustules by hexachlorophane powder, but it is often safer to give systemic antibiotics which are in any case essential in more serious infections. Flucloxacillin (either intravenously or intramuscularly every 24 hours in the first 48 hours of life, then eight-hourly up to two weeks of age, then six-hourly) is the drug of choice as most hospital staphylococci are now penicillin-resistant. It should be given less frequently to the pre-term baby (every 12 hours during the first week, eight-hourly between one and four weeks). Other useful drugs include penicillin (for sensitive organisms) and gentamicin. A five-day course is adequate for simple pustular lesions, but osteomyelitis may need six weeks treatment or more.

Listeriosis

Listeriosis is an increasingly common condition in Great Britain and is an important cause of death in the newborn in many countries where pasteurization of milk is less rigorous (e.g. France). The baby is infected from his mother, who is usually a symptom-free carrier. Sometime previously, she has ingested the bacterium (*Listeria monocytogenes*) in contaminated milk, milk products or undercooked meat.

The organism is a Gram-positive rod, and is not difficult to identify on routine culture.

The fetus may be infected transplacentally. This produces septicaemia and often meningoencephalitis with third trimester infections, but usually fetal death and abortion if the infection is earlier. The baby may be infected by inhaling contaminated meconium during delivery. This leads to pneumonia and septicaemia. Jaundice and purpura often occur, with atypical lymphocytes in the blood.

Mortality is not high provided that appropriate antibiotic treatment is given promptly. In survivors, there is a risk of mental handicap and hydrocephalus.

The antibiotic of choice is ampicillin as some strains appear to be penicillin-resistant. Gentamicin can also be used. It used to be thought that the organism was difficult to eradicate from the mother who was at risk of having recurrently infected fetuses but there seems to be no good evidence for this in humans.

Congenital syphilis

This disease, once common in this country and now again increasing in incidence, is still extremely common in many developing countries. The infecting organism, the spirochaete *Treponema pallidum*, infects the fetus by crossing the placenta after the fourth month of pregnancy. The affected baby may be stillborn or may develop a number of characteristic signs of the disease within the first few weeks of life. It is essential that all pregnant women should have serological tests for syphilis. VDRL and TPHA tests are commonly used.

The clinical signs of congenital syphilis appear after about three weeks and these include snuffles associated with infection of the nasal bones and cartilages, eczema round the mouth with fissures and subsequent scarring at the angles of the mouth (rhagades), hepatosplenomegaly, anaemia, a generalized copper-coloured maculopapular rash with blisters which may be particularly severe over the palms and soles giving rise to 'washerwoman's skin'. There may be general failure to thrive and fever.

It is not uncommon for a syphilitic mother to give birth to a normal infant. In such a situation, the infant's serum tests such as VDRL will be positive, because of positive transfer of maternal antibodies. The presence of characteristic symptoms or signs with positive VDRL, rather than a positive result itself, should therefore be the indication for treatment. However, if the baby's VDRL titre is much higher than the mother's, congenital infection is likely. The IgM specific test may be very helpful; the IgM fluorescent treponemal antibody absorption test (IgM FTA-ABS) indicates that the baby has produced antibodies, as IgM does not cross the placenta. Treatment is with penicillin given as procaine penicillin G, 50 000 units/kg/24 hours for 14 days.

Candidiasis (thrush)

This fungal infection is often acquired from the mother's vagina with subsequent re-infection from the mother's or attendant's fingers. It is also common in babies who are on broad-spectrum antibiotics or whose mothers are careless about sterile preparation of artificial feeds. Commonly, it presents with white plaques on the tongue or inside the mouth which, unlike milk curds, rub off only with difficulty and leave a raw, red bleeding surface underneath. Infection of the perianal, vulval or scrotal skin is also common and may provide a source of re-infection. A candidal napkin rash may often be distinguished from an ammoniacal dermatitis by the fact that it goes down into the skin creases and by the presence of satellite lesions around the area of erythema.

In the ill preterm baby receiving intravenous feeding there is a risk that superficial candidiasis may lead to septicaemia which is usually fatal. Treatment is with nystatin, 100 000 units four-hourly onto the tongue, or by nystatin creams for the nappy area. Gentian violet is messier, but cheaper. Septicaemia is difficult to treat but we have used amphotericin B, miconazole and flucytosine.

Tuberculosis

Very rarely tubercle bacilli are transmitted transplacentally or via infected amniotic fluid from mother to fetus. Less rarely an infant is infected postnatally by a mother with active disease. The incidence of the disease in infants and children in communities with a high rate of adult tuberculosis can be much reduced by immunization with BCG shortly after birth (see Chapter 4). Provided a mother with active disease is started on treatment, she may continue to breast feed her baby. He should be immunized with isoniazid-resistant BCG and started on isoniazid to make doubly sure he does not catch the infection.

Viral infection

Cytomegalovirus (CMV)

This is a virus similar to herpes and is acquired in utero causing severe generalized disease in the baby with enlargement of liver and spleen, jaundice, microcephaly with mental retardation, choroidoretinitis and intracranial calcification. The neonate may present with signs of intra-uterine growth retardation, microcephaly, respiratory distress or encephalitis. The diagnosis may be confirmed by demonstrating a rising titre of serum complement-fixing antibodies, by culturing the virus from the urine or by finding inclusion bodies in renal tubular cells in the urine. This clinical syndrome is rare, but some surveys have shown that cytomegalovirus can often be grown from the urine of apparently normal newborn babies. The prognosis for these infants is still not certain. When giving a blood transfusion it is now our practice only to give blood which does not contain CMV antibodies.

Congenital rubella

Whereas in the child and adult German measles is a mild infection, in the newborn infant it is an extremely serious disease. If it is acquired during the first four weeks of pregnancy, there is a greater than 50% chance of fetal damage, but most commonly intrauterine death occurs. Over the next few weeks, during the phase of organogenesis, there is about a 25% chance of fetal damage, but when damage does occur it naturally involves many organs in the body. These include the eye, leading to microphthalmos, cataract, glaucoma or choroidoretinitis; the brain, leading to mental retardation or microcephaly; the ear, leading to deafness; and the heart, most commonly patent ductus arteriosus, pulmonary stenosis, ventricular or atrial septal defects. In addition, the disease remains active throughout pregnancy and for the early months of extrauterine life so that the infant may be born with osteitis, myocarditis, petechial haemorrhages, anaemia and pneumonia. The virus may be recovered from the urine or throat of an affected infant for several months after birth. The greatest risk of fetal damage occurs, therefore, before the mother knows she is pregnant. In addition, it may follow mild or unrecognized clinical attacks of rubella. After three to four months gestation, there is a less than 2% chance of a fetus suffering damage from cogenital rubella, but the baby must always be checked for deafness.

If a woman develops an illness suggestive of rubella during the first trimester of pregnancy, the diagnosis should be confirmed serologically by examination of paired serum specimens. If over the four weeks between the specimens there is a sharp rise in rubella-specific antibody levels, this is clear evidence of a recent infection. It is common practice in this situation to offer a therapeutic abortion, since the fetus is very likely to be born severely handicapped.

It is now policy in Great Britain to immunize actively all susceptible girls before puberty with attenuated rubella virus, thus making it impossible for such girls to catch the disease during a subsequent pregnancy. The vaccine is extremely effective, but unfortunately many girls are not being immunized at present. One possible alternative is to give rubella vaccine in early infancy (as in the USA) with measles and mumps vaccines. It is not known how long protection given by the vaccine lasts, however.

All babies whose mothers have had serologically confirmed rubella in pregnancy must be followed up carefully. Sometimes there is very little serological evidence of rubella at first in the baby. The IgM specific antibodies may not always be present in an infant with congenital rubella.

Herpes

See above (p. 289).

Acquired immune deficiency syndrome (AIDS)

This disease is caused by the human immunodeficiency virus (HIV), formerly called the human T cell lymphotropic virus type III (HTLV III). There is progressive failure of the body's immune system leading to chronic diarrhoea, malnutrition, wasting, increased suscepti- bility to opportunistic infections with such organisms as toxoplasma, candida and pneumocystis, and death. There is, at present, no cure, so it is giving rise to a lot of anxiety in the community.

About 1% of all AIDS cases have been children under 13 years of age. They have caught the disease either via infected blood products (e.g. haemophiliacs or following exchange transfusion) or from their infected mother (either in utero, at birth, or subsequently). An infected mother, who could transmit the virus to her baby, is likely either to be an intravenous drug abuser or the sexual contact of someone in a high-risk group—a bisexual male or another drug abuser.

It is not yet clear what proportion of babies born to infected mothers will develop AIDS. It is likely to be between 25% and 65%. At birth, babies of infected mothers will have antibody in their circulation. Posi- tive IgM antibody, and/or IgG antibody persisting beyond 6–12 months, indicates that the infant is infected. Not all infected patients will go on to develop the full clinical disease. The proportion of adults may be as low as 10% but may be higher in babies. Certainly progression of the disease seems to be rapid in children. It is likely that the large variety of antigens that the infant meets causes enhanced virus replication in T helper lymphocytes.

It seems very difficult to transmit the infection from infected children to close family contacts or hospital staff. There is no evidence that an infected individual poses a threat to others at home, school or residential institution, and the same is probably true of the newborn nursery.

If a known AIDS sufferer is in labour, staff in the delivery room should wear protective clothing against spillage of blood or secretions. Care must be taken against penetrating injury from needles. The mucous membranes of eyes and mouth should also be protected.

Ideally, the newborn baby should be looked after by the mother as much as possible. She should not breast feed—breast milk is rich in lymphocytes, some of which will be T helper cells. Of course she should not contribute to any milk banks.

The virus is heat labile and inactivated by autoclaving. Any potentially contaminated spillage can be mopped with 10% hypochlorite or 2% activated glutaraldehyde solutions.

Protozoal infections

Congenital toxoplasmosis

Infection in pregnant women may affect the fetus since the protozoon is able to cross the placenta. Characteristic features include encephalitis with a raised protein and lymphocyte count in the CSF, choroidoretinitis, jaundice with hepatosplenomegaly, myocarditis and thrombocytopenic purpura. The diagnosis is made by finding a high concentration of toxoplasma antibody in the newborn baby's blood. There is often associated mental retardation and hydrocephalus, and 'tram-line' intracranial calcification is classically found on skull radiography.

Pneumocystis carinii

Infection by this protozoon is uncommon and is usually found in the preterm or already sick baby or in babies with immune deficiency. The usual presentation is with pneumonia and signs of respiratory distress. Transplacental infection has been described and nursery epidemics may occur. Treatment is with pentamidine isethionate 4 mg/kg/day in divided doses, but it is difficult to make the diagnosis during life and up to two-thirds of affected babies die.

Further Reading

de Louvois, J. (1985) Serious infections in the newborn. *Serious Infections Update No 7*.

Hanshaw, J.B. & Dudgeon, J.A. (1978) *Viral Diseases of the Fetus and Newborn.* Philadelphia: W.B. Saunders.

Hurley, R., de Louvois, J. & Draser, F. (1979) Perinatal and neonatal infection. *J. antimicrob. Chemother.*, 5. Suppl. A.

McCracken, G.K., Jr. & Nelson, J.D. (1977) *Antimicrobial Therapy for Newborns.* New York: Grune & Stratton.

Miller, M.E. (1978) *Host Defences in the Human Neonate.* New York; Grune & Stratton.

Remington, J.S. & Klein, J.O. (1976) *Infectious Diseases of the Fetus and Newborn Infant.* Philadelphia: W.B. Saunders.

Sudden or Gradual Deterioration

The recognition of a particular disease in a newborn baby is often difficult. This is because many conditions affecting, for example, the brain, heart or lungs may produce the same clinical signs. In particular, infections commonly mimic other illnesses. Making an accurate diagnosis depends on the clinical and laboratory evaluation of a relatively small number of non-specific signs and symptoms. In preterm babies, who are at higher risk, the severity of the disease is often greater yet the clinical features are even less specific than in term babies.

If a baby suddenly deteriorates or collapses, it is important to rely on the general principles of resuscitation (see Chapter 3). This will include correcting hypoxaemia with added oxygen and assisted ventilation, correcting acidaemia or hypoglycaemia and, subsequently, treating with antibiotics appropriate for a wide range of possible pathogens.

After initial resuscitation or in the baby who deteriorates insidiously it is very important not to start treatment (especially antibiotics) until adequate base-line investigations have been done: arterial blood gases, blood for culture, haemoglobin and full blood count, sugar and electrolytes, lumbar puncture and urine culture. Treatment should not await the results in an ill baby.

The purpose of Table 17.1 is to provide a quick reference guide to the possible differential diagnoses of some important features of illness in the newborn. Detailed discussion of these conditions will be found in the appropriate chapters elsewhere in this book.

Table 17.1 Possible differential diagnoses of some presenting features of illness in the newborn.

Presentation	Time	Additional symptoms, signs or associated clinical features	Possible cause	Action	See also Chapter
Collapse (sudden illness producing a shocked, grey mottled baby)	Usually after first 48 hours	Cyanotic attacks, diarrhoea or vomiting, weight loss, poor sucking, refusing feeds, minor infection	Septicaemia (especially Gram −ve)	Infection screen including LP; antibiotics before results are available	16
	<48 hours	As above	As above; especially Group B β-haemolytic streptococcal infection	As above. High dose penicillin and gentamicin	16
	<48 hours	Small-for-dates, baby of diabetic mother	Hypoglycaemia	Intravenous glucose	5, 15
	<48 hours	History of hypoxaemia, large volumes of intravenous alkali	Intraventricular haemorrhage (IVH)	Ventilation, transfusion	6
	2–3 weeks	Dehydration, ambiguous genitalia in female	Salt-losing congenital adrenal hyperplasia	Intravenous saline with care	9
Bleeding	<48 hours	Umbilical cord	Slipped clamp	Reclamp, transfuse if necessary	13
	48–72 hours	Umbilical stump, melaena	Haemorrhagic disease	Vitamin K_2, transfuse	13
	generally after 48 hours	Gut haemorrhage, small baby, Rhesus disease	Necrotizing enterocolitis	Plain abdominal X-ray	9
	Any age	Any site including pulmonary in very ill baby	Disseminated intravascular coagulation (DIC)	Treat precipitating illness; fresh frozen plasma	13
Pallor (sudden anaemia)	At birth	Tachypnoea, tachycardia or bradycardia	Fetomaternal haemorrhage, torn velamentous cord vessel	Immediate clamping of cord, transfuse group O −ve blood	13

	History / clinical signs	Condition (usually rhesus disease)	Treatment	Ref
	…pulmonary oedema	(usually rhesus disease)	…change transfusion, paracentesis, digital-ization, diuretics, ventilation	
1st 72 hours	Breech or difficult delivery, erythroblastosis	Intra-abdominal haemorrhage (adrenal, liver or spleen)	General supportive measures, transfusion	13
Any time	Already ill baby	DIC, covert bleeding	Treat precipitating illness; fresh plasma, blood	13
1st 72 hours	Severe RDS, history of hypoxia large volumes of intravenous alkali	IVH	Ventilation, transfusion	6
2nd week	Normochromic blood film, low birth weight (preterm) baby	Anaemia of prematurity	Transfusion	5
Fits 1st 48 hours	Cyanotic attacks, difficult or traumatic delivery	Intraventricular, subarachnoid or subdural haemorrhage, intrapartum asphyxia, anoxic brain damage	General resuscitation. Transfuse if necessary	14
1st 24 hours	Small-for-dates baby; large-for-dates baby; baby of diabetic mother	Hypoglycaemia	Intravenous dextrose after confirming with blood glucose test strips	5, 15
5–8 days	Mother with vitamin D deficiency or hyperparathyroidism	Hypocalcaemia	Calcium and magnesium supplements	14
1st week	Hypotonia	Organic acidaemias	Check plasma and urine by amino and organic acid chromatography	9, 14
Any age	Apnoeic attacks, general illness, bulging fontanelle, very rarely neck stiffness	Meningitis, usually E. coli or Group B β-haemolytic streptococci	Antibiotics, general measures for resuscitation	16

Table 17.1 (contd.)

Presentation	Time	Additional symptoms, signs or associated clinical features	Possible cause	Action	See also Chapter
Cyanotic attacks	1st 48 hours	Fits, history of traumatic delivery	Subdural haemorrhage, anoxic brain damage	General resuscitation transfuse if necessary	14
	After 48 hours	Diarrhoea or vomiting, lethargy, poor sucking	Infection, especially septicaemia	Infection screen, including LP, antibiotics	16
	Any age	Extreme preterm delivery	Apnoeic attacks of prematurity, intraventricular haemorrhage	Stimulation, theophylline, apnoea alarm	5
	Any age	Murmur, tachypnoea, heart failure	Congenital heart disease	Investigations and treatment for heart failure	10
Respiratory distress (tachypnoea/ recession/ gasping/ cyanosis)	1st 4 hours	Preterm, low Apgar scores	RDS	Appropriate ambient O_2 concentration, respiratory support	6
	Birth	Meconium staining of liquor and skin. Fetal distress. Small-for-dates baby	Meconium aspiration	Suck out trachea, appropriate O_2, antibiotics	5

Age/timing	Clinical features	Cause	Management	Ref
Birth	Oligohydramnios; characteristic facies; failed resuscitation	Potter's syndrome (renal agenesis, pulmonary hypoplasia)	Fatal	9
Birth	Thick tube fails to pass down both nostrils	Bilateral choanal atresia	Intubate, ventilate, surgical referral	3, 9
Early days	Retrognathia, glossoptosis, midline cleft palate	Pierre Robin anomaly	Nurse prone	9
Any age	During resuscitation, ventilation	Pneumothorax	Increase inspired O_2 concentration, drain if under tension	3, 6
During feed	Choking, hydramnios, inability to pass tube into stomach	Tracheo-oesophageal fistula	Suck out pouch, refer to surgeon	3, 9
During feed	Choking	Aspiration	Treat pneumonia (oxygen, antibiotics)	6
Any age	Cyanosis, murmur, small heart and/or 'ground glass' lung fields on chest X-ray	RDS, TAPVD especially, but many forms of cyanotic CHD	ECG, 100% O_2, echocardiography	10
On ventilator	Deteriorating hypoxia, struggling	Blocked tube, extubated, tension pneumothorax, worsening pulmonary disease	Change tube reintubate, chest drain, increase ventilation	6
On ventilator	Big baby fighting ventilator	Above causes excluded	Paralyse	6

18

The Mother and Baby in Hospital

Visiting

Hospital visiting for friends and relatives has often been severely restricted. The reasons given include interruption of nursing routine and the need to protect patients from fatigue. There is now no doubt that the visiting of mothers, fathers and siblings of newborn babies to a special care nursery should be unrestricted and encouraged as far as possible (Fig. 18.1). The same should apply to the ordinary postnatal ward. The evidence that such visiting increases the infection risk is poor, especially if those with obvious colds or sore throats stay away. A play-group for children of mothers attending the antenatal clinic or visiting the new baby is also very helpful.

The atmosphere on the unit should be as welcoming and friendly as possible.. Elaborate equipment is necessary but the rooms should not look and feel too clinical to non-medical people: there should be paintings on the walls, nurses wearing patterned smocks and even background music. Mobiles can be hung from or above cots and pretty toys put near the babies.

Animal studies show that there is a sensitive period after birth in which a mother gets to know her baby. If the mother and baby are separated at this time, the baby may be rejected on his return. There is increasing evidence that babies separated from their parents on special care baby units for many days or weeks are more at risk of being subsequently neglected or even battered by their parents. This is because there is no automatic affection between mother and child: the relationship is built up gradually over the early days, weeks and months of life and depends on intimate contact and frequent handling. This needs to be encouraged particularly when the baby is in an incubator. As soon as possible the mother should touch, feed and handle her baby, gradually doing more and more for longer and longer periods. Many studies have now shown that mothers who have extra contact with their babies after birth are more likely to look at them, touch them and talk to them more often. It takes a particular effort by the nurses to achieve this and to make parents feel at home surrounded by all the gadgetry. There are few babies too sick to be touched in the incubator and gradually fed and cuddled by their parents. Small babies often look very strange to their parents; there are now several companies who make specially designed premature baby clothes and these can often make them look prettier and more human. High stools are easy for mothers to get on and off, and give a good view

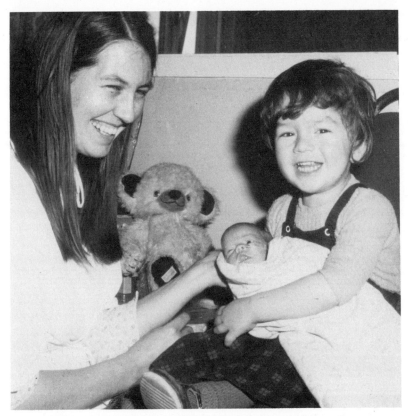

Fig. 18.1   Families should be encouraged to visit the baby in a special care unit

when their baby is in an incubator. Rocking chairs give a homely atmosphere and are more comfortable for a mother with a sore perineum.

Siblings should also be welcomed, not only to show them the new baby, but also because parents are more likely to come if they do not have to worry about baby-sitting arrangements. A playbox full of toys kept in the unit is useful to occupy them during a long visit.

If parents are not to be frightened (Fig. 18.2) time and trouble must be taken to explain what equipment is for and why it is necessary. Such things as eye covers for babies having phototherapy may be taken for granted by nursing and medical staff, yet to the unprepared mother they can be a great shock.

An increasing problem in recent years has been the transfer of the sick newborn baby for intensive care to another hospital (see Chapter 3). Ideally the mother should also be transferred, but this is not always possible. In such cases, it is an excellent idea for an instant photograph of

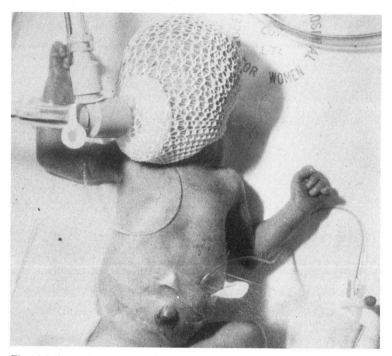

Fig. 18.2 A baby being ventilated via a face-mask. Note how frightening he must look to his mother

the baby to be taken before the baby is transferred (and preferably before too many tubes, catheters or masks are attached) and for it to be left with the mother. This is also valuable if a mother is too ill to visit her baby in the same hospital. If a mother is separated for some time, more photographs should be taken later. Postnatal ward routine must enable the new mother to make frequent visits to her baby in a special care nursery.

Babies often stay in hospital long after their mothers go home. It is important therefore that special care units include parents' rooms where they can stay overnight and thus involve themselves in their baby's care. As well as a bedroom there should ideally be a sitting-room and cooking facilities. Quite often it is possible for the baby to be nursed with his mother in a section of a postnatal ward set aside for the care of small, well babies. The mother who has just had her first baby may particularly benefit from this arrangement by gaining confidence in handling her new baby in such an atmosphere.

It is well known that many very small babies do not survive the neonatal period. Parents are therefore sometimes reluctant to form a close relationship with their baby in case he should die. We suspect that parents who have visited their baby and helped to nurse him when he was ill are more likely to be helped to grieve should the baby die (see below).

Going home

When a preterm baby leaves hospital it is often a time of great excitement —many parents have a small celebration with the staff when they leave —but it is also very worrying for them to have the baby at home with them on their own for the first time.

The discharge needs careful organization. The paediatrician and special care nurses must make a point of informing the general practitioner and health visitor that the baby is going home. It may be difficult to choose a suitable day of the week. Weekends are more convenient for many parents because father is home and a car may be available. On the other hand many districts have no health visitor at weekends and the GP may be away. Discharge during the week is usually preferable.

Some units are now experimenting with liaison staff between hospital and community. We have found it very helpful to have a liaison health visitor who can regularly review the baby's progress in hospital and keep the other health visitors informed. She can also feed back information about the baby's home to the unit so that bad housing, for example, can be brought to the unit's attention. If possible, one of the neonatal nurses from the unit should be available to visit the baby at home shortly after discharge. She can act as a support for the health visitor who may find the care of tiny babies at home very demanding and worrying.

Several controlled trials have shown that earlier discharge than in the past is safe. The criteria for allowing a baby home are:

1 satisfactory feeding and weight gain. They do not include a specific weight which must be achieved. Many babies of 1800 or 1900 g can now be allowed home quite safely.

2 no abnormality on examination.

3 parents who are confident about taking their baby home.

Parents will often have seen apnoea monitors in use in the hospital and ask if they need one at home. The baby should not be discharged if he is having apnoeic attacks. If he is well there is no evidence that present monitors, which alarm when respiration ceases, have anything to offer. In the future, oximeters, which detect cyanosis or hypoxaemia, may be more valuable.

Parents need clear information about vitamin and other supplements which have been prescribed and the time of their next appointment. They should have the telephone number of the neonatal unit but should be encouraged to use their primary care team.

Helping the Parents

There are a number of special situations that make particular demands on staff skills and which doctors and nurses often feel ill-equipped to deal with.

The stillbirth

The mother who has a stillbirth has a great need to grieve over and mourn the loss of her baby. For this reason, it is usually better for the mother to see, hold and name the dead baby. One cannot grieve over something that is treated is if it has never been. Mothers should be encouraged to insist on proper burial for their stillbirth and to know where the baby is buried. The DHSS has advised that all health authorities give financial help with such babies in cases of need. It is essential that parents' involvement is encouraged because denial, with no allowance for mourning, stores up great emotional problems for the future. The well-meant advice to 'forget about it' and 'try for another one as soon as possible' is wrong because it does not allow for the natural and prolonged period of mourning which must, for psychological reasons, take place.

The deformed baby

Much of the above also applies here. In the case of the malformed stillbirth it is usually best for the parents to see the infant. An imagined deformity is usually worse than reality. Even an anencephalic baby can, with judicious use of towels and drapes, look very presentable.

In the case of a non-lethal abnormality, the attitude of nursing and medical staff during the early hours of life is critical. Thoughtless remarks, or even a misguided desire to protect the mother, may easily lead to rejection of the baby or, at the very least, to feelings of guilt and distress. Try to talk to both parents together; it often helps for them to hold the baby while you explain the problem simply and clearly. You will need to repeat the explanations several times because parents in their panic often do not take in what you say. Ensure that the consultant obstetrician and paediatrician are informed so that they can visit the mother. Do not forget to inform the general practitioner and health visitor and to arrange and coordinate any necessary follow-up. Parents who have had abnormal babies should be encouraged to attend for genetic counselling so that the possible risks of recurrence can be explained to them and advice given about further children.

Some hospitals now have pre-pregnancy clinics. We have been impressed by their usefulness both in preparing worried or bereaved parents for a new pregnancy and, for example, in advising diabetic women who wish to have a baby (see Chapter 15).

The neonatal death

Every effort must be made to establish contact between the critically ill baby and his parents. If he dies, mourning is then easier; if he survives, the relationship so established is crucial. Many mothers are able to talk about their pain and grief while still in hospital. Others need more time, or blame themselves, the doctors or the nurses for what has happened.

Discussing baptism and inviting the relevant religious minister is often a great source of comfort to distressed parents in times such as when a baby is critically ill or dying. Close liaison with the hospital chaplain and local churches means priests and ministers become familiar with the unit and with performing blessings and baptisms amongst intensive care equipment. Very often this helps parents feel that they are doing something special for their sick baby.

In many cases an autopsy is necessary to establish the precise cause of death or particular syndrome of abnormalities present. This is to advise parents on the risk of abnormality in subsequent pregnancies. If this is explained to parents in a sensitive and compassionate manner, most will agree.

Parents should be invited back a few weeks after losing their baby, not only for such genetic counselling, but also to talk through their experience with the obstetrician or paediatrician. This is often extremely helpful.

Parents who have had a previous stillbirth or neonatal death will naturally be very anxious during a subsequent pregnancy. Even the excitement of having a normal baby will be mixed with grief at the memories of the previous loss. They should be helped to welcome and love the new baby in his own right and not as a replacement for someone else.

If a previous baby died suddenly and unexpectedly without obvious reason (sudden infant death syndrome, SIDS, cot death), parents will be particularly fearful that the same thing could happen again. They will need particular support and attention from obstetrician, paediatrician, general practitioner and health visitor.

The handicapped child

Sometimes it is obvious to the midwives or doctor that the newborn baby has a congenital abnormality or syndrome which is likely to give rise to handicap in the future. It is important in this situation that parents are told the truth, but give the mother a chance to accept her child beforehand. It is usually possible for a sensitive midwife or junior doctor to prepare the ground for the senior paediatrician to confirm the diagnosis and explain the implications to the mother and father. A mother who is not allowed to handle her child, or who is told it is handicapped before she has had a chance to cuddle and feed it, may reject the child despite all subsequent efforts of medical and nursing staff. This is not in the best interests of the baby and seldom in the best interests of the parents.

It is important that long-term support is given to the parents of handicapped children once mother and baby leave hospital. This is best done by someone who has already established a trusting and close relationship with the family. The general practitioner could take on this role, but a senior paediatrician is usually the most suitable person; he also has the advantage of being able to coordinate ancillary help whether in terms of physiotherapy, speech therapy, surgery or community care.

Helping the Staff

Working on a special or intensive care neonatal unit looking after ill babies is very stressful for nurses and doctors. Stillbirth, the care of handicapped babies or neonatal death causes considerable additional stress. It is often useful for staff to provide mutual support for each other so that they can cope with such situations. Regular ward meetings or discussions or discussion groups are often valuable. Parents who seem demanding or difficult to deal with are frequently very anxious. Often they are too frightened or emotionally involved to take in explanations about their baby's illness or procedures which must be carried out. The same information and explanation may need to be given on several occasions and this can also add to the pressure on staff. A regular meeting of paediatricians, child psychiatrists, midwives, obstetricians, special care nurses, health visitors, general practitioner, and other community workers is very useful in emphasizing the team approach and providing mutual support. It may be helpful for there to be a specific counsellor to whom staff can convey their feelings. It is quite normal for staff to grieve at the death of a baby. They may also feel that they have failed when a baby does not survive. It is often very difficult to find the right words when talking to newly bereaved parents. If nurses and doctors can be helped to understand and come to terms with their own feelings they will be better able to help the parents.

Further Reading

Brimblecombe, F.S.W., Richards, M.P.M. & Roberton, N.R.C. (1978)

Separation and Special Care Baby Units. *Clinics in Development Medicine, 68.*
London: Spastics International Medical Publications and Heinemann Medical.

Klaus, M.H. & Kennell, J.H. (1976a) *Maternal Infant Bonding.* St Louis: C.V. Mosby.

Klaus, M.H. & Kennell, J.H. (1976b) Parent to infant attachment. In *Recent Advances in Paediatrics,* 5, ed. D. Hull. Edinburgh and London: Churchill Livingstone.

McFarlane, A. (1977) *The Psychology of Childbirth.* London: Open Books.

Prince, J. & Adams, M.E. (1978) *Minds, Mothers and Midwives.* Edinburgh and London: Churchill Livingstone.

Richards, M.P.M. (1982) Low birth weight babies. Family repercussions. *British Journal of Hospital Medicine, 28,* 480–486.

─19─

Perinatal Care in Developing Countries

Of all low birthweight infants born worldwide, 95% are in developing countries. Of all small-for-dates infants, 98% are in developing countries. The care of newborn babies in the third world is clearly a different problem from that in industrialized countries. It is not possible here to give a complete account of the difficulties to be faced, so this chapter is only an introduction to the care of the vast majority of the world's babies.

Many of the principles of perinatal care in the developing countries apply equally to those countries that are still developing. However, in those parts of the world where the infant mortality rate is the same as that in the UK a century ago, and where the money available per head is often less than 80p (or 1 US dollar) per year, priorities must clearly be very different.

Preventive medicine is especially important. Efforts must be concentrated against malnutrition and infection, the two biggest killers in developing countries. But progress can only be made if local customs, rituals and taboos are taken into account. In addition, political instability will undermine even the most sophisticated medical aid programme.

In many developing countries children make up nearly 50% of population, yet a high proportion of the children will not live to reach adult life. Before family planning advice will be acceptable in such communities, it is probably essential to reduce the infant mortality rate. Only then can parents accept family planning, and the perinatal mortality will eventually fall. Even in developed countries, where the perinatal mortality rate has fallen greatly, there are still considerable differences betwen social classes. In Africa and Asia, 75% of the population is dispersed in rural areas, where perinatal mortality is higher, but most doctors work in the towns. In many countries periurban slums and shanties are expanding at an alarming rate.

Antenatal Care

It is difficult to establish the relationship of maternal diet to the outcome of pregnancy (see also Chapter 2). There is almost certainly a wide range of nutritional intake which is compatible with a successful result. Experience from occupied countries during the Second World War, where the population suffered undernutrition, showed that their babies tended to be shorter and weigh less and had an increased chance of being born early. The rate of growth in man is greatest and most critical during fetal life and the first year of life, by which time most brain growth has occurred. It is therefore very important to improve maternal and therefore fetal nutrition as well as infant nutrition. Birth weight is a major determinant of infant mortality. The underweight fetus is usually born into an environment which is totally unsuitable for his subsequent satisfactory growth. In areas where undernutrition is common, there is evidence that supplementation of total energy will improve the baby's birth weight. However, food supplementation can be expensive and the results from carefully supervised feeding trials may be better than can be achieved in national programmes. Protein supplementation, which is more expensive, may not be as effective.

Prenatal care is good preventive medicine and is therefore very worthwhile. In order to reduce infant mortality we need to know more about the nature, aetiology and prevention of low birth weight in developing countries. Anaemia can be recognized and treated—routine iron and folate supplements should be given; it may be due to such things as malnutrition, malabsorption, hookworm or haemolysis. Osteomalacia should be detected and treated with vitamin D supplements and chronic parasitization with malaria treated (parasites cross the placenta). Good antenatal care means a certain number of visits to outlying communities and it is important that the people visiting have basic training in what to look for so that the quality of care is adequate. Once high-risk cases are identified, they should be encouraged to move to hospital for delivery. The training of a primary health care team–midwives, nurses, auxiliary helpers and, perhaps most important, the traditional birth attendants— in the basic skills of modern medicine and community health should have high priority. Active immunization with tetanus toxoid, even with only one injection in pregnancy (although two are much more effective), will save many babies' lives.

Labour

Elaborate equipment is usually neither possible nor desirable. The local 'wise women' or traditional birth attendants should be educated in simple sterile techniques including hand washing, antiseptics and such procedures as episiotomies and stitching. In this way, it is usually possible to make use of the positive features of the culture to good effect, while discouraging harmful customs such as packing the vagina with rock salt or dressing the cord with animal dung. The Sudan is a good example of a place where such progress has been made.

Trained midwives should recognize that a most important factor in reducing perinatal (and also maternal) mortality is the prevention of

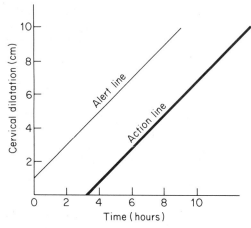

Fig. 19.1 A cervicograph. From R.H. Phillpot & W.M. Castle (1972) *Journal of Obstetrics and Gynaecology of the British Commonwealth*, 79, p.595, by permission of the authors and editor

prolonged labour. This can be due to cephalopelvic disproportion (not uncommon in communities where there is widespread rickets and osteomalacia leading to a deformed pelvis). Some prolonged labours will be due to malpresentation, but an important and common cause is abnormal uterine action and this may be easily recognized and treated without sophisticated apparatus or drugs. The principles of management involve early recognition of inert labour (by doing a vaginal examination as soon as the patient presents and subsequently at least every four hours), an active first stage which should be no longer than six to 12 hours and, finally, avoiding delay in the second stage. Progress is assessed both by dilatation of the cervix and by the level of the presenting part in relation to the pelvic brim. The cervix normally dilates at about 1 cm per hour. If a simple tool like a cervicograph is used it is easy to spot at once where action needs to be taken so a midwife may seek a doctor's help. The addition of an alert line to the cervicograph (Fig. 19.1) has proved a simple and effective way of detecting primigravidae with reduced pelvic size and inefficient uterine action in all parts of the world, and is especially valuable in rural areas where there are fewer doctors and X-ray facilities. The patient's cervical dilatation is plotted successively on the cervicograph. If the rate of dilatation is too slow, the plot will cross the alert line. Arrangements are then made to transfer the patient to a central intensive care obstetric unit so that the active management can be started within four hours. This usually involves stimulating the uterus by oxytocin for as long as there is progress in the absence of fetal distress. For a detailed account of the use of such guide-lines, see Philpott (1979).

Fetal distress or well being can be detected without sophisticated monitoring equipment. It is usually adequate for a midwife to listen to fetal heart rate through a metal trumpet to detect danger signs. In addition, the use of subsequent fetal movements may be very useful. It has been noticed that fetal movements stop about two days before the death of the fetus. If, therefore, the mother subjectively counts less than 10 movements per day, the fetus should be considered in danger of imminent demise.

This will not prevent deaths due to intrapartum asphyxia. If there is delay in the second stage it is often safer to use the ventouse than to try and get forceps into a small African pelvis. In Africa, however, the caesarean section rate may need to be high because of the high incidence of maternal hypertension and pre-eclampsia.

Birth

If a baby is born asphyxiated, the principles laid down in Chapter 3 apply. Only simple equipment is required: a laryngoscope, endotracheal tube, some form of suction and an operator who understands the principles of what is required. It is important to realize that air is perfectly good for resuscitating the baby; 100% oxygen is not required. If intubation is not possible, mouth-to-mouth resuscitation is acceptable, although if it is available a bag and mask will be less likely to lead to infection of the baby (see Chapter 3). In either case a control must be maintained of both the volume of air administered and its pressure (less than 30 cm water). Simple pressure monitoring equipment can be made cheaply and easily. The contents of the resuscitator's mouth are all that is required and it is useful to practise blowing up a sphygmomanometer in this way to see what sort of pressures are generated (but remember that the sphygnonamometer gives pressures in millimetres of mercury, not centimetres of water). If mouth-to-mouth resuscitation is given, a cotton or nylon square acting as a filter will reduce the infection rate. Perhaps the most important thing is the teaching of the difference between blue and white asphyxia, thereby reducing greatly the incidence of iatrogenic problems. Resuscitation may be greatly aided by receiving the baby onto a suitably firm surface on which the head may be easily extended.

The delivery room itself needs no special facilities. It may be a simple hut heated by a stove and humidified by evaporating water from a wet cloth.

Feeding

The best prophylaxis against subsequent infant mortality from infective diarrhoea and protein-energy malnutrition is breast feeding. It is particularly unfortunate that commercial advertising in the developing countries, coupled with a not unnatural desire in mothers to mimic their more sophisticated sisters in urban areas or the developed world, has led to a decline in breast feeding. In rural India, Nigeria and Ethiopia nearly all mothers still breast feed when their babies are 9 months old. In urban areas the proportion is only 20–60%, with the smaller proportion being in those relatively better off. The advantages of breast feeding are set out in Chapter 7. Protection against infection and the establishment of adequate intervals between births are particularly important advantages in the developing countries. Frequent suckling and prolonged lactation postpone the return of menstruation and ovulation because prolactin is released from the anterior pituitary gland in response to suckling and inhibits ovulation in the ovary. Supplementary milk or other foods significantly reduce the contraceptive effect of breast feeding.

Children who are breast-fed suffer fewer episodes of infection than those who are artificially fed. In rural Africa, Asia or South America, infection resulting from the inability of the mother to make up or keep feeds in a sterile way is a major cause of infant death. Her inability to afford the expensive powdered milks also means that she may make them up in too dilute a concentration, thereby leading to a protein-energy malnutrition and an even greater susceptibility to infection. It is probable that failure of lactation is extremely rare in such communities, compared with more sophisticated and regimented maternity units. In such circumstances wet nursing is more valuable, but there are taboos against this in many societies. It is likely that cup and spoon feeding is a safer alternative to the bottle because of reduced risk of infection and it is therefore always used in special care units in the third world.

A most important advance in recent years has been the use of the indwelling plastic nasogastric tube for feeding infants too ill or too immature to suck. Such tubes are cheap, easy to place in position after a little practice and straightforward in use provided simple precautions are taken. If there is not enough expressed breast milk to use in this situation it is probably best to use a simply modified cow's milk preparation in which carbohydrate is added but the milk is otherwise unmodified. If the baby is fed to give his appropriate energy intake, he will automatically receive a reduced protein and mineral load as compared to ordinary cow's milk, which will reduce the incidence of such problems as hypocalcaemic convulsions, hypernatraemic dehydration and renal failure. The intrinsic anti-infective qualities of breast milk (lactoferrin, secretory IgA, polymorphs and lymphocytes) are irreplaceable, however. For this reason, breast feeding should be continued for as long as possible and this will also have the important effect of spacing pregnancies adequately since, as we have seen, the mother is less likely to conceive whilst breast feeding her baby.

From about 4–6 months of age other foods should be given and increased to supplement the breast milk.

General Neonatal Care

It is often not realized that even in the tropics babies need to be kept warm at night as the temperature can fall very sharply. The principles of the neutral thermal environment apply (see Chapter 5), but in many ways temperature control becomes more difficult in developing countries as incubators can be positively dangerous. This is because they are a potent source of infection if not looked after properly. They are expensive to buy in the first place and resources are better spent elsewhere; they are complex pieces of equipment, which frequently go wrong and are expensive in time, money and trained personnel to put right. The best heat source for these babies is their own mother. This has the additional advantage of promoting the mother–infant relationship, a field in which the developing countries are far in advance of the West. When a baby is nursed in a cot it is important that it is deep so that there are no draughts over the sides. Additional heat can be provided by one or two guarded electric light bulbs under or over the cot. Perspex heat shields are relatively inexpensive and simple to make locally and considerably cut down evaporative heat loss. Expanded bubble plastic packing material is an extremely cheap way of providing good insulation when wrapped around a baby. As indicated in Chapter 4, situations in which the baby is particularly at risk from heat loss include immediately after birth, during nappy changing, and bathing. It is very important to dry and swaddle the baby immediately after birth and the first bath should be delayed for at least three days even in large mature infants.

Care of the umbilical cord is a matter frequently surrounded by traditional practices, rituals and taboos in may communities. The high incidence of neonatal mortality from tetanus acquired following cutting of the cord with an unclean instrument or treatment of the cord with cow dung may be reduced greatly. This is best done firstly by immunizing pregnant mothers with tetanus toxoid during the last trimester of pregnancy. This produces an IgG antibody response which passively protects the neonate from acquired tetanus. Secondly, education must be given in cord care: this means giving either packs containing a blade (which village midwives are instructed to boil before use), some swabs and a simple tie or rubber bands, which are cheap and effective. Treatment of established neonatal tetanus is by high doses of penicillin, heavy sedation (sufficient to abolish the spasms) and tube feeding; paralysis and ventilatory support are used in some sophisticated units. Anti-tetanus serum (ATS) also has a place. Mortality rates remain high.

When to use antibiotics and which antibiotic to use are difficult problems in communities where there are absent or inadequate bacteriological services. A good rule of thumb is that any deterioration of the baby's condition after about 48 hours of life is due to infection, and the threshold for the use of antibiotics in a given clinical situation must be low. Cheap and useful antibiotics in this context are penicillin and chloramphenicol. Chloramphenicol when used for short courses in appropriate dosage (50 mg/kg per day for the first 48 hours, then 25 mg/kg per day) is a very safe drug as well as being very effective against a wide range of bacterial infections. The incidence of the 'grey baby' syndrome when the drug is correctly used is extremely rare. It is also very cheap, much more so than possible alternatives such as gentamicin.

The treatment of conjunctivitis in tropical countries is important. Any purulent discharge should be assumed to be gonococcal and treated with systemic and topical penicillin. Silver nitrate (Credé) drops are potentially dangerous as they become concentrated due to evaporation in high temperatures and cause chemical burns. Sulphacetamide of collodial silver drops are both cheap and effective and may be used for nongonococcal infections.

In the management of jaundice, it is not necessary to have sophisticated phototherapy units. Reflected sunlight provides very adequate phototherapy, although care must be taken not to allow the baby to be burned. Recent evidence that intermittent phototherapy for 15 minutes out of every hour is as effective as continuous treatment makes this object easier to achieve.

There are few specific neonatal tropical diseases. However, diphtheria, whooping cough, polio and measles are still common, dangerous and largely preventable by an active immunization programme. Chronic malaria is a widespread cause of babies being born small. Smallpox is now eradicated. As mentioned above, tetanus may be prevented by giving 1 ml of tetanus toxoid intramuscularly to the mother on her first antenatal visit and repeating the dose during the seventh or eighth month of pregnancy. It may be useful to give the baby BCG at birth (intradermally). This may also protect against atypical mycobacterial infections which are common. Polio vaccine is also often given very early, and it is now clear that breast feeding has no inhibitory effect on the antibody response of infants to oral polio vaccine beyond the newborn period, and there is, therefore, no need to interrupt it to allow the vaccine to be taken up. The reason for the generally poor uptake in the tropics remains unclear.

Future Priorities

There is no doubt that the high perinatal mortality rate in many developing countries is associated with a high incidence of low birth weight babies (less than 1500 g). This is largely due to intrauterine growth retardation rather then preterm delivery and is probably related to the low standard of nutrition and health in the community as a whole. Priority must be given to improving the nutritional standards of the people. Mothers and babies particularly at risk should be detected early and transferred to large centres for care. Local customs should be encouraged except when they are harmful and education of traditional birth attendants in the principles of modern midwifery is particularly valuable. Mothers should be educated in the importance of antenatal care. It may be particularly difficult to build up their confidence if the person giving advice is Western.

Breast feeding should be actively encouraged as a means of preventing infant malnutrition, infection and death, and as a way of spacing pregnancies adequately. Available resources must be spread in the most effective possible way: priority cannot be given to babies severely malformed, injured or retarded. Much can be done with simple, cheap and locally made aids such as light bulbs as an overhead source of heat and plastic bubble sheeting as swaddlers. Many 'disposable' items such as feeding and suction catheters and endotracheal tubes can be used several times if they are resterilized on each occasion. For example 'butterfly' cannulae can be reused as follows: rinse with saline, wash out and store in aqueous iodine, rinse and drop into boiling water for one minute, and then cool before putting up the next drip. This is much cheaper than throwing them away after only their first use. It is important that sophisticated equipment such as incubators and ventilators is not imported to copy what is useful in a sophisticated neonatal unit. In addition, the Western practice, still too widespread, of separating mothers from their babies and bottle feeding should be strongly discouraged.

It is unfortunate that the implementation of any medical programme for improving perinatal care depends as much on political stability and political decisions as on strictly medical implications. It is this which most limits progress in many developing countries at present.

Further Reading

Cutting, W.A.M. & Ludlam, M. (1984). Making the best of breast feeding. *Family Practice*, *1*, 69–78.

Ebrahim, G.J. (1977) *Care of the Newborn in Developing Countries.* London: Macmillan.

Hamiza, M.H. & Segall, M.M. (1975) *Care of the Newborn Baby in Tanzania* Dar es Salaam: Tanzania Publishing House.

King, M., King, F & Martodipoero, S. (1980) *Primary Child Care.* Oxford: Oxford University Press.

Morely, D. (1973) *Paediatric Priorities in the Developing World.* London: Butterworths.

Philpott, R.H. (1979) The management of labour. In *Recent Advances in Obstetrics and Gynaecology*, ed. J.A. Stallworthy & G.L. Bourne. Edinburgh & London: Churchill Livingstone.

Philpott, R.H. & Castle, W.M. (1972) Cervicographs in the management of labour in primigravidae. *J. Obstet. Gynaec. Br. Commonw.*, 79, 592.

Warely, M.A. (1978) Care of the newborn. In *Diseases of Children in the Subtropics and Tropics*, 3rd ed, ed. D.B. Jellife & J.P. Stanfield. London: Edward Arnold.

Appendix

Normal Values in the Newborn

Blood

pH	7.3–7.4
$Paco_2$	4.6–6.0 kPa (35–45 mmHg)
Pao_2	7.3–12.0 kPa (55–90 mmHg)
Bicarbonate	18–25 μmol/l
Base excess	−7 to −2 mmol/l
Ammonia	50–100 μmol/l (may be higher in preterm or jaundiced babies)
Calcium	1.9–2.7 μmol/l (tendency to lower values in preterm babies)
Creatinine	9–62 μmol/l (day 2) (higher in cord blood)

Electrolytes
  Sodium   135–150 mmol/l (may be lower in preterm babies)
  Potassium   4.0–6.0 mmol/l
  Chloride   95–105 mmol/l

Glucose	2.0–6.0 mmol/l (lower in the first few hours)

Immunoglobulins
  IgA   none–0.05 g/l ⎫
  IgM   less than 0.2 g/l ⎬ cord blood
  IgG   4–15 g/l ⎭

Iron	20–50 μmol/l
Magnesium	0.7–1.2 mmol/l
Osmolality	280–305 mosmol/kg water
Phenylalanine	<0.37 mmol/l

Protein
  Total   50–70 g/l
  Albumin   30–40 g/l
  Globulins   10–30 g/l

T_4 125–275 nmol/litre ⎫ Higher than adult normal range during
TSH   <3 mu/l ⎬ first week of life. Decreases to adult nor-
                  ⎭ mal range by 8–10 days

Urea	3.4–8.4 mmol/l

Haemoglobin (capillary blood levels are 2–3 g/dl higher than those of blood obtained by venepuncture)

day 1	16–20 g/dl	1 month	11–17 g/dl
1 week	13–23 g/dl	3 months	10–14 g/dl

Packed cell volume		Reticulocytes	
day 1	52–58%	day 1	2–8%
2 weeks	46–54%	1 week	0.5–5%
3 months	35%	1 month	0–0.5%

White cell count		Platelets (see also Chapter 13)	
day 1	$6–35 \times 10^9/l$	day 1	$350 \times 10^9/l$
1 week	$8–16 \times 10^9/l$	2 weeks	$300 \times 10^9/l$
1 month	$6–14 \times 10^9/l$	3 months	$250 \times 10^9/l$

Neutrophils		Fibrinogen	1–3.5 g/l
day 1	50–80%		
day 4	35–60%		
3 months	25–45%		

Urine

Creatinine clearance	0.6–1.1 ml/sec/1.73 m²
VMA	up to 10 μmol/24 hours

Cerebrospinal fluid

Glucose	3.8–5 mmol/l
Total protein	100–1200 mg/l (higher in preterm babies)
Cells	up to 20/μl (lymphocytes)

Categories of Babies Receiving Neonatal Care*

1 Introduction

1.1 Three broad levels of infant care may be identified in the neonatal period—normal care, special care and intensive care.

1.2 The purpose of this memorandum is to describe these levels of care, and to categorize the infants who require each level of care so as to provide an audit of the workload.

1.3 The memorandum also details the staffing and facilities currently recommended for proper care.

2 Definitions of neonatal care

2.1 *Intensive Care*
Care given in a special or intensive care nursery which provides continuous skilled supervision by nursing and medical staff.

2.2 *Special Care*
Care given in a special care nursery or on a postnatal ward which provides

* From the statement of the British Paediatric Association and the British Association for Perinatal Paediatrics.

observation and treatment falling short of intensive care but exceeding normal routine care.

2.3 *Normal Care*
Care given, usually, by the mother in a postnatal ward, supervised by a midwife and doctor but requiring minimal medical or nursing advice.

3 The use of categories of neonatal care in hospital

3.1 The list of categories in paragraph 4 should not be regarded as exhaustive but serves as a guide. The categories allow a nursing officer to count the number of babies receiving each level of care at a particular time. It must be understood that Intensive Care includes the categories described under Special Care, and there is therefore a hierarchy of care.

3.2 Some units may find it useful to subdivide intensive and special care to allow a more detailed audit of their workload.

3.3 The babies to be counted are those using the facilities or staff of the unit. This would include babies who are in an operating theatre or being transferred between hospitals when the count is made.

3.4 In order to obtain a complete picture of the workload it will be necessary to collect returns from the postnatal wards for those babies receiving special care. Babies who clearly require a level of care which cannot be provided because of shortage of staff or facilities should be included in the category reflecting the level of care required.

3.5 It may be necessary to undertake a count several times within a 24 hour period to demonstrate that there are times, for instance during the night, when the workload is not matched by the available resources.

4 Clinical categories

4.1 *Intensive care*
4.1.1 Babies receiving assisted ventilation (intermittent positive pressure ventilation (IPPV), intermittent mandatory ventilation (IMV), constant positive airway pressure (CPAP) and in the first 24 hours following its withdrawal).
4.1.2 Babies receiving total parenteral nutrition.

(Some units may wish to record these first two categories as a special and major subdivision of intensive care).

4.1.3 Cardiorespiratory disease which is unstable, including recurrent apnoea requiring constant attention.
4.1.4 Babies who have had major surgery, particularly in the first 24 postoperative hours.
4.1.5 Babies of less than 30 weeks gestation during the first 48 hours after birth.
4.1.6 Babies who are having convulsions.
4.1.7 Babies transported by the staff of the unit concerned. This would usually be between hospitals, or for special investigations or treatment.
4.1.8 Babies undergoing major medical procedures, such as arterial catheterization, peritoneal dialysis or exchange transfusions.

4.2 *Special care*
(Some units may find it useful to make a sub-division, for example into high and

low dependency special care to allow more detailed audit of their workload).

4.2.1 Babies who require continuous monitoring of respiration or heart rate, or by transcutaneous transducers.
4.2.2 Babies who are receiving additional oxygen.
4.2.3 Babies who are receiving intravenous glucose and electrolyte solutions.
4.2.4 Babies who are being tube fed.
4.2.5 Babies who have had minor surgery in the previous 24 hours.
4.2.6 Babies with a tracheostomy.
4.2.7 Dying babies.
4.2.8 Babies who are being barrier nursed.
4.2.9 Babies receiving phototherapy.
4.2.10 Babies who receive special monitoring (for example frequent glucose or bilirubin estimations).
4.2.11 Other babies receiving constant supervision (for example babies whose mothers are drug addicts).
4.2.12 Babies receiving antibiotics.
4.2.13 Babies with conditions requiring radiological examination or other methods of imaging.

5 Resources required for neonatal care

5.1 These are the present recommendations of the BPA.

5.2 *Intensive care*
5.2.1 *Medical staff.* Minimum medical staff should consist of both an experienced paediatric registrar and SHO on duty and available in the intensive care area at all times with an appropriately trained consultant in charge.
5.2.2 *Nursing staff.* There should be an establishment to allow a ratio of four *trained* nurses (with neonatal intensive care experience) to each cot. This ratio allows for 24 hours cover and leave. The optimum ratio is 5:1.
5.2.3 *Equipment.* The following equipment must be avilable for each baby receiving intensive care:

1 intensive care incubator, or unit with overhead heating
1 respiratory, or apnoea, monitor
1 heart rate monitor
1 intravascular blood pressure transducer or surface blood pressure recorder
1 transcutaneous Po_2 monitor or intravascular oxygen transducer
1 transcutaneous Po_2 monitor
2 syringe pumps
2 infusion pumps
1 ventilator
1 continuous temperature monitor
1 phototherapy unit
1 ambient oxygen monitor
Facilities for frequent blood gas analysis using micromethods
Facilities for frequent biochemical analysis including glucose, bilirubin and electrolytes by micromethods.
Access to ultrasound equipment for visualization of organs such as the brain
Access to equipment for radiological examination

5.3 *Special care*
5.3.1 *Medical staff.* Minimum medical staff for 24 hour cover: an appropriately experienced SHO should be on duty, and an experienced more senior member of staff should be on call, with a consultant paediatrician in charge.
5.3.2 *Nursing staff.* There should be an establishment to allow a ratio of 1.25 nurses (with neonatal experience) to each cot. This ratio allows for 24 hour cover and leave. The optimum ratio is 1.5:1.
5.3.3. *Equipment.* The following equipment must be available for each baby:

1 incubator, or cot adequate for temperature control
1 ambient oxygen analyser
1 apnoea alarm
1 heart rate monitor
1 infusion pump
1 phototherapy unit
1 ventilator to be used for short-term ventilation
Access to frequent blood gas analysis using micromethods
Access to biochemical analysis (including glucose, bilirubin and electrolytes) by
    micromethods.
Access to equipment for radiological examination
5.3.4 Special care may take place on a post-natal ward, particularly in an area specially set aside for the purpose.

5.4 *Normal care*
Minimal requirements are a low reading thermometer, facilities for clearing the upper airway, for cord and skin care, and for weighing the baby. Emergency resuscitation equipment must be readily available.

Minimum Standards in Neonatal Care*

1 Introduction

1.1 It is of great importance that *minimum* standards should not be regarded as *optimum* standards.

2 Medical records

2.1 As recommended by the Körner Committee, every newborn baby must be given an independent identification number at birth and a personal medical record.

3 Types of maternity units

3.1 *Unit in a district general hospital.* We would expect such a unit to have 1500–3000 births every year. They would accept a cross-section of obstetric deliveries including high-risk mothers. They would require:
(a) Skilled resuscitation at birth. A member of the paediatric junior staff must be on duty 24 hours a day and could be called to the labour ward to provide resuscitation by intubation.
(b) A special care baby unit.

* Statement of the British Paediatric Association

(c) Facilities for short-term intensive care would be provided for babies who are ill for only a short time or until they can be transferred to a neonatal intensive care unit.

(d) In order for this to operate efficiently the paediatric unit should be on the same site as the maternity unit.

3.2 *Small maternity units.* Here the work load could not economically justify resident paediatric staff. Such units must not deliver high-risk mothers, but there must be some arrangements for emergency paediatric care to be provided.

(a) Facilities for the resuscitation of the newborn must be available. The resuscitation can be given by a midwife, or a doctor if one is available, and either a bag and mask or intubation may be used. Those undertaking the care of an asphyxiated baby must have been given instruction in the techniques of resuscitation and have used it in practice.

(b) Paediatric on-call cover must be provided from the nearest paediatric unit. Resources, including medical or nursing, must be available to transfer an ill baby immediately to a special care baby unit.

3.3 *Designated regional intensive care units.* These are situated in units which deliver high-risk mothers and also accept referrals of severely ill babies requiring ventilation. They undertake the special training of paediatricians in neonatal care and conduct research. All neonatal intensive care units accepting referrals must provide a flying squad service.

4   Distribution of special and intensive care cots

4.1 Five special care cots and one intensive care cot must be provided for each 1000 deliveries every year.

4.2 Some special care cots may be provided at the mothers' bedside rather than in the special care baby unit.

4.3 The distribution of intensive care cots should be decided following regional surveys of perinatal care by regional perinatal working parties.

5   Medical staff

5.1 *District general hospital.*

(a) Any hospital with a special care baby unit must have at least two consultant paediatricians on the staff.

(b) A special care baby unit must have a resident paediatrician in the hospital throughout the 24 hours. Such a paediatrician would usually be a senior house officer or a registrar.

5.2 *Small maternity units.* Cover must be provided from the nearest paediatric unit by a consultant paediatrician or a member of the junior staff (the establishment must permit this).

5.3 *Designated regional neonatal care units.*

(a) Such units must have two whole time equivalents of consultant paediatricians.

(b) At any time the hospital must have two paediatricians on duty in the building. At least one of these paediatricians must already be experienced in neonatal care.

6 Nursing and midwifery staff

6.1 Every special or intensive care baby unit must have a recognized nurse/ midwife establishment of its own.

6.2 The recommendations of the Sheldon Committee that there should be one nurse per special care cot and three per intensive care cot must be regarded as the minimum. At least two experienced nurses able to resuscitate babies should be on duty on each shift in a special or intensive care unit.

7 Medical examinations

7.1 Every newborn baby must be fully examined within 24 hours of birth by a doctor with experience of newborn care. The baby must be examined again at discharge either on leaving hospital or at seven to 10 days. The results of these examinations must be recorded in the infant's record.

8 Resuscitation

8.1 At all times, in all maternity units, there must be someone available in the labour ward (or able to reach there within two minutes) capable of starting expert neonatal resuscitation by intubation or bag and mask.

9 Equipment and laboratory services

9.1 Every labour ward must have equipment for resuscitating an asphyxiated baby and some special means of keeping newborn babies warm.

9.2 Every special care baby unit providing continuous oxygen therapy must have a blood gas analyser on site, the ability to X-ray an infant and the equipment to provide at least short-term mechanical ventilation within the unit.

9.3 All special care baby units must have access to a full laboratory service; in particular, the results of urgent investigations such as blood glucose, plasma bilirubin, haemoglobin and CSF examination should be available within three hours.

10 Family support

10.1 The admission of a newborn baby to a special care baby unit is an emotional and stressful time for the family and makes the emotional attachment of a mother to her baby very difficult indeed. Every effort must be made to encourage good relationships within the family.

10.2 Parents must be allowed to visit their babies at any time throughout the day and night.

10.3 Every special or neonatal intensive care unit must have resident accom- modation for mothers either within the unit or very close to it.

10.4 There should be at least one designated social worker for every special or intensive care unit.

Drug Dosages

Drug dosages are discussed in the appropriate chapter but this table also provides a useful summary of those most commonly used.

Drug	Route	Dose	Frequency	Comments
Calcium gluconate	i.m. or i.v. slowly	20 mg/kg (0.2 mg/kg of 10% solution)	6-hourly as necessary	If i.v., dilute to 2.5% i.m. best avoided because of risk of sterile abscess formation. Extravasation may cause local tissue necrosis. Cardiac monitoring desirable (danger of bradycardia or arrest)
	Oral	100 mg/kg (1 mg/kg of 10% solution)	6-hourly or with feeds	
Chloral elixir paediatric BPC	Oral	7.5 mg/kg	6-hourly	
Cyclopentolate eye drops 5% BPC	Local	1–2 drops	30 minutes before examination	
Diazepam injection (10 mg in 2 ml)	i.m. or i.v. slowly	0.25 mg/kg	8-hourly	Care if jaundiced (see Chapter 12)
Diazepam elixir (2 mg in 5 ml)	Oral	0.25 mg/kg	6-hourly	
Digoxin elixir or injection	Oral, i.m. or i.v.	0.005 mg/kg	12-hourly	Maintenance. See p. 228 for digitalization
Dopamine hydrochloride	i.v.	5 µg/kg/min in 5% dextrose	continuous infusion	
Ferrous sulphate (60 mg in 5 ml)	Oral	30 mg	Twice daily	
Folic acid	Oral	0.1 mg	Once weekly	

Frusemide (20 mg in 2 ml)	i.m. or i.v.	1 mg/kg	Up to twice daily	Potassium supplements may be needed
Hydrocortisone sodium succinate	i.m. or i.v.	2.5 mg/kg	6-hourly	
Magnesium sulphate 50% solution	i.m.	0.2 mg/kg	Once daily	Watch for hypotonia: reversible with calcium gluconate
Mannitol	i.v.	1 g/kg (5 ml of 20% solution per kg given over 30 minutes)	repeated as necessary	
Morphine sulphate	i.v. or i.m.	0.1–0.2 mg/kg	6 hourly as necessary	
Naloxone	i.v. or i.m.	0.01 mg/kg	Once	Repeat up to three times after 3 minutes if necessary. May need to be repeated 1–2-hourly for several hours
Pancuronium	i.v.	0.02 mg/kg	repeat as necessary	
Paraldehyde	i.m. (deep)	0.1 ml/kg	6-hourly as necessary	
Phenobarbitone injection	i.m. or i.v.	2 mg/kg	8–12-hourly	See Chapter 14
Phenobarbitone elixir PBC (5 mg/ml)	Oral	1.25 mg/kg	6-hourly	
Phytomenadione (vitamin K)	i.m., i.v. or oral	1 mg	Once	
Sodium bicarbonate (8.4%)	i.v.	0.3 ml/mEq base deficit/kg		
Theophylline	Oral	4 mg/kg	6–8-hourly	Maintenance. Measure blood levels. See p. 132
Thyroxine	Oral	10 µg/kg 24 hours	Once daily	
Tolazoline	i.v.	1–2 mg (bolus) or 2 mg/kg/h in 5% dextrose	Continuous infusion	

Neonatal Special Care Chart

Hospital Name _____

Name: No: DOB :

Date																						
Time																						

Temp (> 38°C ... < 31°C): 38, 37.5, 37, 36.5, 36, 35, 34, 33, 32, 31

Heart rate (> 170 ... < 100): 170, 160, 150, 140, 130, 120, 110, 100

B.P. →

Resp. rate (> 100 ... < 20): 100, 90, 80, 70, 60, 50, 40, 30, 20

Colour
Recession
Grunting

Weight
Type mls/Kg
Cont mls/hr
Int (....hrly)
(....mls)
Supplements
Vits/iron

TcPO$_2$
PH
PO$_2$
PCO$_2$
HCO$_3$
BE
TcPO$_2$
Hb/PCV
U&E/Ca
D.Stix/B.sugar
SeBILI

Intake 24hr
Aspiration
Urine vol
Urine S.G.
Bowels

Comments on progress

Name				Details of baby i.e. Name, Number, DOB.	
Date Time				Each day should be separated by a vertical red line	
Temp	> 38°C 38 37.5 37 36.5 36 35 34 33 32 31 < 31°C				Incubator, skin and rectal temperatures may be recorded in different colour codes Temperatures of greater than 38°C and less than 31°C should be recorded in numerical form
Heart rate	> 170 170 160 150 140 130 120 110 100 < 100				Heart rates of greater than 170 and less than 100 beats per minute should be recorded in numerical form
B.P.					Systolic and diastolic blood pressure recordings
Resp. rate	> 100 100 90 80 70 60 50 40 30 20 < 20				Respiratory rates greater than 100 and less than 20 breaths per minute should be recorded in numerical form
Colour Recession Grunting					P = Pink C = Cyanosed J = Jaundice 0 = None + = Mild + + = Moderate + + + = Severe 0 = None + = Mild + + = Moderate + + + = Severe
					} Spare for the recording of other observations e.g. Abdominal girth
Weight				,	Daily weight
F E E D	Type mls/Kg Cont mls/hr Int (....hrly) (....mls)				Feed -- Type and amount in mls/Kg/day A = Artificial milk B = Breast milk Feed -- Continuous (mls/hr) and whether N/G or N/J G = Gastric J = Jejunal Feed -- Intermittent...Interval between feeds hrs and mode (T = Tube / Bo = Bottle / Br = Breast) ...mls in each feed
Supplements					Feed supplements e.g. Caloreen
Vits/iron					Vitamins = V Iron = I
					} Spare Other feed Other medication
TcPO₂					Transcutaneous PO_2 recordings noted by nursing staff
PH PO₂ PCO₂ HCO₃ BE TcPO₂					Blood gas recordings N.B. Source of blood must be stated e.g. Capillary, Radial etc Transcutaneous PO_2 at the time of blood sampling for correlation
Hb/PCV U&E/Ca D.Stix/B.sugar SeBILI					Haemoglobin/packed cell volume Urea and electrolytes, and serum calcium Blood glucose Serum bilirubin
					} Spare for the recording of other laboratory investigations
Intake 24hr Aspiration Urine vol Urine S.G. Bowels					Separate fluid charts required for hourly recordings Gastric aspirates Urine volumes Urine specific gravities Bowel function
Comments on progress					

Neonatal Intensive Care Chart

Hospital Name _____

Name: No: DOB: Day:

Date: Date:

Temp	> 38°C / 38 / 37.5 / 37 / 36.5 / 36 / 35 / 34 / 33 / 32 / 31 / < 31°C		
Heart rate	> 170 / 170 / 160 / 150 / 140 / 130 / 120 / 110 / 100 / < 100		
B.P. →	> 100		
Resp. rate	100 / 90 / 80 / 70 / 60 / 50 / 40 / 30 / 20 / < 20		
Colour			
Recession			
Grunting			
Ventilator rate			
F_1O_2			
P. Insp.			
P. Exp.			
i.e. Ratio			
Flow			
Lav/Suction			
$TcPO_2$ or PaO_2			
PH			
PO_2			
PCO_2			
HCO_3			
BE			
$TcPO_2$ or PaO_2			
Hb/PCV			

U&E/Ca	Time	Na	K	Urea	Ca	Time	Na	K	Urea	Ca
D.Stix/B.sugar										
SeBILI										

Intake 24hr			I.V.		I.A.		Oral		WT	
Aspiration										
Urine vol										T Vol
Urine S.G.										
Bowels										

Comments on progress

	13	14	15	Time of recordings

Details of baby i.e. Name, Number, DOB, Day of life

Date at beginning and the end of the 24 hr chart

Temp	> 38°C			
	38			
	37.5			Incubator, skin and rectal temperatures may be recorded in different colour codes
	37			
	36.5			Temperatures of greater than 38°C and less than 31°C should be recorded in numerical form
	36			
	35			
	34			
	33			
	32			
	31			
	< 31°C			

Heart rate	> 170			
	170			
	160			
	150			
	140			Heart rates of greater than 170 and less than 100 beats per minute should be recorded in numerical form
	130			
	120			
	110			
	100			
	< 100			
B.P.→				Systolic and diastolic blood pressure recordings

Resp. rate	> 100			
	100			
	90			
	80			
	70			Respiratory rates greater than 100 and less than 20 breaths per minute should be recorded in numerical form
	60			
	50			
	40			
	30			
	20			
	< 20			

Colour				P = Pink C = Cyanosed J = Jaundice +++ = Severe
Recession				0 = None + = Mild ++ = Moderate +++ = Severe
Grunting				0 = None + = Mild ++ = Moderate
				Spare for the recording of other observations e.g. Abdominal girth
				Positioning L = Left R = Right B = Back F = Front

Ventilator rate				Ventilator rate
F₁O₂				Fractional inspired oxygen concentration
P. Insp.				Peak inspiratory pressure
P. Exp.				Positive end expiratory pressure or continuous positive airways pressure
i.e. Ratio				Inspiratory to expiratory time ratio
Flow				Total flow of gas to ventilator
				Spare space for other ventilator recording e.g. Inspiratory gas temperature
Lav/Suction				Bronchial lavage/endotracheal suction
				Spare space for other recordings e.g. Secretions C = Clear Y = Yellow + = Scanty ++ = Moderate +++ = Profuse
				e.g. Hourly transcutaneous PCO₂ (TcPCO₂) recording noted by nursing staff
TcPO₂ or PaO₂				Hourly transcutaneous or arterial PO₂ (delete as appropriate) recording noted by nursing staff

Changes in ventilator settings should be indicated in red by the medical staff

PH				
PO₂				
PCO₂				Blood gas recordings
HCO₃				N.B. Source of blood must be stated e.g. UAC, radial, capillary etc
BE				
TcPO₂ or PaO₂				Transcutaneous or arterial PO₂ (delete as appropriate) at the time of blood sampling for correlation

Hb/PCV				Haemoglobin/packed cell volume
U&E/Ca	Time		Na	Urea and electrolytes, and serum calcium - space for two timed samples
D.Stix/B.sugar				Blood glucose
SeBILI				Serum Bilirubin
				Spare for the recording of other laboratory investigations

Intake 24hr				Separate fluid charts required for hourly recordings
Aspiration				Gastric aspirates
Urine vol				Hourly urine volumes
Urine S.G.				Hourly urine specific gravities
Bowels				Bowel function

24 hr urine output
mls

Comments on progress				e.g. pneumothorax
				chest drain insertion
				etc., etc.

Useful Names and Addresses

The Association of Breastfeeding Mothers
71 Hall Drive
London SE26 6XL
Tel. 01–788 4381

Association of Paediatric Nurses
c/o Miss D. MacCormack
Children's Hospital
Western Bank
Sheffield S10 2TH
Tel. 0742 7111

Association for Spina Bifida and Hydrocephalus
Tavistock House North
Tavistock Square
London WC1 9HJ
Tel. 01–388 1382

BLISS (Baby Life Support System)
(a charity raising money for neonatal units)
Chairman: Susanna Cheal
50 Sumatra Road
London NW6 1PR
Tel. 01–435 6867

British Heart Foundation
57 Gloucester Place
London W1H 4DH
Tel. 01–935 0185

British Paediatric Association
5 St. Andrews Place
Regents Park
London NW1 4LB
Tel. 01–486 6151

Cystic Fibrosis Research Trust
5 Blyth Road
Bromley
Kent BR1 3RS
Tel. 01–464 7211

Down's Babies Association
Queenbourne Community Centre
Ridgacre Road
Quinton
Birmingham B32 2PW
Tel. 021–427 1374

Foundation for the Study of Infant Deaths
5th Floor, 4–5 Grosvenor Place
London SW1X 7HD
Tel. 01–235 1721 or 01–245 9421

Gingerbread (for one-parent families)
35 Wellington Street
London WC2E 7BN
Tel. 01–240 0953

Haemophilia Society
16 Trinity Street
London SE1 1DB
Tel. 01–407 1010

Invalid Children's Aid Association
126 Buckingham Palace Road
London SW1W 9SB
Tel. 01–730 9891

La Leche League of Great Britain
(for help with breast feeding)
BM 3424
London WC1V 6XX
Tel. 01–404 5011

National Association for Deaf/Blind and Rubella Children
164 Cromwell Lane
Coventry
Tel. 0203 23308

National Association for Hospital Play Staff
Thomas Coram Foundation
40 Brunswick Square
London WC1
Tel. 01–278 2424

National Association for Maternal and Child Welfare
1 South Audley Street
London W1Y 6JS
Tel. 01–491 1315

National Association for the Welfare of Children in Hospital (NAWCH)
Argyl House, Euston Road
London NW1
Tel. 01–261 1738

National Childbirth Trust (education for parenthood)
9 Queensborough Terrace
London W2 3TB
Tel. 01–221 3833

National Deaf Children's Society
45 Hereford Road
London W2 5AH
Tel. 01–229 9272

National Society for Brain-damaged Children
35 Larchmere Drive
Hall Green,
Birmingham

National Society for Mentally Handicapped Children
123 Golden Lane
London EC1Y 0RT
Tel. 01–253 9433

National Society for Phenylketonuria and Allied Disorders
58A Burton Road,
Melton Mowbray
Leicester LE13 1DJ

Prenatal Diagnosis Group
Dr Alan McDermott
(Editor of Newsletter)
S.W. Regional Cytogenetics Centre
Southmead Hospital
Bristol

Royal National Institute for the Deaf
224 Great Portland Street
London W1N 6AA
Tel. 01–388 1266

Royal National Insitute for the Deaf
105 Gower Street
London WC1 6AH
Tel. 01–387 8033

Spastics Society
12 Park Crescent
London W1N 4EQ
Tel. 01–636 5020

Stillbirth and Neonatal Death Society (SANDS)
Argyle House
29–31 Euston Road
London NW1
Tel. 01–833 2851

The Stillbirth and Perinatal Death Association
37 Christchurch Hill
London NW3 1LA
Tel. 01–794 4601

Gestational Assessment

For best results the assessment should be carried out when the baby is between 4 and 48 hours of age. The assessments are least accurate when the baby is ill.

1 Dubowitz score

This has proved a reliable method of assessing the gestational age of a baby in the early days of life (see p. 90). With practice it is quick to perform and accurate to within about two weeks either way provided the baby is examined at least a few hours after delivery and is not ill.

Score each external sign and neurological criterion (pp. 349–351). Add up the scores obtained. Read off the baby's gestational age from the vertical axis of the chart on p. 352 where the total score (horizontal axis) meets the diagonal line.

External (superficial) Criteria

EXTERNAL SIGN	SCORE				
	0	1	2	3	4
OEDEMA	Obvious oedema hands and feet: pitting over tibia	No obvious oedema hands and feet: pitting over tibia	No oedema		
SKIN TEXTURE	Very thin, gelatinous	Thin and smooth	Smooth: medium thickness. Rash or superficial peeling	Slight thickening. Superficial cracking and peeling esp. hand and feet	Thick and parchment-like; super-ficial or deep cracking
SKIN COLOUR (Infant not crying)	Dark red	Uniformly pink	Pale pink: variable over body	Pale. Only pink over ears, lips, palms or soles	
SKIN OPACITY (trunk)	Numerous veins and venules clearly seen, especially over abdomen	Veins and tributaries seen	A few large vessels clearly seen over abdomen	A few large vessels seen indistinctly over abdomen	No blood vessels seen
LANUGO (over back)	No lanugo	Abundant; long and thick over whole back	Hair thinning especially over lower back	Small amount of lanugo and bald areas	At least half of back devoid of lanugo
PLANTAR CREASES	No skin creases	Faint red marks over anterior half of sole	Definite red marks over more than anterior half; indentations over less than anterior third	Indentations over more than anterior third	Definite deep indentations over more than anterior third
NIPPLE FORMA-TION	Nipple barely visible; no areola	Nipple well defined; areola smooth and flat diameter <0.75 cm.	Areola stippled, edge not raised; diameter <0.75 cm.	Areola stippled, edge raised diameter >0.75 cm.	
BREAST SIZE	No breast tissue palpable	Breast tissue on one or both sides <0.5 cm. diameter	Breast tissue both sides; one or both 0.5–1.0 cm.	Breast tissue both sides; one or both >1 cm.	
EAR FORM	Pinna flat and shapeless, little or no incurving edge	Incurving of part of edge of pinna	Partial incurving whole of upper pinna	Well-defined incurving whole of upper pinna	
EAR FIRMNESS	Pinna soft, easily folded, no recoil	Pinna soft, easily folded, slow recoil	Cartilage to edge of pinna, but soft in places, ready recoil	Pinna firm, cartilage to edge, instant recoil	
GENITALIA MALE	Neither testis in scrotum	At least one testis high in scrotum	At least one testis right down		
FEMALE (With hips half abducted)	Labia majora widely separ-ated, labia minora protruding	Labia majora almost cover labia minora	Labia majora completely cover labia minora		

(Adapted from Farr et al., *Develop. Med. Child Neurol.* (1966) **8**, 507)

Neurological Criteria

NEURO LOGICAL SIGN	SCORE					
	0	1	2	3	4	5
POSTURE						
SQUARE WINDOW	90°	60°	45°	30°	0°	
ANKLE DORSI FLEXION	90°	75°	45°	20°	0°	
ARM RECOIL	180°	90–180°	<90°			
LEG RECOIL	180°	90–180°	<90°			
POPLITEAL ANGLE	180°	160°	130°	110°	90°	<90°
HEEL TO EAR						
SCARF SIGN						
HEAD LAG						
VENTRAL SUSPEN-SION						

Some notes on techniques of assessement of neurological criteria

Posture. Observed with infant quiet and in supine position. Score 0; Arms and legs extended; 1: beginning of flexion of hips and knees, arms extended; 2: stronger flexion of legs, arms extended; 3: arms slightly flexed, legs flexed and abducted; 4: full flexion of arms and legs.

Square window. The hand is flexed on the forearm between the thumb and index finger of the examiner. Enough pressure is applied to get as full a flexion as possible, and the angle between the hypothenar eminence and the ventral aspect of the forearm is measured and graded according to diagram. (Care is taken not to rotate the infant's wrist while doing this manoeuvre.)

Ankle dorsiflexion. The foot is dorsiflexed onto the anterior aspect of the leg, with the examiner's thumb on the sole of the foot and other fingers behind the leg. Enough pressure is applied to get as full flexion as possible, and the angle between the dorsum of the foot and the anterior aspect of the leg is measured.

Arm recoil. With the infant in the supine position the forearms are first flexed for 5 seconds, then fully extended by pulling on the hands, and then released. The sign is fully positive if the arms return briskly to full flexion (Score 2). If the arms return to incomplete flexion or the response is sluggish it is graded as Score 1. If they remain extended or are only followed by random movements the score is 0.

Leg recoil. With the infant supine, the hips and knees are fully flexed for 5 seconds, then extended by traction on the feet, and released. A maximal response is one of full flexion of the hips and knees (Score 2). A partial flexion scores 1, and minimal or no movement scores 0.

Popliteal angle. With the infant supine and his pelvis flat on the examining couch, the thigh is held in the knee–chest position by the examiner's left index finger and thumb supporting the knee. The leg is then extended by gentle pressure from the examiner's right index finger behind the ankle and the popliteal angle is measured.

Heel to ear manoeuvre. With the baby supine, draw the baby's foot as near to the head as it will go without forcing it. Observe the distance between the foot and the head as well as the degree of extension at the knee. Grade according to diagram. Note that the knee is left free and may draw down alongside the abdomen.

Scarf sign. With the baby supine, take the infant's hand and try to put it around the neck and as far posteriorly as possible around the opposite shoulder. Assist this manoeuvre by lifting the elbow across the body. See how far the elbow will go across and grade according to illustrations. Score 0: Elbow reaches opposite axillary line; 1: Elbow between midline and opposite axillary line; 2: Elbow reaches midline; 3: Elbow will not reach midline.

Head lag. With the baby lying supine, grasp the hands (or the arms if a very small infant) and pull him slowly towards the sitting position. Observe the position of the head in relation to the trunk and grade accordingly. In a small infant the head may initially be supported by one hand. Score 0: Complete lag; 1: Partial head control; 2: Able to maintain head in line with body; 3: Brings head anterior to body.

Ventral suspension. The infant is suspended in the prone position, with examiner's hand under the infant's chest (one hand in a small infant, two in a

Graph for reading gestational age from total score (Dubowitz method)

$$y = 0.2642x + 24.595$$

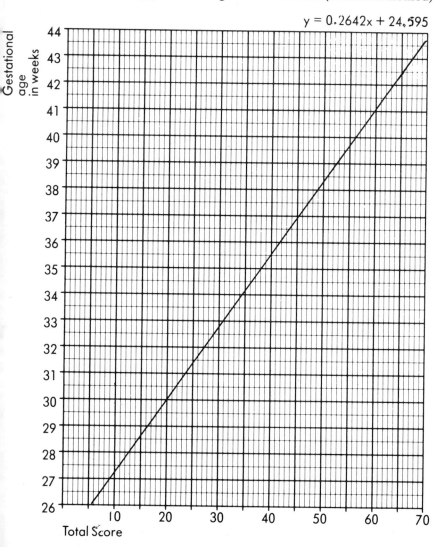

large infant). Observe the degree of extension of the back and the amount of flexion of the arms and legs. Also note the relation of the head to the trunk. Grade according to diagrams.

If the score for an individual criterion differs on the two sides of the baby, take the mean. *For further details see Dubowitz et al., 1970.*

2 Parkin, Hey and Clowes score

This is quicker to perform but may not be quite so accurate.

Skin texture. Tested by picking up a fold of abdominal skin between finger and thumb, and by inspection.

0 very thin with a gelatinous feel
1 thin and smooth
2 smooth and of medium thickness, irritation rash and superficial peeling may be present
3 slight thickening and stiff feeling with superficial cracking and peeling especially evident on the hands and feet
4 thick and parchment-like with superficial or deep cracking

Skin colour. Estimated by inspection when the baby is quiet.

0 dark red
1 uniformly pink
2 pale pink, though the colour may vary over different parts of the body, some parts may be very pale
3 pale, nowhere really pink except on the ears, lips, palms and soles

Breast size. Measured by picking up the breast tissue between finger and thumb.

0 no breast tissue palpable
1 breast tissue palpable on one or both sides, neither being more than 0.5 cm in diameter
2 breast tissue palpable on both sides, one or both being 0.5–1 cm in diameter
3 breast tissue palpable on both sides, one or both being more than 1 cm in diameter

Ear firmness. Tested by palpation and folding of the upper pinna.

0 pinna feels soft and is easily folded into bizarre positions without springing back into position spontaneously
1 pinna feels soft along the edge and is easily folded but returns slowly to the correct position spontaneously
2 cartilage can be felt to the edge of the pinna though it is thin in places and the pinna springs back readily after being folded
3 pinna firm with definite cartilage extending to the periphery and springs back immediately into position after being folded.

Score each external sign in turn. Add them up. Read off the baby's gestational age on the following chart:

Score	Gestational age days	weeks	
1	190	27	
2	210	30	
3	230	33	
4	240	34½	
5	250	36	
6	260	37	
7	270	38½	
8	276	39½	
9	281	40	
10	285	41	
11	290	41½	
12	295	42	

Further Reading

Brazelton, T.B. (1984) *Neonatal Behavioural Assessement Scale*, 2nd ed., Spastics International Medical Publications. London: Blackwell.

Buckler, J.M.H. (1979) *A Reference Manual of Growth and Development*. Oxford: Blackwell Scientific.

Dubowitz, M.S. & Dubowitz, V. (1977) *Gestational Age of the Newborn*. Reading, Mass.: Addison-Wesley.

Dubowitz, L., Dubowitz, V. & Goldberg, C. (1970) Clinical assessment of gestational age in the newborn infant. *Journal of Pediatrics* 77, 1.

Insley, J. & Wood, B.S.B. (1982) *A Paediatric Vade-Mecum*, 10th ed. London: Lloyd Luke.

Parkin, J.M., Hey, E.N. & Clowes, J.S. (1976) Rapid assessment of gestational age at birth. *Archives of Disease in Children, 51,* 259.

Index

Umbilical (*cont.*)
  cord bleeding, 265
    blood sampling, 54–55
    care in developing countries, 329
    examination of, 70
    occlusion, sequence of events
        following, (Fig. 3.1) 47
  examination, 70, 79
  hernia, 178
  vein, 210
    catheter insertion into, 54
Urethral
  obstruction, male, 73
  valves, 166, 200, (Fig. 9.25) 201
Urinary
  oestrogen analysis, maternal, 29
  reducing substances tests, 242
  tract infection, 299
    follow-up examination for, 80
Urine
  culture, 242
  normal values, 334
  passage of, 84
Urticaria, neonatal, 196

Vaccines
  in developing countries, 330
  pertussis, 277
  polio, 330
  rubella, 308
  tuberculosis, 85
Vaginal, neonatal
  bleeding, 264
  examination, 74
  infections, ascending, 289
Valvular lesions, cardiac, 226–7
Vamin, 152, (Table 7.8) 154
Van den Bergh reagent, 238
Venous cannulation in parenteral feeding,
    156–7
Ventilation
  in apnoea, 52–53, (Fig. 3.4) 54, 132
  mechanical, for meconium aspiration,
      127
    problems following, 129
    in RDS baby, 117–20
Ventricular
  hypertrophy, 215
  obstruction, 222–3
  septal defect, 218–19

Viral infections, 307–9
Virilization, 197–9
Vision tests, 88
Vitamin A deficiency, congenital
      abnormalities and, 164
Vitamin B supplements in preterm babies,
    101–110
Vitamin C supplements in preterm babies,
    101
Vitamin D deficiency, maternal, 101
Vitamin E deficiency in preterm babies,
    100
Vitamin K
  levels, neonatal, 262
  synthetic water-soluble analogues, 9
  therapy, 268, 269
    during surgery, 167
Vitamin supplements
  neural tube defects and, 187
  in parenteral feeds, 152–3
  for preterm babies, 100–1
Vitlipid, 153
Vomiting, transfer to special care unit for,
    82

Warfarin side-effects, (Table 2.5) 40
Washerwoman's skin, 305
Water-borne infection, 302
Webbing, 193
Weighing babies, 83–84
Weight
  at birth, 13
    low *see* Birth weight, low; Preterm
        baby; Small-for-dates baby
  chart, (Fig. 4.1) 64, 65
  gain, 83–84
    during pregnancy, fetal growth and,
        23
Werdnig–Hoffman progressive spinal
      paralysis, 271, 277–8
Wilson–Mikity syndrome, 129–30
  diagnosis, 108
Withdrawal symptoms, 280–2
Wolf's syndrome, 206

X-linked recessive disorder incidence,
    (Table 8.2) 162

Zinc deficiency, maternal, 18